D1035274

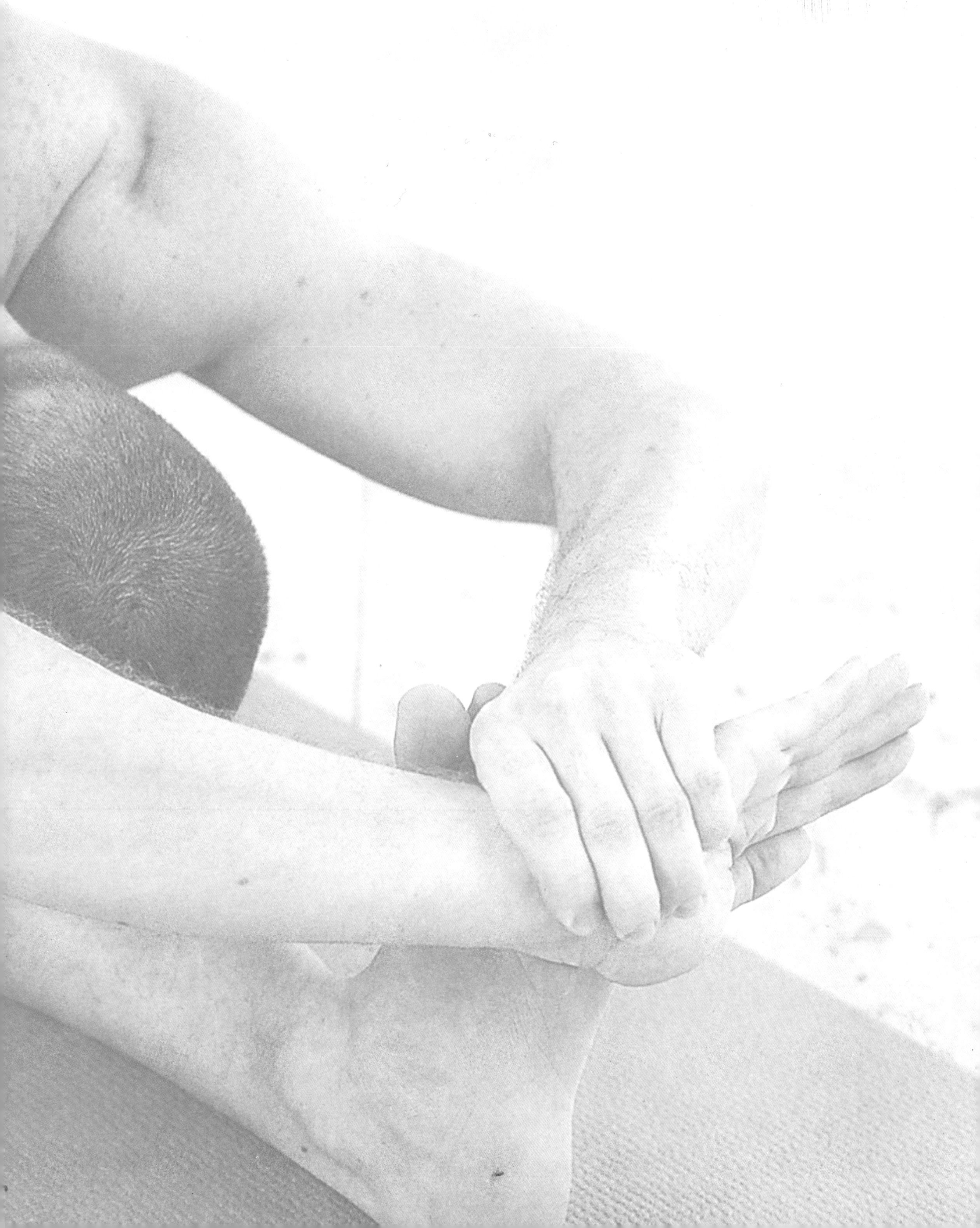

Iyengar | YOGA

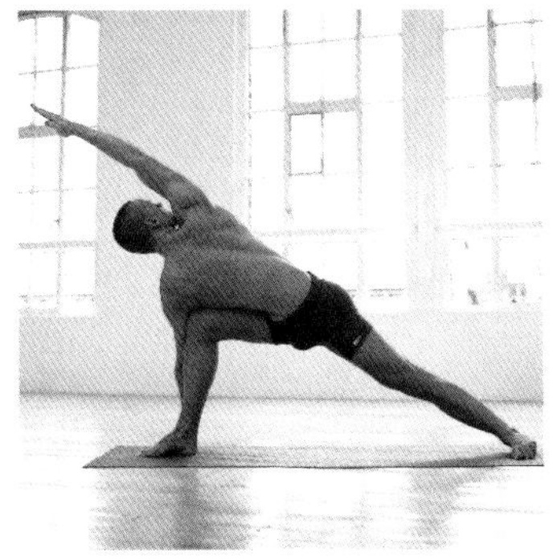

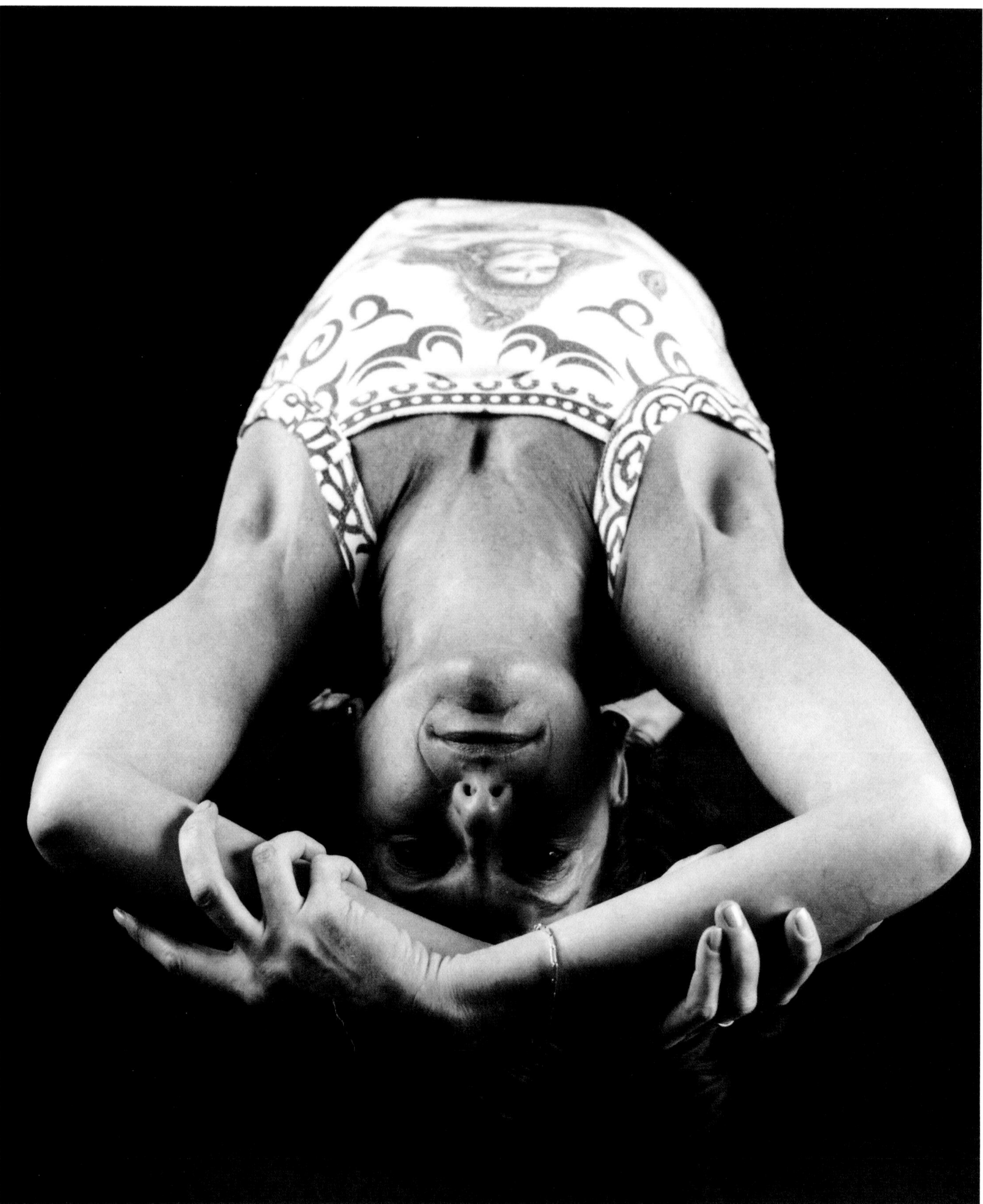

Iyengar | YOGA

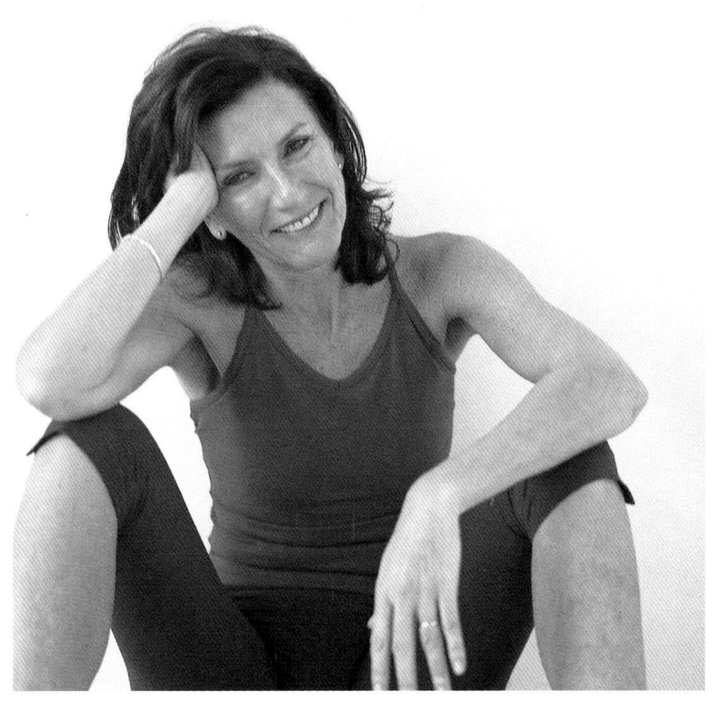

Judy Smith | CLASSIC YOGA POSTURES FOR MIND, BODY AND SPIRIT

PHOTOGRAPHY BY CLARE PARK

LORENZ BOOKS

This edition is published by Lorenz Books

Lorenz Books is an imprint of Anness Publishing Ltd
Hermes House, 88–89 Blackfriars Road, London SE1 8HA
tel. 020 7401 2077; fax 020 7633 9499
www.lorenzbooks.com; info@anness.com

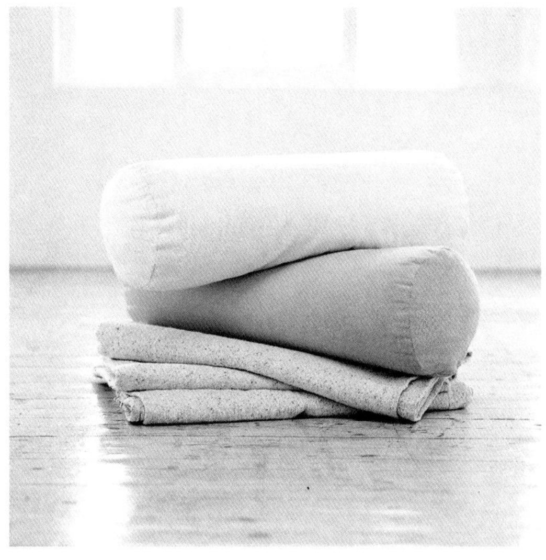

UK agent: The Manning Partnership Ltd, 6 The Old Dairy,
Melcombe Road, Bath BA2 3LR; tel. 01225 478444;
fax 01225 478440; sales@manning-partnership.co.uk

UK distributor: Grantham Book Services Ltd, Isaac Newton Way,
Alma Park Industrial Estate, Grantham, Lincs NG31 9SD;
tel. 01476 541080; fax 01476 541061; orders@gbs.tbs-ltd.co.uk

North American agent/distributor: National Book Network,
4501 Forbes Boulevard, Suite 200, Lanham, MD 20706;
tel. 301 459 3366; fax 301 429 5746; www.nbnbooks.com

Australian agent/distributor: Pan Macmillan Australia, Level 18,
St Martins Tower, 31 Market St, Sydney, NSW 2000;
tel. 1300 135 113; fax 1300 135 103; customer.service@macmillan.com.au

New Zealand agent/distributor: David Bateman Ltd, 30 Tarndale Grove,
Off Bush Road, Albany, Auckland; tel. (09) 415 7664; fax (09) 415 8892

A CIP catalogue record for this book is available from the British Library.

Publisher: Joanna Lorenz
Managing Editor: Judith Simons
Project Editor: Katy Bevan
Designer: Anita Schnable
Main Photography: Clare Park
Additional Photography: Bonieventure Bagalue
Production Controller: Darren Price
Yoga Positions: Juliet Byrne, Laura Dymock, David Johnston, Peter Oakley,
Jenny Roche, Judy Smith
Photographs on page 15 courtesy of Gerry Clist and Michael Rabe.

10 9 8 7 6 5 4 3 2 1

Contents

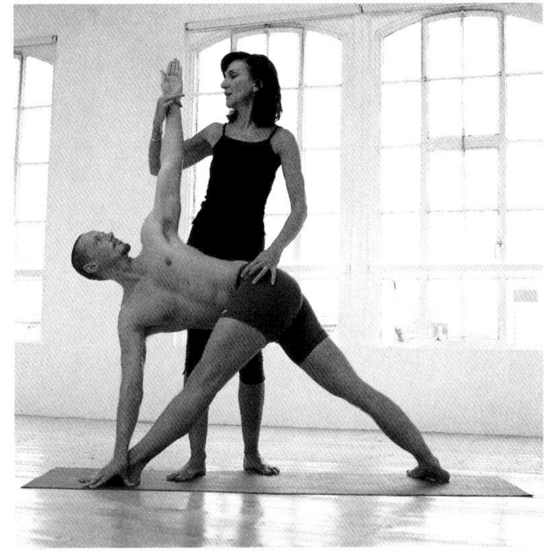

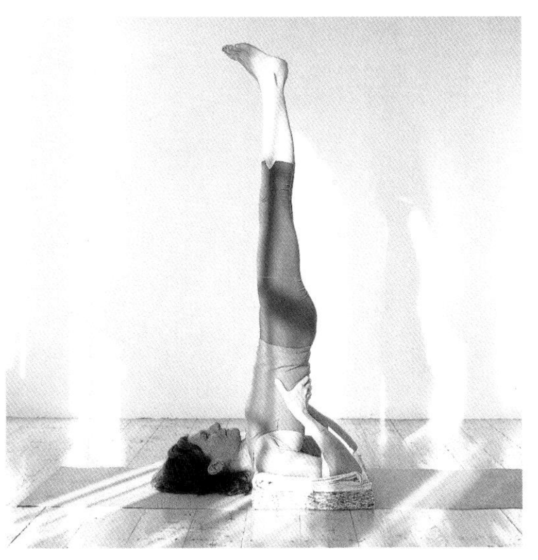

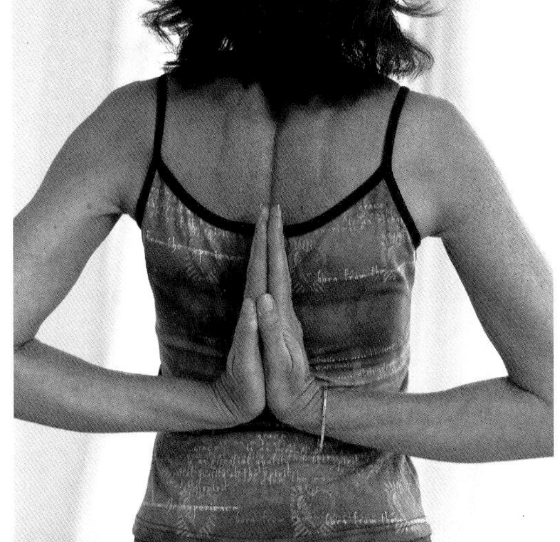

Foreword

This illustrated book on Iyengar yoga provides the reader and practitioner with detailed instructions for beginners and experienced students alike. It follows the classical Iyengar asanas as detailed in *Light on Yoga*, written by Yogacharya Mr B.K.S. Iyengar (Guruji) in 1966. Guruji's dedication to his own practice inspires everyone who meets him or comes into contact with his ideas, to strive and follow in his footsteps.

Guruji has always encouraged those among his pupils, who are gifted in demonstrating his methods of yoga, or in public speaking or in writing articles or books to go forth and spread his art, and so has approved Judy's venture.

Since the opening of the Ramamani Iyengar Memorial Yoga Institute in Pune, India, by B.K.S. Iyengar in January 1975, I have attended many classes at the Institute with Mr Iyengar, Geetaji and Prashanti (his daughter and son). I have also had the honour and privilege of welcoming Guruji to Crystal Palace where 1,000 of his pupils stood on their heads during his impeccable teaching at the EuroYoga Convention in 1993.The most memorable occasion for me, was when Guruji came to Manchester during the 1980s and 1,000 of his pupils from the North of England performed a short demonstration in welcome and appreciation of his visit. On that occasion Guruji remarked that although he had demonstrated his art to thousands of people around the world, this was the first time 1,000 of his pupils had performed in front of him.

In May 2002 I had the privilege of welcoming Geetaji to Crystal Palace in London for the celebration of the Iyengar Yoga Jubilee. It was Geetaji's first visit to Europe, where she taught 1,000 participants during many days of teaching.

Judy has recently assisted in the Therapeutic Class run by Guruji and Geetaji in Pune and she teaches in the Remedial Class at the Maida Vale Iyengar Institute London. Through constant practice and visiting the home institute, Pune, and with the help of Guruji, Geetaji and Prashanti, Judy has been able to correct her own posture with the teachings of Iyengar yoga.

Below left and right Students practising standing postures and inversions under Geetaji's watchful eyes at the Iyengar Jubilee, Crystal Palace, 2002.
Opposite Namaste is the traditional greeting among yogis.

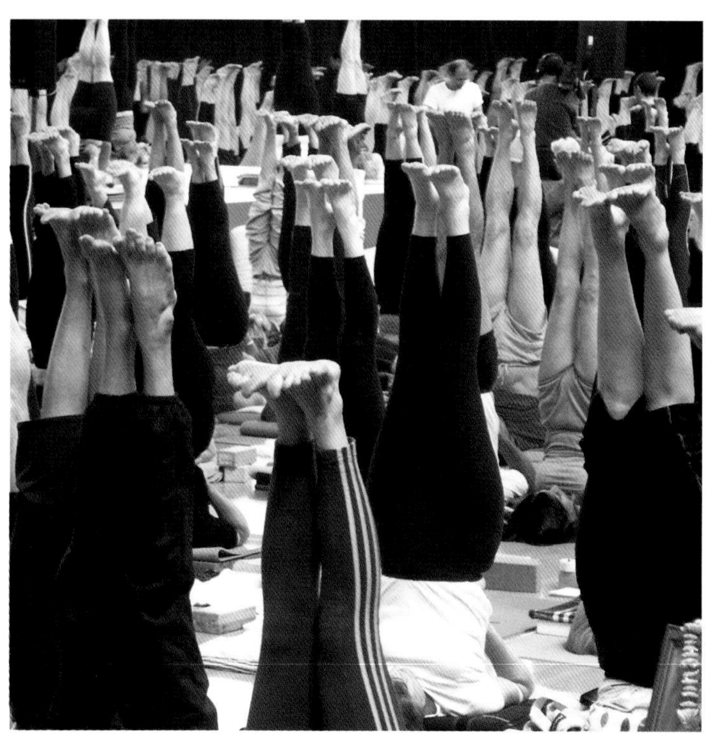

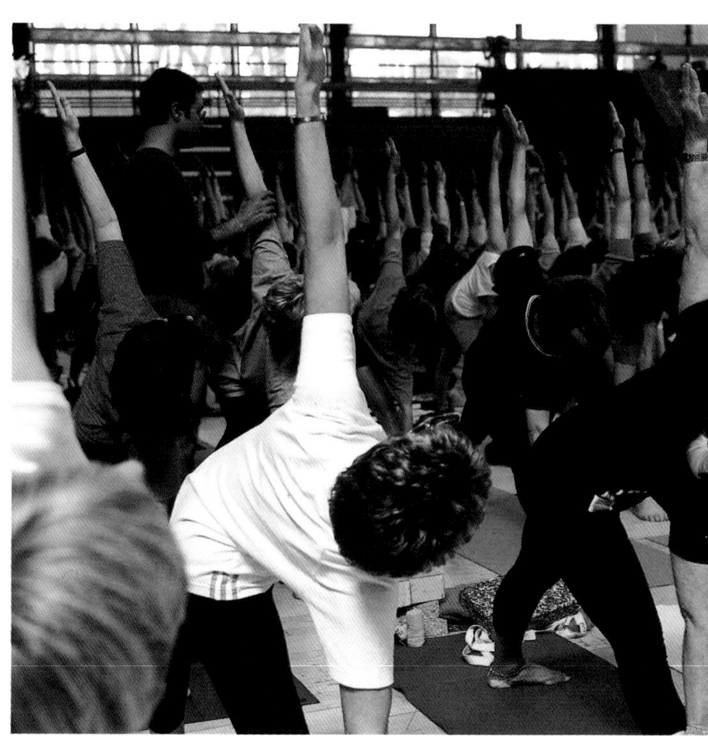

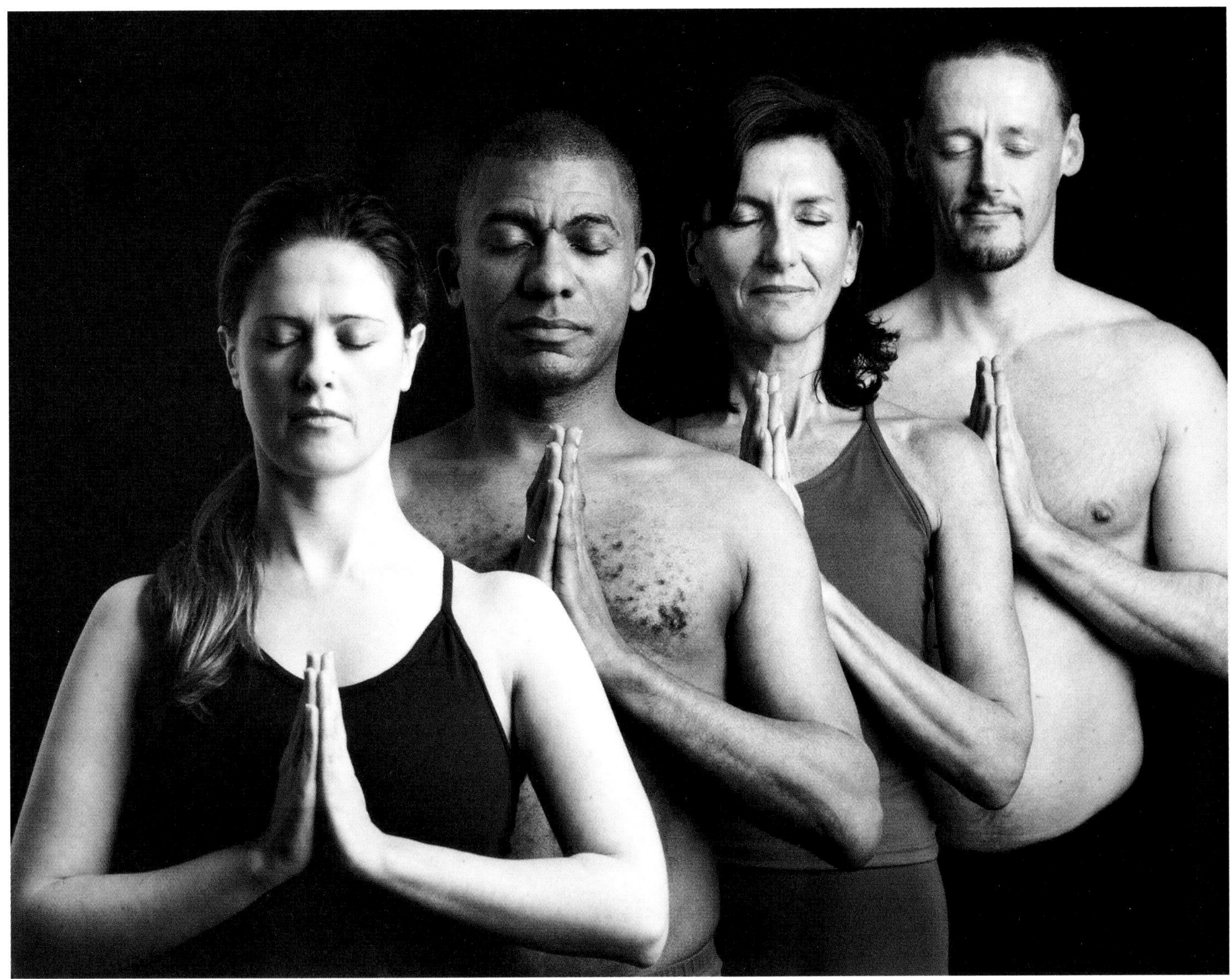

Judy has written a thorough introduction to the history and philosophy behind Iyengar yoga. Here she explains that yoga is very much a practical philosophy, focusing essentially on correct alignment of the body so that it can develop harmoniously.

The section on the asanas is clearly laid out in order of their importance to learning and practice: Standing Asanas, Seated Asanas, Twists, Inverted Asanas, Supine and Prone Asanas. The section on basic Pranayama and Savasana that follows has easy-to-understand instructions that can then be practised at home, without a teacher. This book also provides a useful reference for students already attending classes.

The section on Routine Practice is very well laid out for sequence practice using thumbnail photographs with minimal instructions. I particularly applaud Judy's comment: "Remember to consolidate and not be in too much of a hurry to get to the last routine. It is not about how fast you work, but about the quality, understanding and proficiency of your work."

The Yoga Therapy section shows how to use the props, and shows sequences of selected asanas to treat specific minor ailments. I feel sure that all teachers of yoga will find this section of the book a wealth of information.

Although I have practised and taught Iyengar yoga for 37 years, and read many books that have been produced by Guruji's western students, in my opinion, very few have specifically been structured in keeping with Iyengar's methods. I hope that I have been able to encourage you all to not only read this book, but to practise, practise, practise.

I am very pleased to recommend Judy's book on Iyengar yoga to all those who wish to follow the one true path to a healthy life.

Jeanne Maslen
Previously Chair of the Manchester and District Institute of Iyengar Yoga (the oldest Iyengar institute), and second-chair of the BKS Iyengar Teacher's Association.

Introduction

Yoga is a practical philosophy, not a religion, and requires no allegiance to any particular system of belief. The word "yoga" comes from the Sanskrit word "yug", meaning to join, yoke or unite. It is a traditional Indian philosophy that involves the integration of the physical and spiritual in order to achieve a sense of well-being. This synthesis and inseparability of the body and mind leads to a greater connection to one's consciousness.

In the practice of yoga, the body is linked to the movement, mind and breath to bring about a feeling of balance, relaxation and harmony. The practitioner uses the physical self to refine the mind. Through this thorough training of the body and thought, one is taught to awaken every cell of one's self and one's soul.

The practice of asanas (postures) improves a variety of ailments, strengthens and tones muscles and develops flexibility. Various movements in the postures result in blood saturating, nourishing and cleansing the remotest parts of the body. Psychologically, yoga increases concentration, stills the mind and promotes a feeling of balance, tranquillity and contentment.

There is a difference between yoga and other physical exercises. Asanas are psycho-physiological, while physical jerks are purely external. Asanas develop body awareness, muscles and flexibility, as well as generating internal awareness and stabilizing the mind. In physical exercises, body movements may be done with external precision, whereas in yoga, together with the precision, a deeper awareness is awakened, which brings about balance in body and spirit.

My journey with yoga began over 20 years ago. As a child and a teenager I was extremely tall, and to compensate for this I had very bad posture, which resulted in rounded shoulders, backache, lethargy and a pessimistic outlook on life. Iyengar yoga, with its attention to detail, appealed to me, as it challenged both the head and the physical frame, and enabled me to exercise control and discipline in all aspects of my life. Not only did my posture and flexibility improve, but I became physically stronger, calmer and a more balanced and centred human being.

I practise every day for however much free time I have. It is advisable to set aside a similar time each day or night to practise and to make this part of your daily routine. In order to satisfy my thirst for knowledge, I attend regular classes, workshops and seminars both in the UK and abroad. My studies are also greatly enhanced by my visits to Mr Iyengar's Yoga Institute in Pune, India, where I spend a month at a time under his watchful eyes and those of his daughter and son, who help to run the institute.

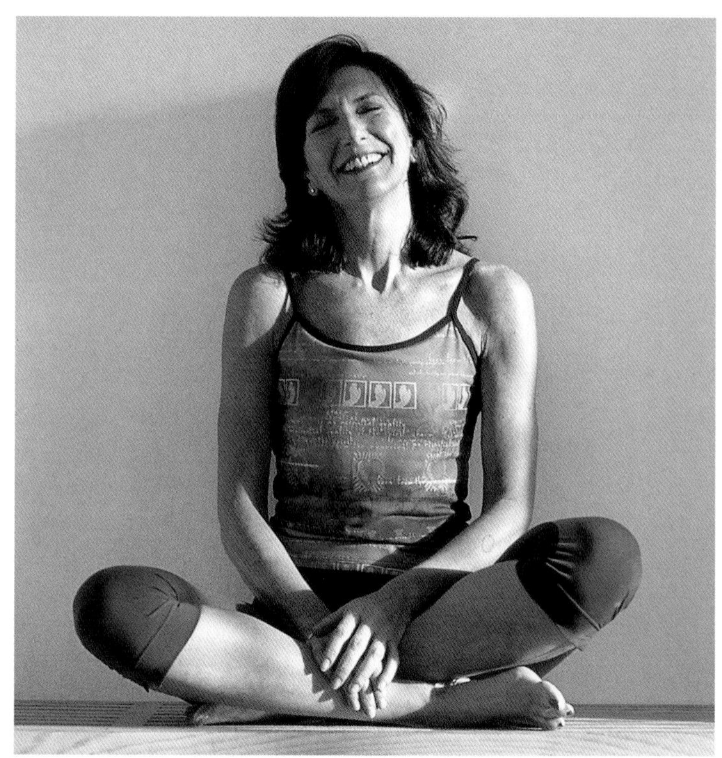

Above Judy Smith first began learning Iyengar yoga to help herself, and has since gained much satisfaction from helping numerous students to help themselves.

I have been teaching Iyengar yoga for 15 years and have trained to a senior level with some inspirational teachers. My students include both the elderly and children, people with mixed abilities, minor complaints and various problems, both physical and mental. When they arrive for the class, their bodies and minds are stiff and unyielding; when they leave, they walk out taller and their entire being radiates serenity and peace.

Right When first learning the more challenging postures, it is a great support to have an attentive teacher.
Below The constant practice of yoga brings flexibility, freedom from tension and peace of mind.

Teaching yoga has been both a satisfying and rewarding experience. Through this book I hope to inspire people to begin or rekindle their yogic journey.

Practising the asanas (postures) and pranayama (breathing) with honesty and diligence, intelligence and awareness, will bring about clarity, energy and serenity in all aspects of one's life.

The asanas and programmes offered are suitable for both beginners and more experienced practitioners and should be repeated and practised as often as circumstances allow, anything from an hour a week to several hours a day.

I wish you joy, light and happiness as you travel along your path to enlightenment.

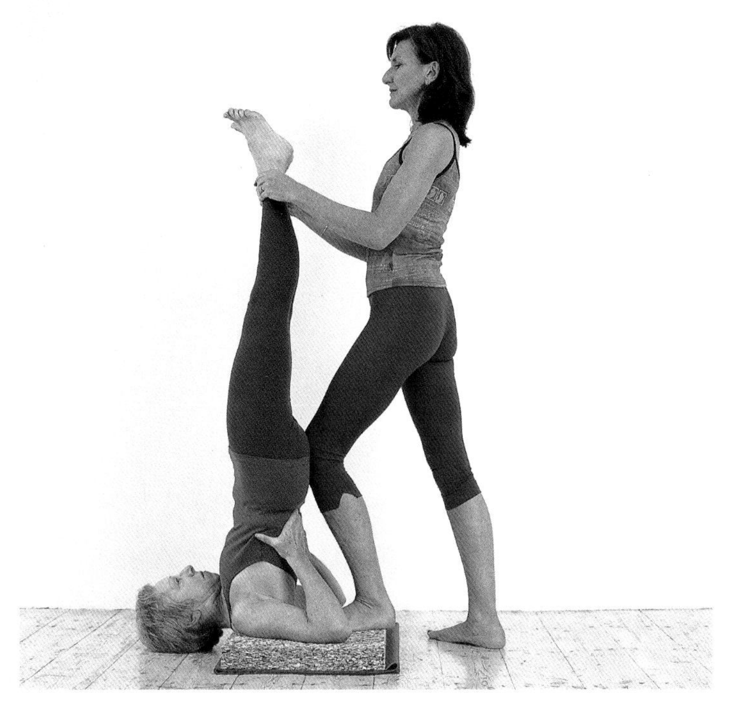

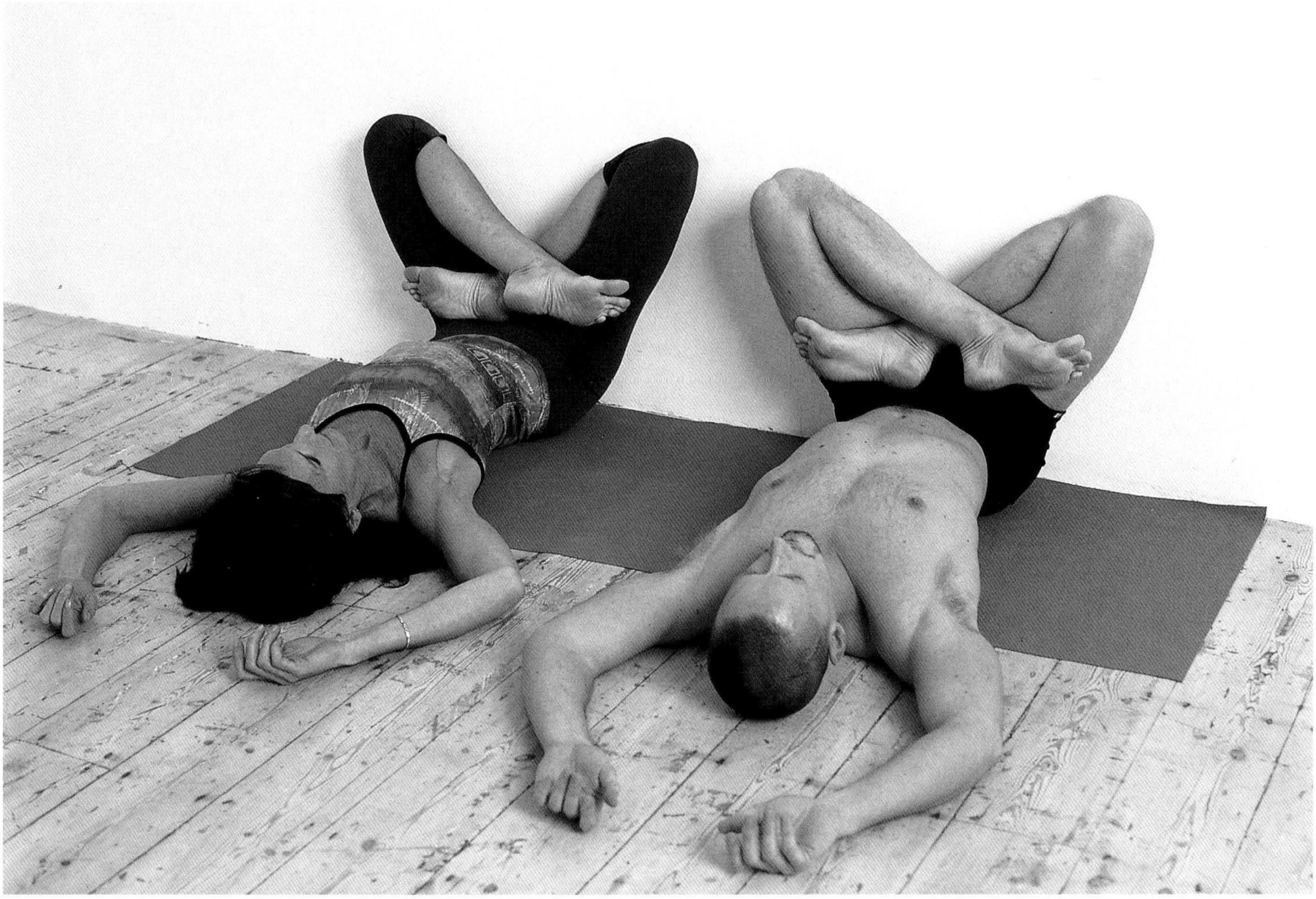

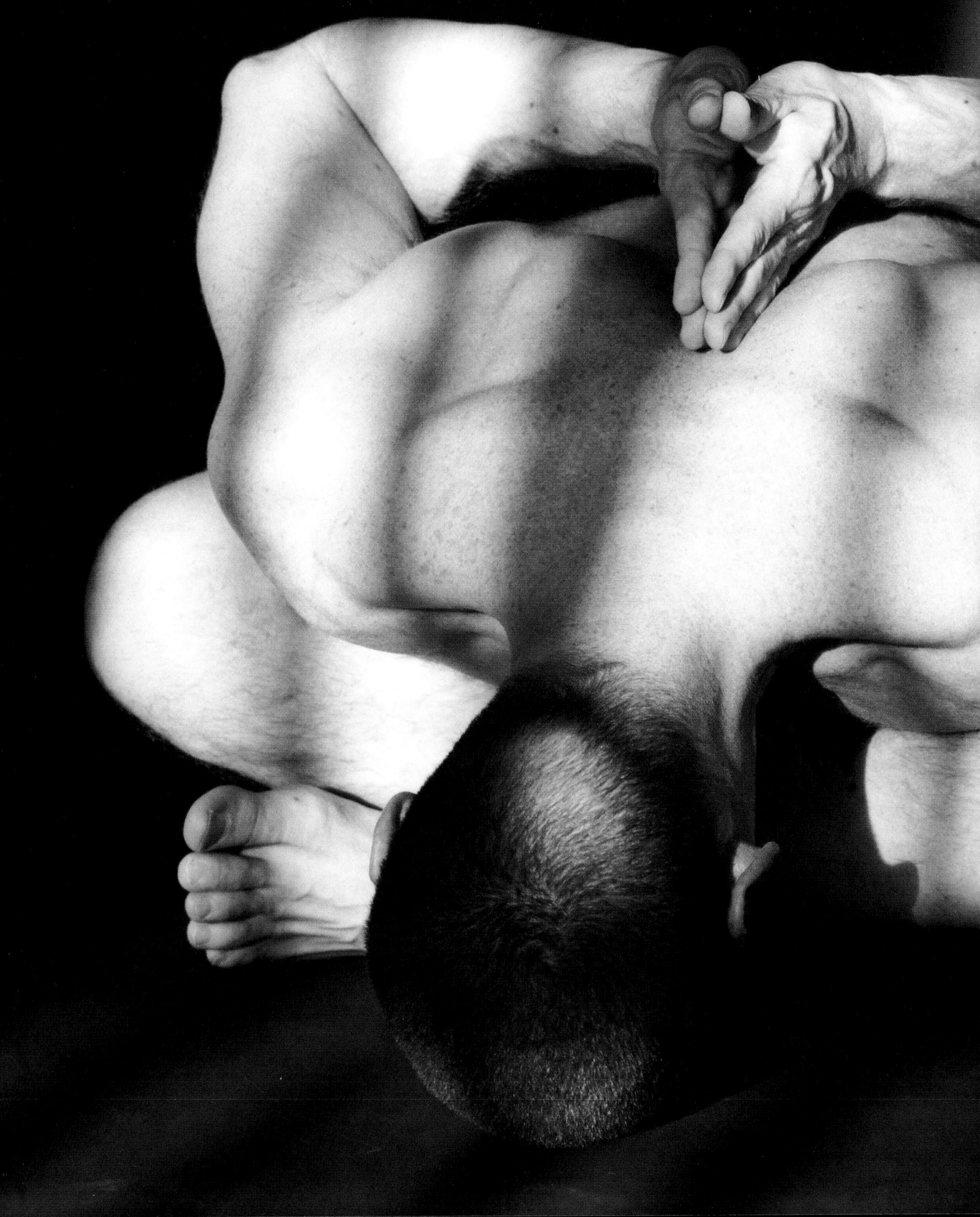

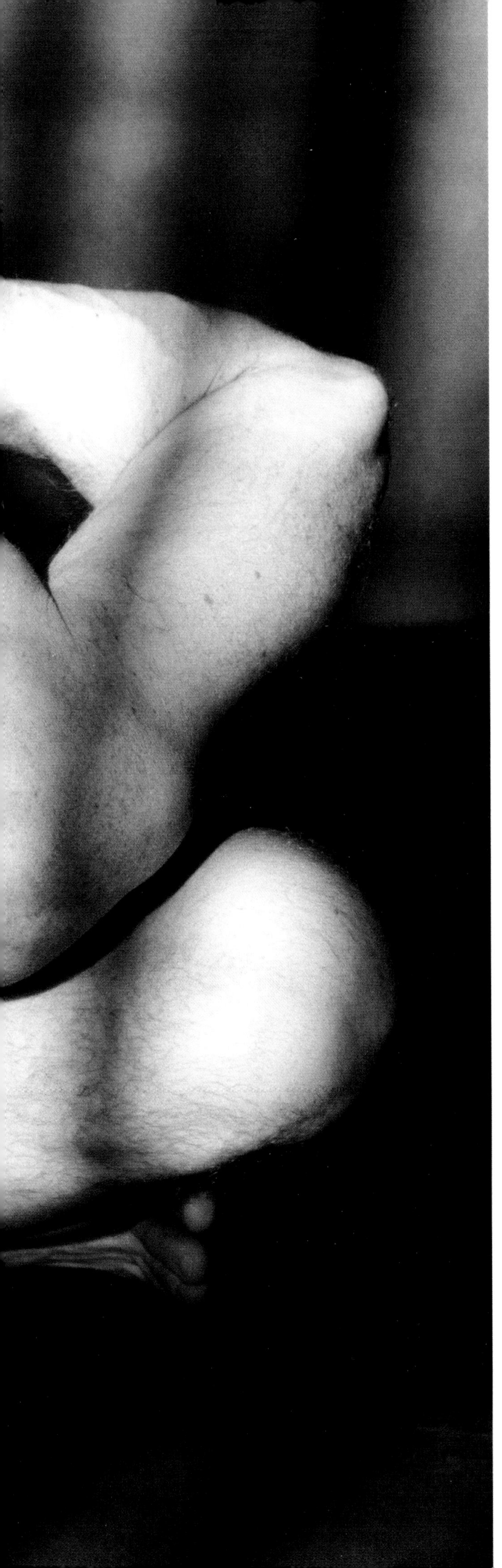

Iyengar Basics

"Yoga is a practical philosophy. It shows, from moment to moment, the way to face the world and at the same time to follow a spiritual path. Yoga strikes a balance between the happiness of the world, that is self-centred happiness, and the happiness which extends beyond one's own self." B.K.S. Iyengar

Mr Iyengar has systematized over 200 classical yoga postures, the result of which is Iyengar yoga. This method of practising yoga is methodical and progressive, and emphasizes precision, detailed correctness and absolute safety. The postures have been structured and categorized to allow students of all levels of fitness and ability to progress surely and safely from basic to more challenging postures and, by so doing, to gain flexibility, strength and sensitivity in mind, body and spirit.

History and Philosophy

Iyengar yoga focuses on correct alignment of the body so that it can develop harmoniously and anatomically perfect. If the student practises with intelligence and awareness, there is little chance of injury or pain. As all bodies are different and people have specific weaknesses and difficulties, Iyengar yoga makes use of props to help students achieve the best possible poses within their limited capacity.

The Iyengar method, which is renowned for its precision and attention to detail, involves the practice of asanas (postures) and pranayama (breathing). Because of the intense concentration required to position parts of the body, both skeletally and muscularly, the mind becomes focused and sharp, and this results in a form of "meditation in motion". Practitioners strive for this state of total physical awareness, mental clarity and ultimate serenity.

A vital aspect of Iyengar yoga is the sequencing of postures. There is a cumulative effect when poses are practised in a particular order, and when this is adhered to there is less chance of injury and incorrect practice. Iyengar yoga can also be used therapeutically to treat a variety of ailments.

There are numerous styles of yoga, of which Iyengar is one. It was developed by Yogacharya B.K.S. Iyengar, one of the world's most respected experts on yoga. As a child he suffered from various illnesses, and at the age of 16 was introduced to yoga by his sister's husband, Sri T. Krishnamacharya, who was a teacher in Mysore. Iyengar began practising yoga to regain his health and strength, and in 1936 his guru sent him to Pune for 6 months to teach.

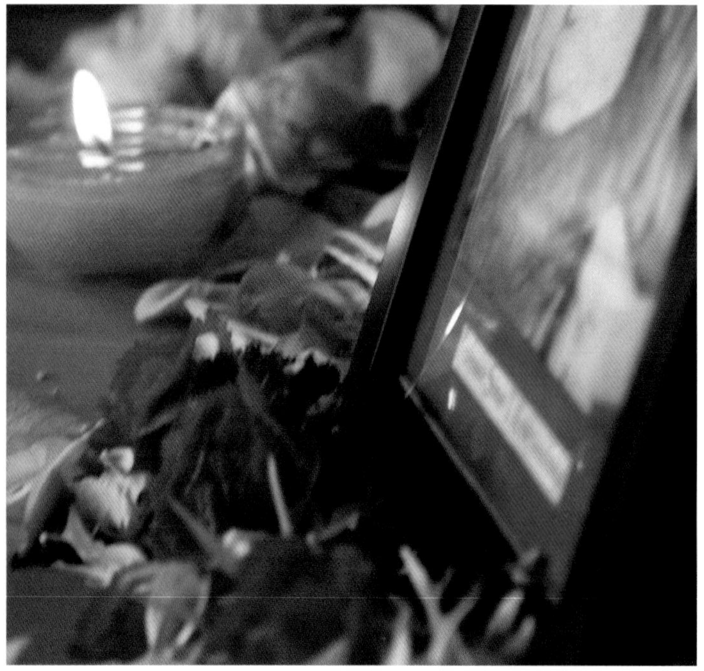

The precision and perfection in his practice was reflected in his teaching, and the number of students grew. He became recognized and respected as a yoga teacher, and in 1952 he met Yehudi Menuhin. This encounter was instrumental in introducing yoga and Mr Iyengar to the Western world. Menuhin was a dedicated student and invited Mr Iyengar to England to teach him. Many people joined in these classes, and soon a large number of Westerners became his students and invited him back the following year.

Back in Pune, he decided that he wanted the masses to experience yoga but was restricted by the size of the rooms and halls in which he taught. In 1975 he opened his own institute, the Ramamani Iyengar Memorial Yoga Institute, named in memory of his wife, who died just before his dream was realized. Students from all over the world regularly visit Pune and spend a month being taught by his daughter, Geeta, and son, Prashant, with their father keeping a watchful eye on everybody. Mr Iyengar is in his mid-80s, and to see him carry out some of the asanas is a real inspiration to his devoted followers. There are hundreds of Iyengar yoga institutes training students in his method of yoga around the world, including Europe, America, Japan, Israel, Australia, New Zealand, South Africa and Canada, as well as Bombay, Bangalore, Delhi, Madras and Rishikesh.

Mr Iyengar's comprehensive book *Light on Yoga* was published in 1966. This work has been acknowledged as the Bible of yoga and has been widely translated. Other books written by Mr Iyengar are *Light on Pranayama*; *The Art of Yoga*; *The Tree of Yoga* and *Light on Yoga Sutras of Patanjali*.

Left The founders of yoga and gurus past and present are venerated and admired.

Opposite It is through the dedication and hard work of B.K.S. Iyengar himself that Iyengar yoga has become such a popular form of yoga.

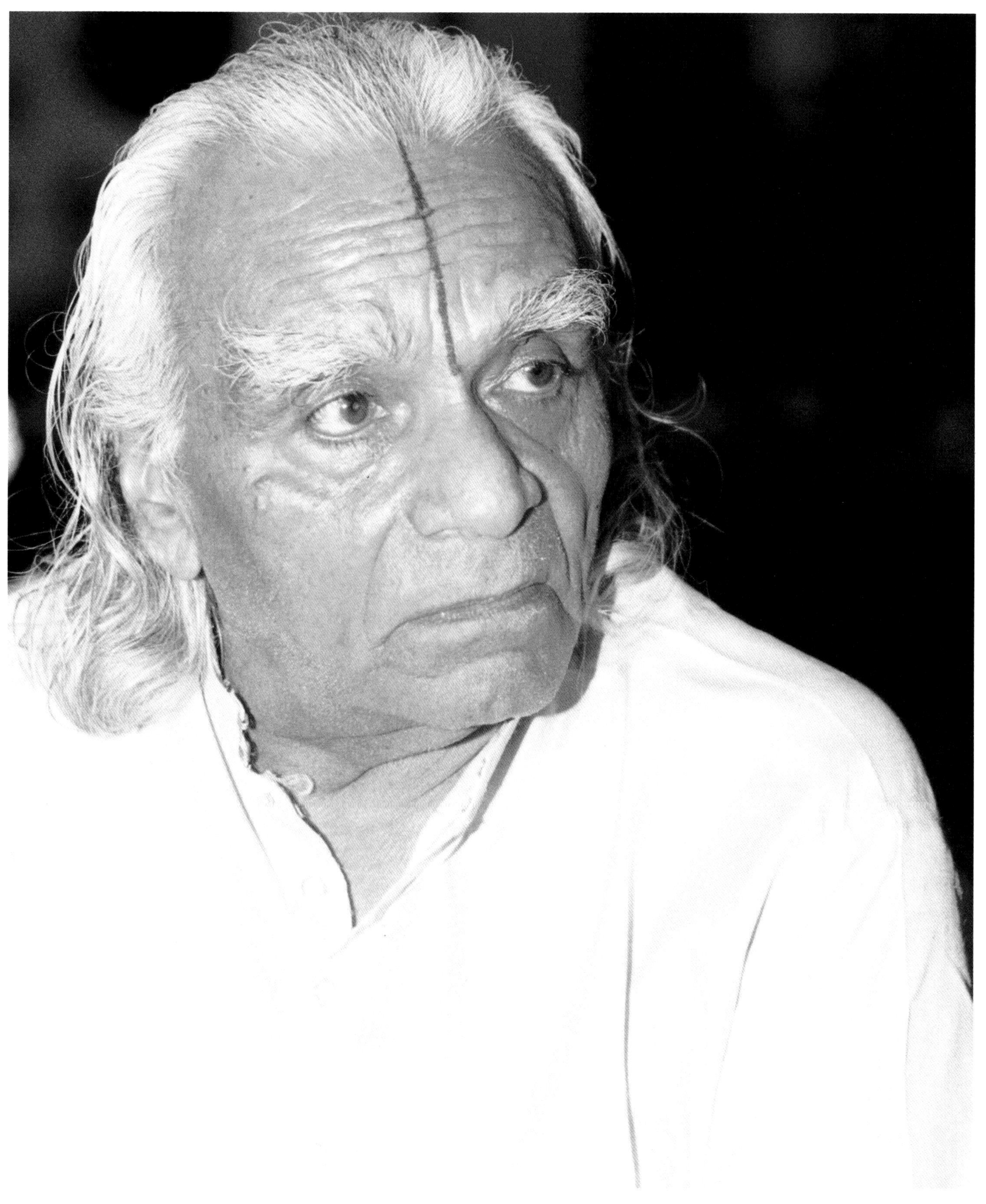

The Yoga Sutras

The philosophy followed by B.K.S. Iyengar is that of Patanjali, a sage who lived in India around 300BC. Patanjali is depicted as a statue with a man's torso and the coiled tail and seven-headed crown of a serpent. In the traditional symbolism of ancient India, this represents infinity. Two of his hands are folded in prayer, representing a meditative state, while the other two hands are holding a conch and discus of light. The conch reminds us of our yoga practice and the discus represents the wheel of time or the law of cause and effect. One half of his face is smiling, the other is serious. Patanjali is known as the founder of yoga and he codified a set of 196 aphorisms called the Yoga Sutras. This work systematizes the principles and practices of yoga by bringing together all the various strands of the theory and practice, and presenting them in one concise, comprehensive text.

These aphorisms cover all aspects of life, beginning with a code of conduct and ending with man's vision of his true self. Patanjali shows how, through the practice of yoga, we can transform ourselves, gain control over the mind and emotions, overcome obstacles hindering our spiritual enlightenment and attain the goal of yoga.

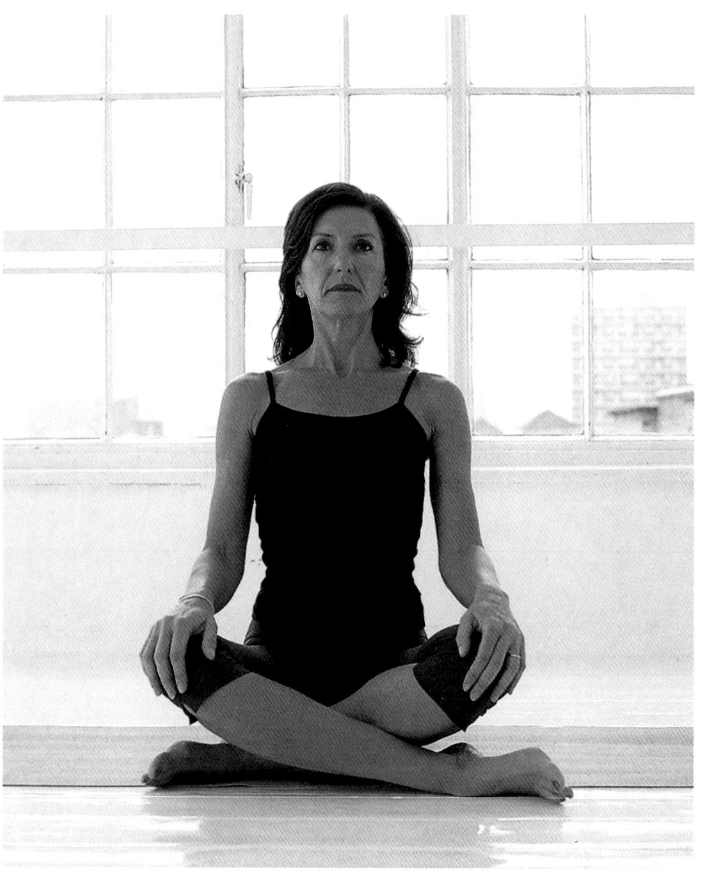

THE EIGHT LIMBS OF YOGA

According to Patanjali, yoga consists of eight limbs. Each of these limbs has its own separate identity, but all form part of a whole, and when they are integrated, the eight stages become true yoga. The eight aspects of yoga are:

1 **Yama** (Social discipline)
These five universal laws include: non-violence; truthfulness; non-stealing; sexual restraint and freedom from desire. As codes of ethical behaviour, they should be followed in everyday life to promote harmony and understanding in society.

2 **Niyama** (Individual discipline)
These five principles of personal conduct are cleanliness; contentment; austerity; study of one's own self and devotion to God. While the yamas apply to universal morals, the niyamas are rules of behaviour that apply to one's physical and mental discipline.

3 **Asana** (Postures)
According to Patanjali's Sutras, **"**Postures bring about stability of the body and poise of the mind.**"** Practising asanas improves flexibility, vitality and health, and activates the organs (heart, lungs, kidneys, liver, spleen and pancreas). However, the true importance of postures is the connection between body and mind, so the two become interwoven, initiating the path from physical to spiritual awareness.

4 **Pranayama** (Breath control)
Patanjali states that pranayama should be practised only after a firm foundation in asana has been established. Practising pranayama releases tension in the body, calms the nervous system and keeps the mind tranquil.

5 **Pratyahara** (Withdrawal and control of the senses)
This withdrawal of the senses from objects of desire is the link between the first four limbs and the last three. After following the rules for universal and personal ethics (yama and niyama) and practising asanas and pranayama, one can turn one's senses inwards and achieve complete tranquillity.

Left Sukhasana, or simple cross legs position, is a comfortable pose in which to meditate. Choose a posture you will be able to stay in for a long time.

6 **Dharana** (Concentration)
After work on the body in asanas, refinement of the mind though pranayama and internalization of the senses of perception in pratyahara, the sixth stage, dharana, is reached. Here the mind is in a state of total absorption and is concentrated on a single point or task in which it is totally engrossed. The longer the mind remains in this state of focus, the more powerful it becomes.

7 **Dhyana** (Meditation)
When the practitioner maintains uninterrupted focus of attention in dharana, it becomes dhyana. In this state of deep concentration and undisturbed meditation, the mind, body and breath become one and merge into a single state of being.

8 **Samadhi** (Self-realization)
This is this the culmination of yogic achievement – a true sense of communion and peace. This settling of the mind is the essence of yoga, where one has risen above the senses as a result of the complete refinement of both body and mind. The body and senses are at rest as if asleep, the mind and reason are alert as if awake, yet everything has gone beyond consciousness.

The first five limbs (yama, niyama, asana, pranayama and pratyahara) are known as the disciplines of yoga. They prepare the body and clear the mind and senses in readiness for the next three limbs (dharana, dhyana and samadhi), which are known as the attainments of yoga. Patanjali says, "The study of the eight limbs of yoga leads to the purification of the body, the mind and the intellect; the flame of knowledge is kept burning and discrimination is aroused."

The demands of modern life can bring about stress, which leads to illness as well as mental anguish. Good health is the harmony between body, mind and soul. It is a result of a balanced diet, exercise and a mind that is stress free. In yoga, the asanas revitalize the body and pranayama brings about a sense of calmness. This helps to free the mind of negative thoughts caused by the fast pace of today's world. It is encouraging to know that in this age of pressure, there are well-established techniques in yoga to restore health and help contribute to a life of happiness and harmony.

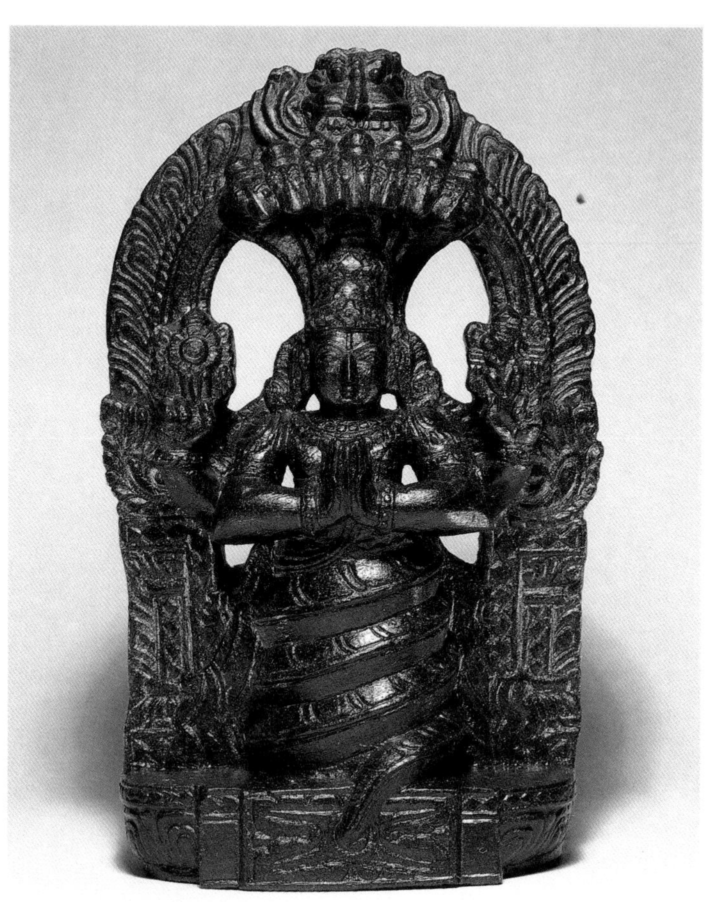

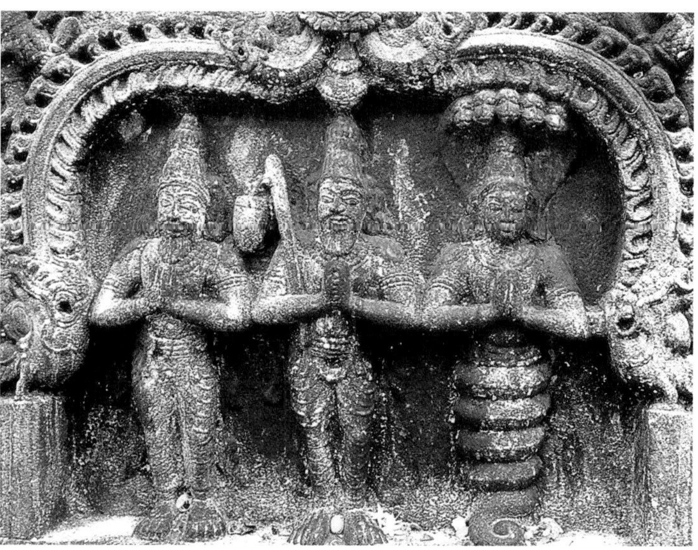

Top This is a statuette representing Patanjali, the ancient Indian sage acknowledged as the founder of yoga. His sutras, or writings, have been translated from Sanskrit and interpreted by many.
Bottom Here on the right is Patanjali as the serpent god, and one of a trinity of devotees witnessing the dance of the god Natajara at his temple in Chidambaram. The other figures are Vyaghrapada, a rishi or sage, with the feet of a tiger, and Simhavarman, an early king.

How to Use the Book

Here you will find a basic introduction to Iyengar yoga for both beginners and more experienced students. It offers a selection of postures from each of the asana groups – standing postures for vitality; seated postures for serenity; twists, which are cleansing; inverted poses for developing mental strength; supine poses, which are restful, and prone poses, which are energizing. There is also a section on relaxation and pranayama (breathing).

Generally, the asana groups and the individual postures within each group are listed in the order in which they should be learned and practised as outlined by Mr Iyengar. The postures are also graded according to their level of difficulty from 1 to 5, with 5 being the most challenging. This grading is represented by the number of highlighted stars at the start of each asana.

Instructions are given for each posture, and photographs show the final posture, as well as the various stages leading to it. There are also tips on how to improve the posture and how props can help less flexible students. (See overleaf for details of props and how to use them.)

The Routine Practice chapter provides over 20 suggested programmes that vary in degree of difficulty and duration. Students should begin with Sequence 1 and proceed at their own pace, remembering to consolidate and not be in too much of a hurry to get to the last routine. It is not about how fast you work, but about the quality, understanding and proficiency of your practice.

The Yoga Therapy chapter provides programmes and advice for students with minor medical conditions. Props are used in most of these sequences to help less able students attain the best pose possible within their personal physical constraints.

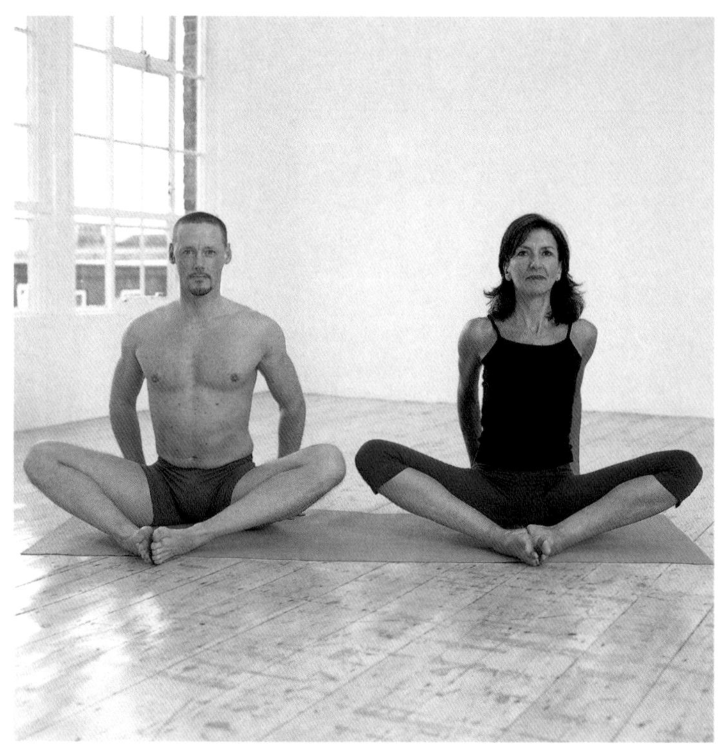

Above Baddhakonasana, a seated posture. Practising yoga in company, or in an organized class with a qualified teacher, is a motivating way to begin, and continue, to learn.

APPROACHING YOGA PRACTICE

"An asana is not a posture which you assume mechanically. It involves thought, at the end of which a balance is achieved between movement and resistance." B.K.S. Iyengar

Practice is essential for improving both physical and mental discipline. There are no rules for when, how often or how long you should do this, but obviously the more regular the practice, the greater the benefit to the practitioner. Practice must be adapted to suit one's circumstances, and the intensity and level of each session should reflect this. For example, if you feel tired after a long day at the office, practise restful/calming postures; if you feel stiff and lethargic, practise standing poses. Listed below are some general guidelines for practice:

- The best time to practise is on an empty stomach. If this is not possible, wait 4–5 hours after a heavy meal and 2–3 hours after a snack.

- Wear light, loose, comfortable clothing that allows free and uninhibited movement.

- Practise with bare feet on a non-slip mat or floor. A carpet is not good as the feet slide and cannot grip the surface.

- Practise in a warm, airy room out of direct sunlight.
- Remove hard contact lenses.
- In each group of asanas, first practise the easier version before attempting the more difficult one. It is advisable to gain proficiency in the simpler version over a period of a few days before progressing to the final pose.
- Practise with full concentration and awareness of the parts of the body involved in each asana. The postures should be done slowly, smoothly and with full understanding.
- Pay attention to accuracy and alignment. When the body is correctly aligned, the flow of energy is uninterrupted.
- It is important to breathe while in the postures. Where no specific instructions are given, breathe normally. Generally one inhales on upward movements, where the chest and abdomen are expanded and broad, and exhales on downward/forward movements, where the chest and abdomen may be compressed.
- Maintain the pose for as long as is possible without causing any physical or mental strain. Keep the eyes, mouth, throat and abdomen relaxed throughout.
- The eyes should be kept open and the mouth shut in all postures, unless otherwise instructed.
- If adverse physical or mental effects are felt during or after practice, seek the advice of a qualified Iyengar teacher.
- This book should be used in conjunction with, not instead of, attending classes. It is important to be instructed and corrected by a teacher.
- Each practice session should be followed by 5 minutes relaxation in Savasana (Corpse pose).

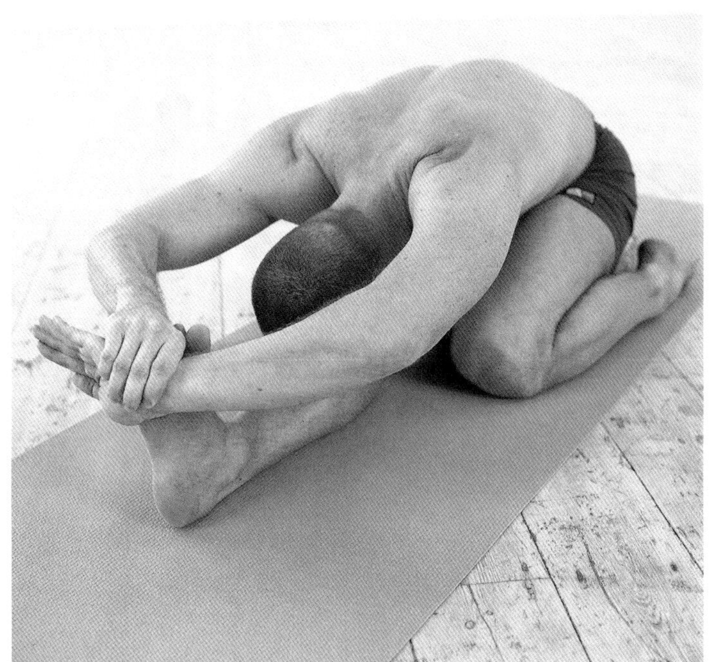

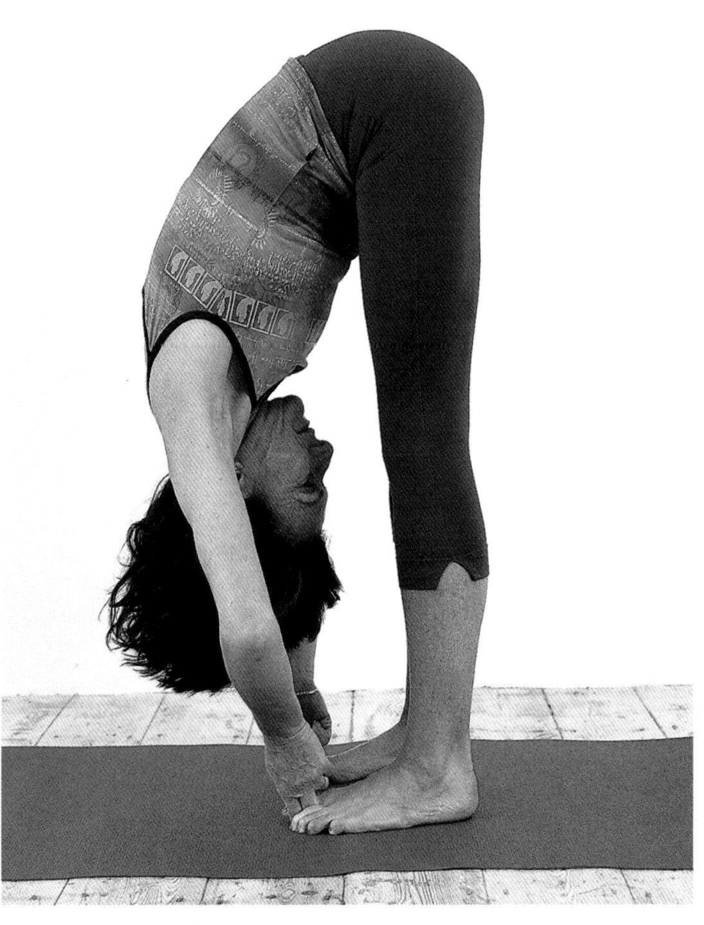

Above right One of the five basic forward bending postures, Trianga Mukhaikapada Pascimottanasana.
Right Padangusthasana, or Finger to Toe pose, strengthens the legs and makes the spine more flexible. Both standing and sitting forward bends aid digestion and tone the abdominal organs.

Equipment

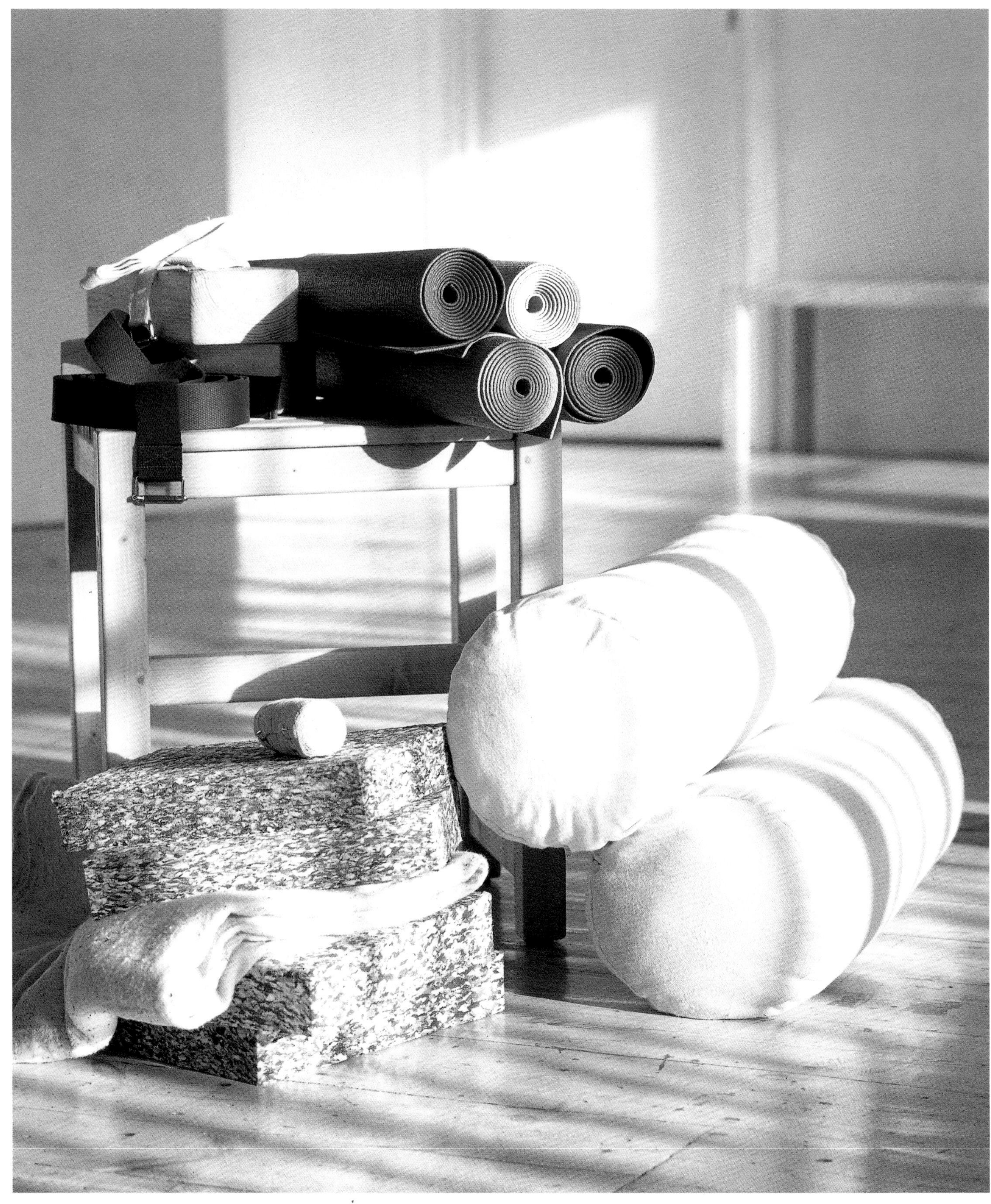

Historically, yogis used logs of wood, stones and ropes to help them practise asanas effectively. Mr Iyengar has invented a variety of props that allow the postures to be held easily and for longer, without strain. The use of props makes the asanas more accessible to all yoga students, whether they are stiff or flexible, young or old, weak or strong, beginners or advanced. They may also be used by those who wish to conserve their energy because of fatigue or injury. Props allow muscular extension to take place while the brain remains passive. Mr Iyengar refers to this as practising "with effortless effort".

Non-slip mats These prevent the feet from sliding during standing poses. It is helpful to draw or fold a line down the centre of the mat to assist with alignment.

Chair A chair is used for easy twisting postures, e.g. Bharadvajasana (Chair pose), or as a support for the body in Chair Sarvangasana and Ardha Halasana.

Wooden blocks These are used when stiffer students find that they cannot reach the floor with their hands. In sitting and standing postures, they can be used to support the legs or hands and to help with twisting poses.

Foam blocks Many students find it difficult to lift the spine in seated poses. Sitting on one or two foam blocks helps to achieve this spinal lift. Blocks are used to support the neck and shoulders in Salamba Sarvangasana, and in restorative poses the blocks are used to support the student's head.

Bolsters Used mainly in restorative and recuperative postures, bolsters support the head or the spine. A couple of cushions or rolled-up blankets can be substituted.

Eyebags These are small bean bags used to calm the eyes in recuperative poses. Also used is the traditional crêpe bandage, that should be lightly wrapped around the head and eyes, helping to release tension around the eye area.

Straps Use straps around the feet in straight-legged postures where the hands cannot catch the toes or foot. The strap is used in Salamba Sarvangasana to prevent the arms sliding apart, and in Supta Baddhakonasana to secure the feet together, close to the pelvis.

Opposite A selection of props used to help students. Furniture and other objects in the home can be adapted and used as props, or they can be purchased from yoga centres.
Right Bolsters and blankets are useful. You may already have similar items at home.
Far right Blocks are made of wood, cork or foam.

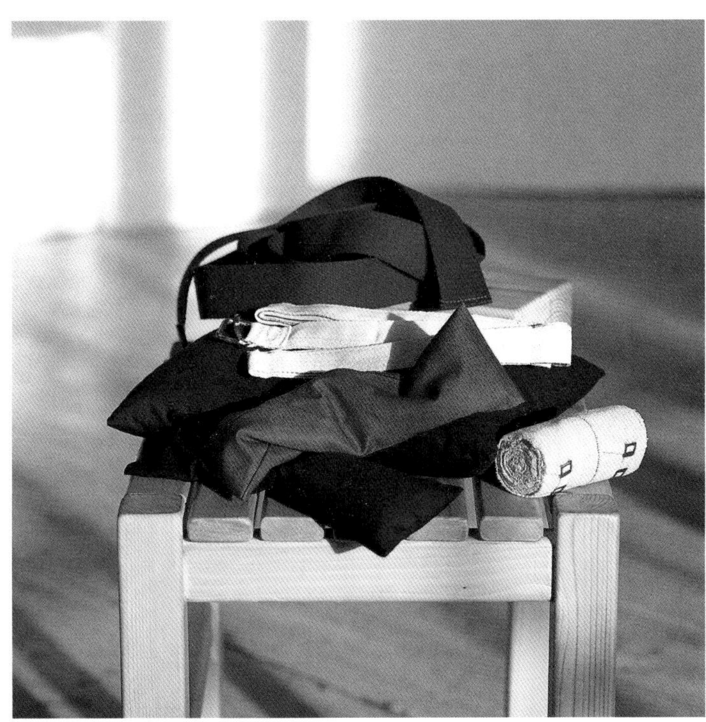

Above Halasana stools come in different heights for all shapes of body. Bandages and bean bags are useful aids to calm the eyes and keep the mind quiet.

Halasana stool This stool is used to support the thighs in Ardha Halasana. In standing twists, the raised foot is supported on a stool or chair. The head may be supported on the Halasana stool in restorative poses.

Blankets Folded blankets may be used instead of foam blocks. They are used to support the head in Savasana, pranayama and restorative postures. They give additional lift to the spine in seated and twisting asanas. A rolled-up blanket can be used to support the feet in Virasana. On a practical note, in Savasana the body temperature is lowered, so cover up and use the blanket for warmth.

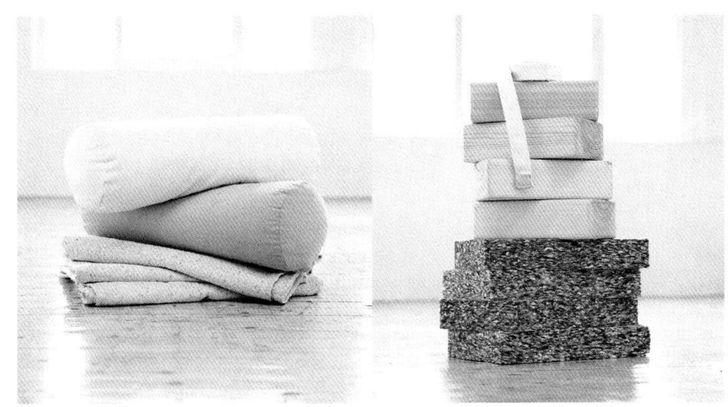

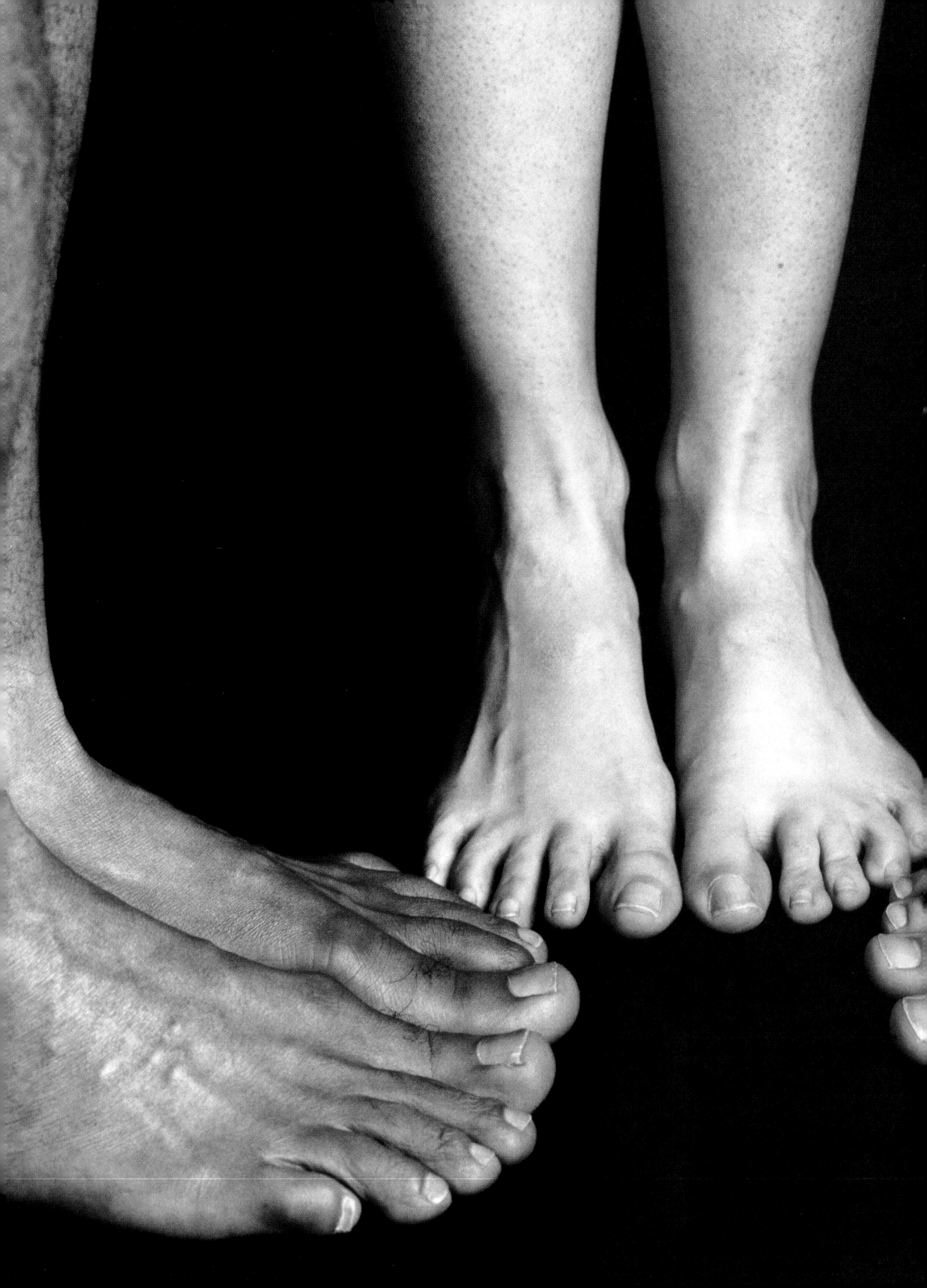

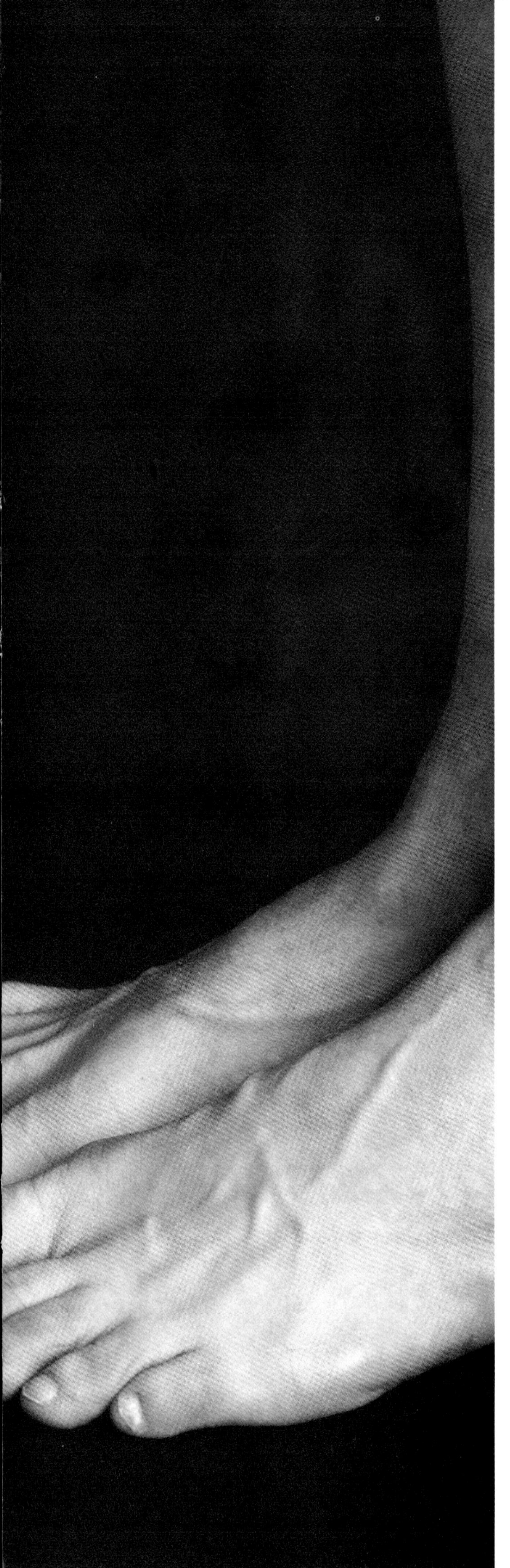

Standing Asanas

Standing postures are dynamic and energizing and form the basis of all other postures. Through them practitioners become familiar with various parts of the skeletal and muscular body and learn to use their intelligence to bring action and awareness to these parts. Standing postures develop strength, stamina and determination.

Tadasana | MOUNTAIN POSE

In this pose we are taught how to stand correctly. It brings attention to our posture and makes us aware of how the legs and feet have to work in order to stand up straight. All standing poses begin and end with Tadasana.

★

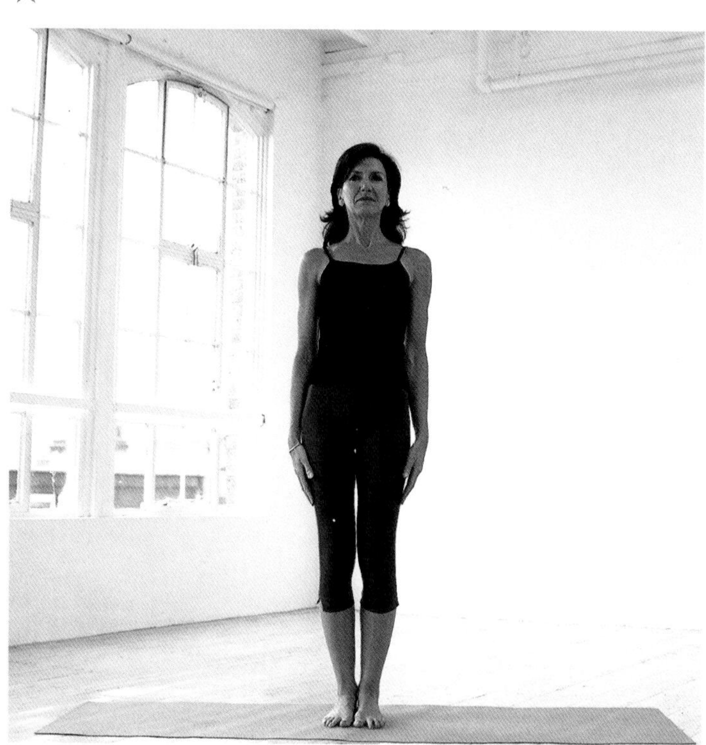

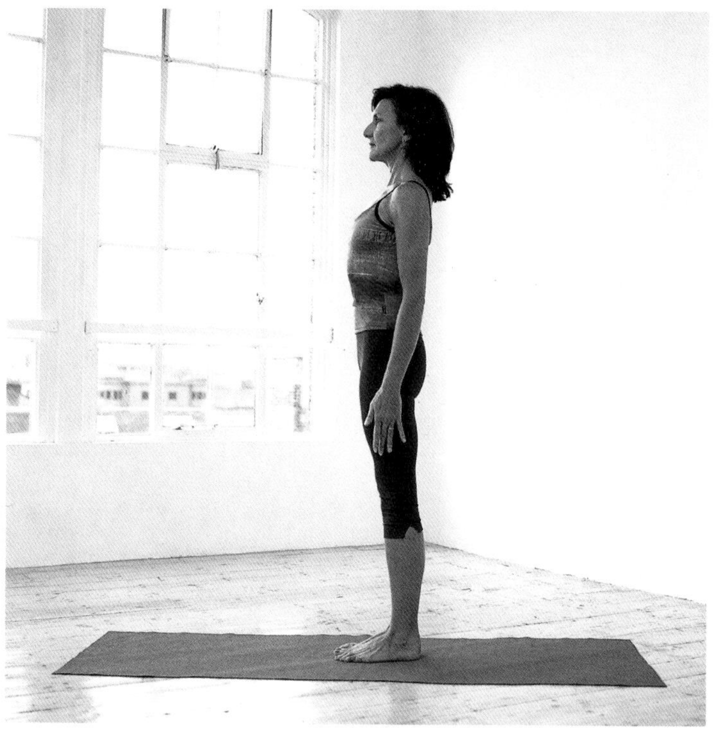

1 Stand with the feet together – big toes, inner ankles and inner heels touching. Spread the body weight evenly over the feet, keeping the inside edges of the feet parallel.

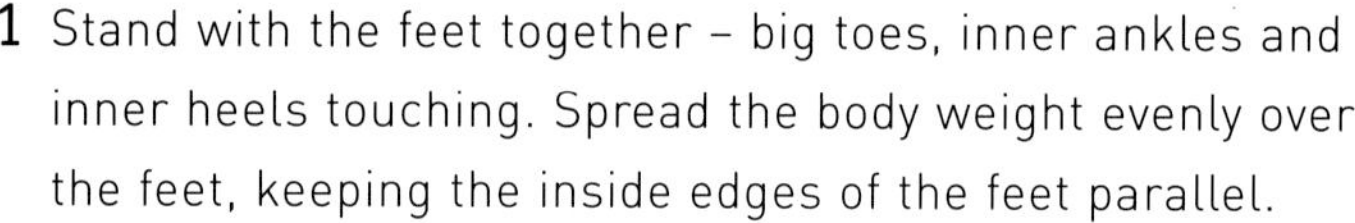

Tighten/lift the kneecaps and pull up the thigh muscles so the legs stretch strongly. Feel the spine extending upwards and the lift in the front of the body. Roll the shoulders back and take the shoulder blades into the body to open the chest.

Focus on Tadasana

• Although relatively simple, this posture is crucial as it teaches awareness of the body and the recognition of any postural difficulties. Try to perfect this posture before moving on to the next pose.
• Press the feet firmly into the floor and extend the crown of the head towards the ceiling.
• Extend the sides and back of the neck, balancing the head on the top of the spine.
• Feel the front body "opening" from pubis to chin.
• Project the breastbone towards the front of the chest.
• Ensure that the body is stretching evenly on all sides – front, back, left and right. Strain is caused to the body by leaning habitually to one side or the other.

2 Allow the arms to hang down the sides of the body with the palms facing the legs.

Extend the neck up, relax the face and look straight ahead. Hold for 30–60 seconds.

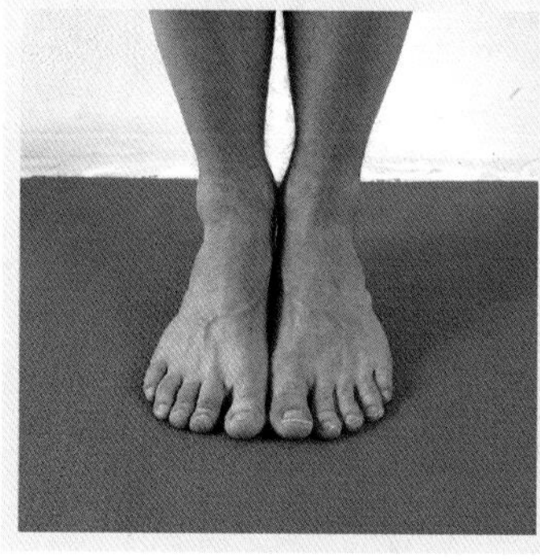

Focus on feet

• It is important to keep the inside edges of the feet parallel, and the big toes and ankle bones together Weight should be evenly spread over the heels and soles of the feet.

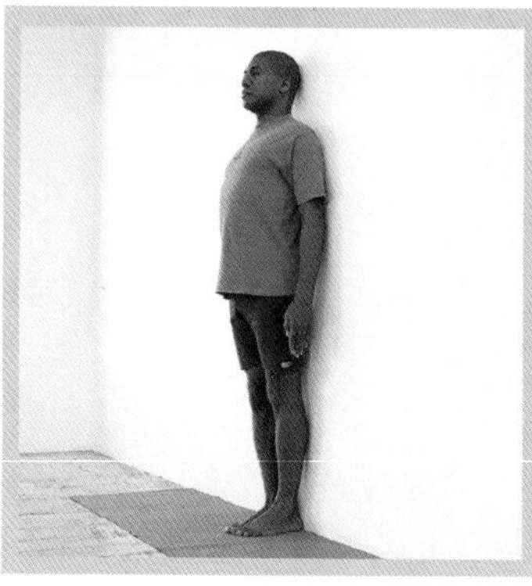

Modification

• If you find it hard to balance, try Tadasana standing against a wall. This is also helpful to ensure that you are standing straight, and not leaning forwards or backwards.

Vrksasana | TREE POSE

This posture tones and stretches the leg muscles and teaches balance. Consistent practice of the balancing postures will improve your concentration and increase muscle tone and general poise.

★

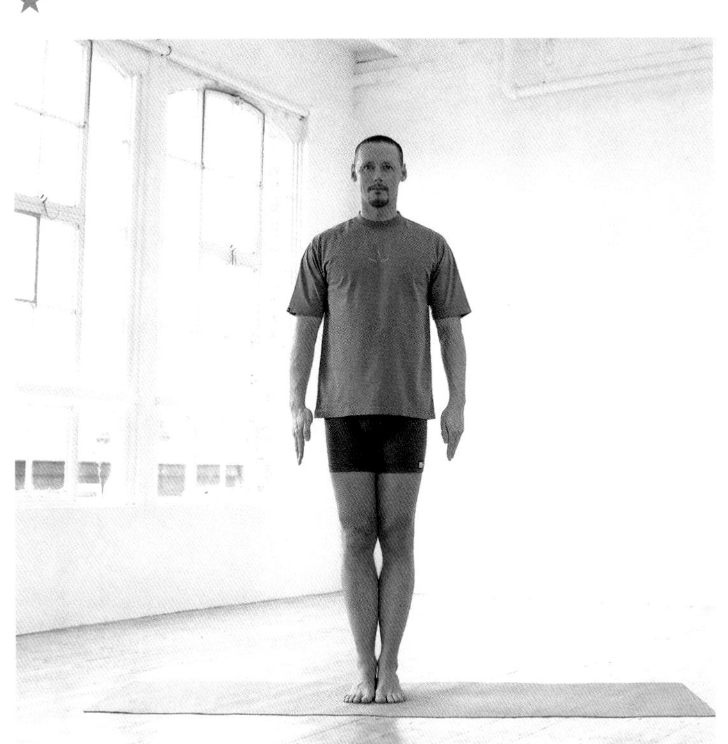

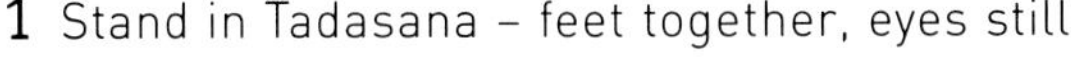

1 Stand in Tadasana – feet together, eyes still.

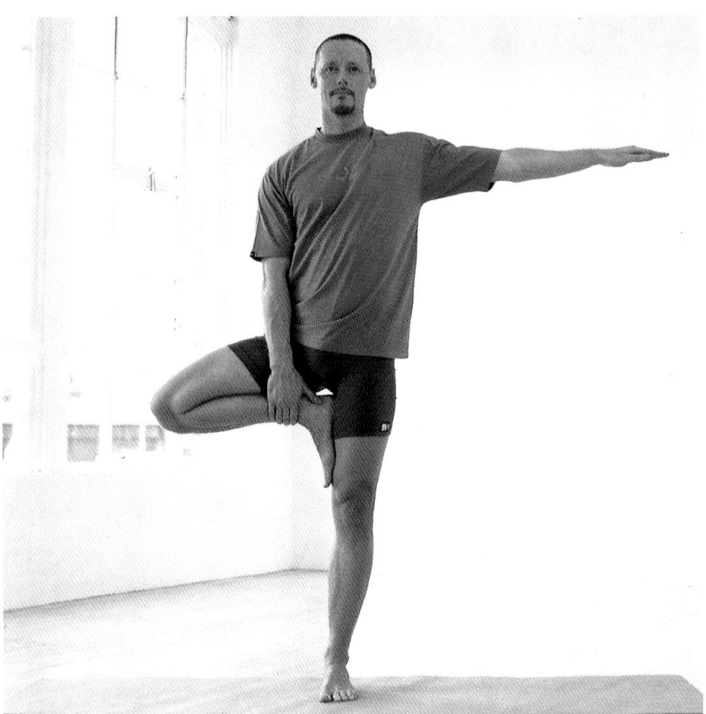

2 Bend the right knee to the side (without disturbing the left leg). Hold the ankle and place the sole of the right foot high on the left inner thigh with the toes pointing towards the floor. Keep the bent (right) knee back in line with the left leg and keep the left leg steady.

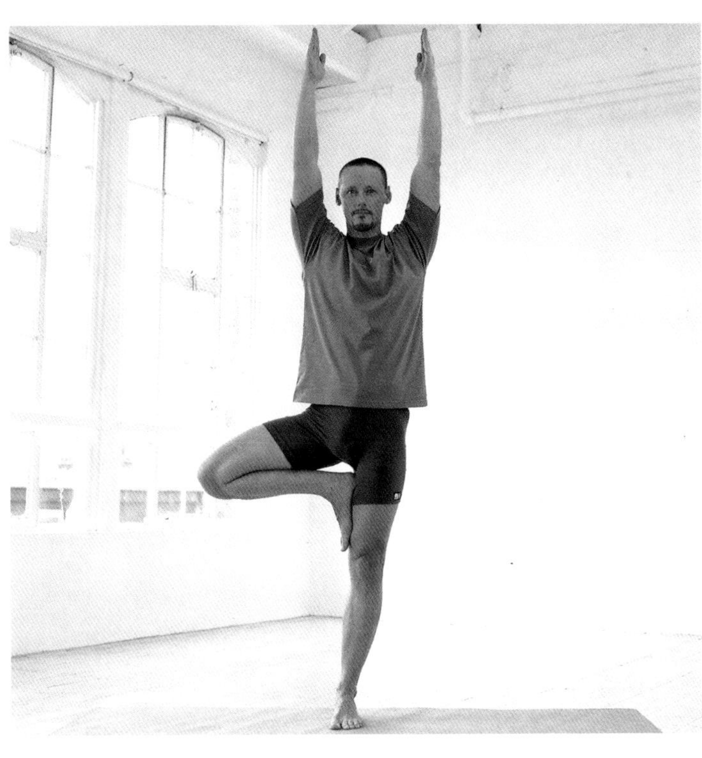

3 Inhale and stretch the arms over the head with palms facing one another. Straighten the elbows and extend the arms and trunk up.

Join the palms if you can do so without bending the elbows, otherwise keep them apart. Hold for 30–60 seconds. Exhale, then lower the arms and the right leg and repeat on the other side.

Focus

• To help maintain balance, try to focus the eyes on an object in the middle distance. Balancing poses such as Vrksasana can contribute to improving concentration in the long term.

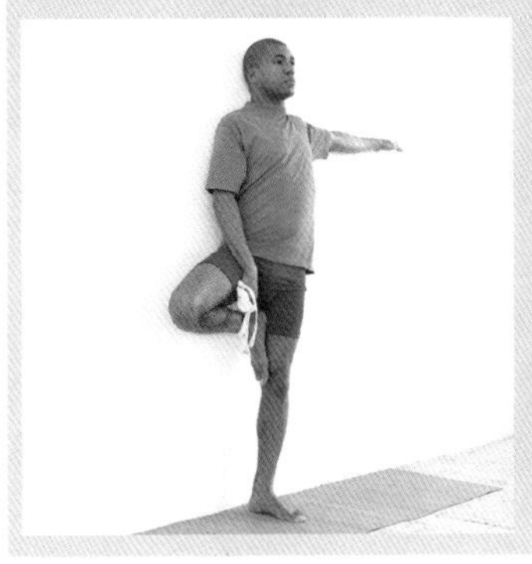

Modification

• To help with balance, use the wall for support and hold the foot up with a strap.
• Keep the grounded foot pressing firmly into the floor.
• Don't allow the left leg to bow to the side.

Utthita Trikonasana | EXTENDED TRIANGLE POSE

This pose strengthens the legs, makes the hips more flexible and relieves backache. In this posture, when turning the feet, it is important not to turn the hips as well. Start on the right side, then repeat the posture to the left.

★

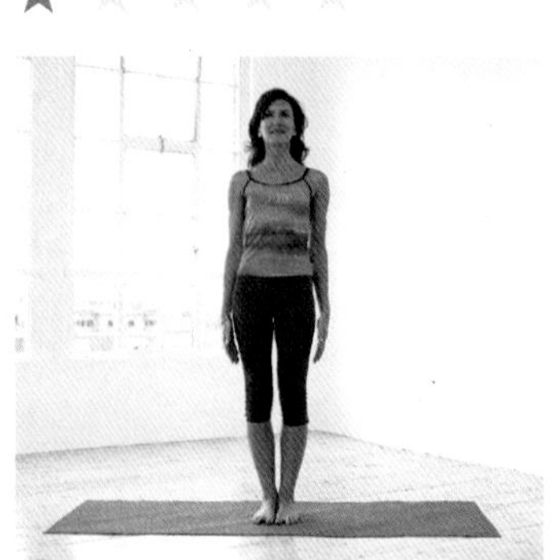

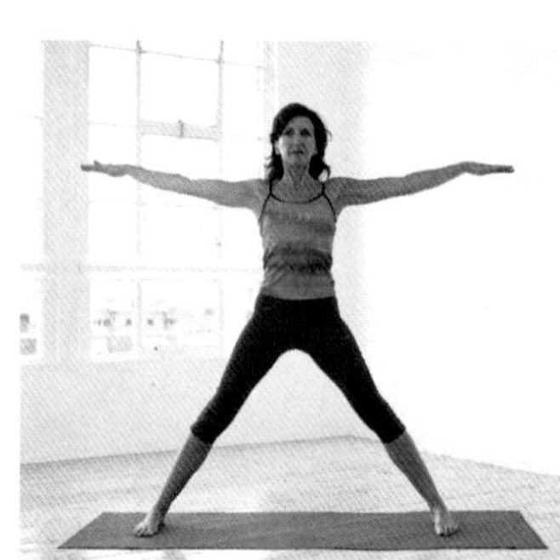

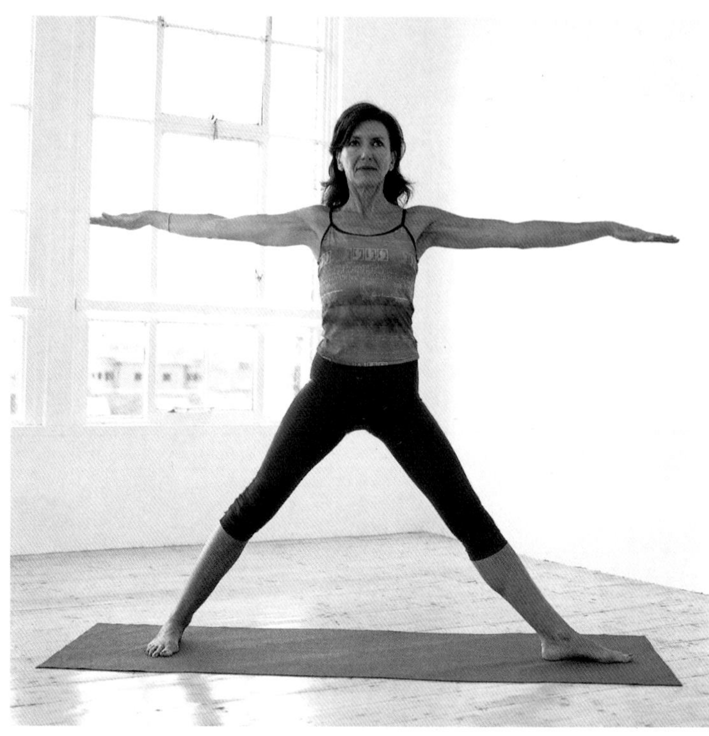

1 Stand in Tadasana.

2 Inhale deeply, jump or step* your feet 1–1.2m/3–4ft apart and extend the arms out to the side, keeping the palms facing the floor (* students with back problems should step their feet apart).

Ensure that both feet are level with one another, legs extended and straight, knees lifted.

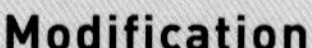

3 Turn your left foot out about 90 degrees (so that it is parallel to the side of your mat), and turn your right foot slightly inwards (about 15 degrees). The left heel should be in line with the instep of the right foot. As you turn the right foot in, rotate the right leg outwards, and as you turn the left foot outwards, rotate the whole leg to the left, so that the legs are rotating away from one another. Keep the left knee pulled up and facing in the same direction as the left foot.

Modification

- The final aim is to reach the floor, with the palm face down. If you cannot reach, place the hand on the ankle. If you need more help, use a brick standing on its end under the left hand to get more extension in the spine and to allow the chest to turn towards the ceiling.
- Students who are less flexible can do this posture with the back against the wall to aid balance. In this case, place the brick next to the wall to keep it steady. or try the posture with the back foot against the wall.
- If the neck aches when turning the head, either look straight ahead or look towards the left foot.

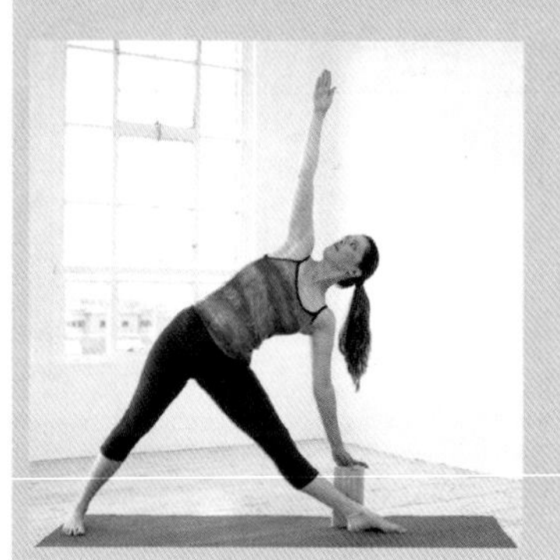

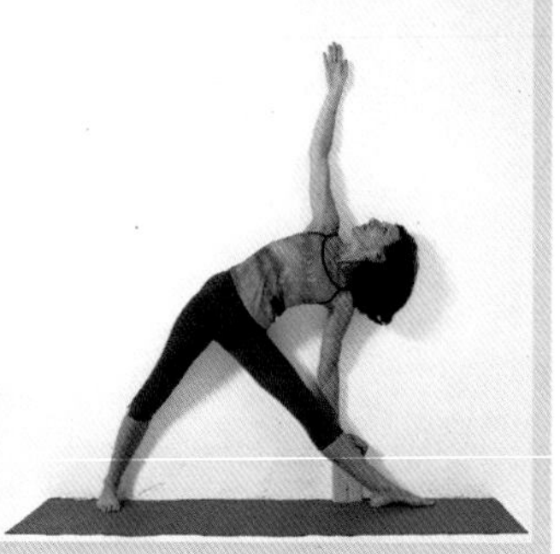

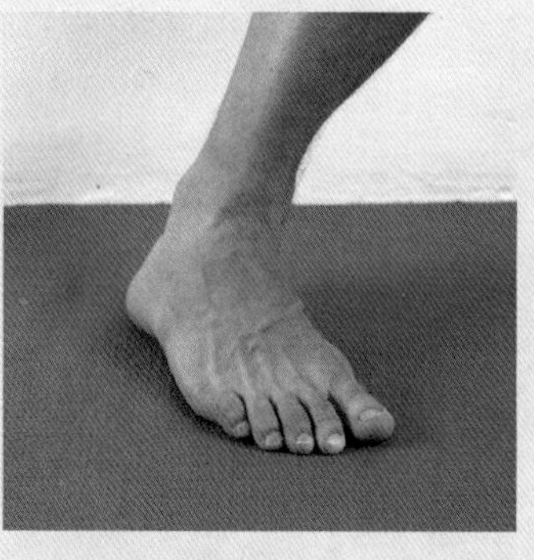

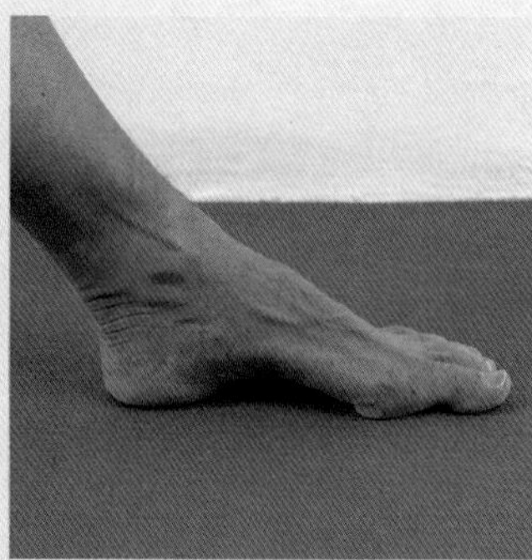

Focus

- Turn the back foot in 15 degrees. Press the corners of both feet into the floor and lift the instep.
- Stretch the toes forwards and the heels back to lengthen the soles of the feet.

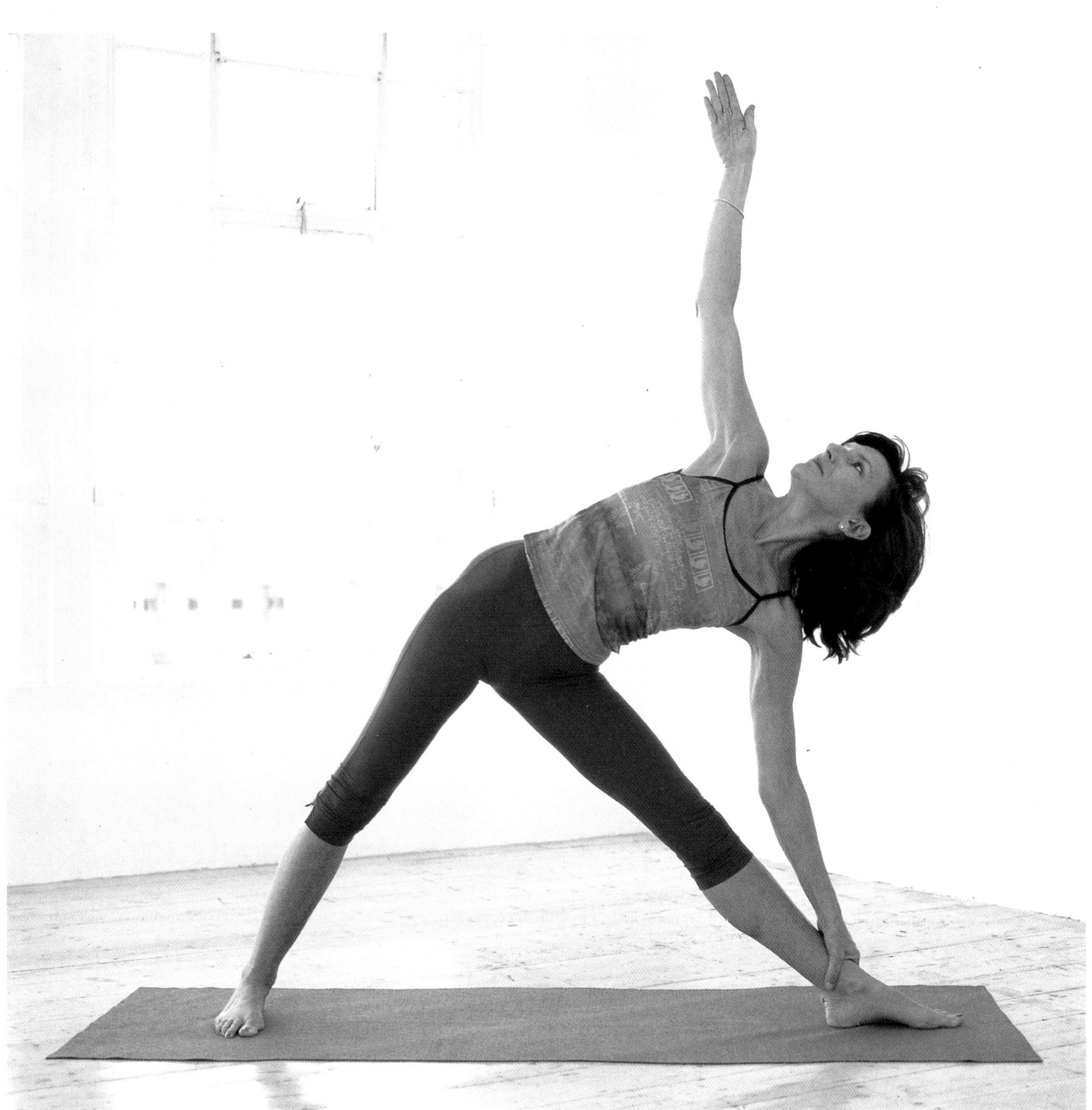

4 Lift the trunk, extend the arms further and then exhale and stretch the trunk sideways to the left. Hold the left ankle with the left hand.

Extend the right arm upwards, keeping the palm facing forwards and keeping it in line with the left arm. Turn the head and look towards the right thumb.

Extend both legs strongly and rotate the navel forwards and upwards.

Hold for 30–40 seconds, inhale and come up, then turn the right foot out and the left foot inwards and repeat on the other side. After doing both sides, come back to the centre of the mat in Tadasana.

Utthita Parsvakonasana | EXTENDED LATERAL ANGLE POSE

This posture strengthens legs and spine, and helps to open the chest. The full lunge twists the body, stimulating the organs inside the body, aiding digestion and the elimination of toxins.

★ ★

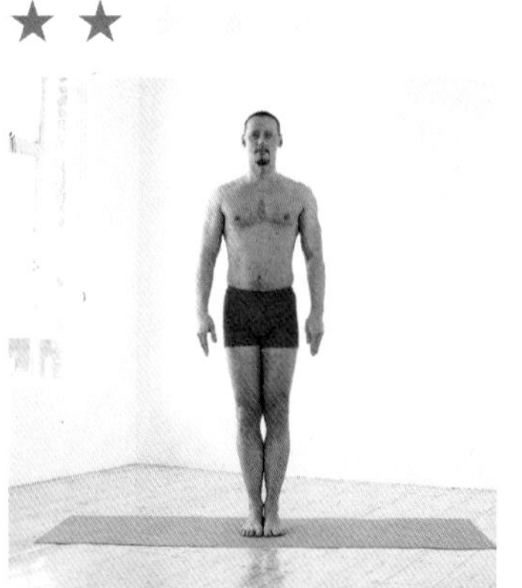

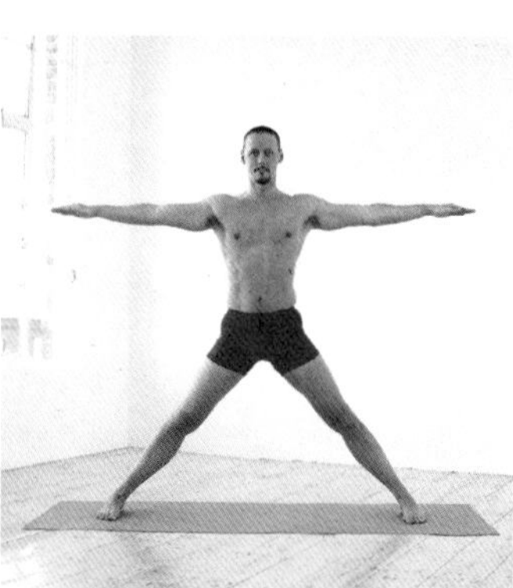

1 Stand in Tadasana with feet together.

2 Inhale deeply, jump or step your feet 1.3m/4.5ft apart and extend the arms out to the side, keeping the palms facing the floor. Next, turn the right foot inwards 15 degrees and the left foot outwards 90 degrees. Broaden the palms and extend the whole arm from the tops of the shoulders to the fingertips. Move the shoulders away from the ears.

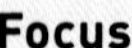

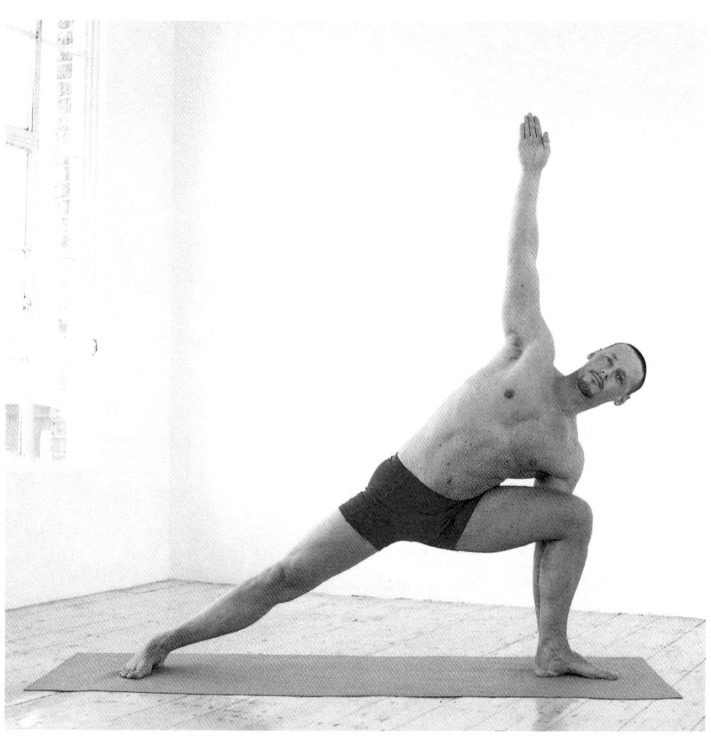

3 Keep the right leg firm and straight, and bend the left knee to 90 degrees – keeping the shin perpendicular and the thigh parallel to the floor. Exhale and extend the trunk sideways, placing the fingertips of the left hand on the floor by the outer edge of the left foot. Keep the right leg stretched and firm – to do this press the outer edge of the right foot into the floor.

Focus

- As with all directional postures, begin with the right side first, then continue with the left for balance.
- If the neck is uncomfortable, look straight ahead not towards the ceiling.
- Move the buttock of the left (bent) leg forwards towards the left inner thigh and, at the same time, keep the left knee moving back slightly, thus keeping the groin open.
- Keep the top arm pointing towards the ceiling, as this will help to keep the chest open and lifted.
- Make sure that the back foot is turned in by 15 degrees and the instep is in line with the heel of the front foot.

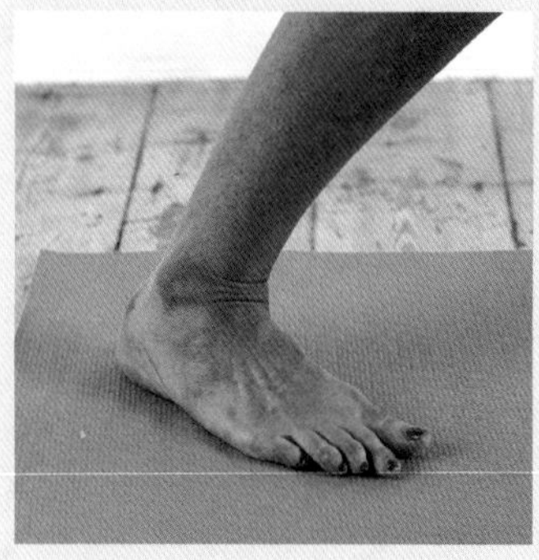

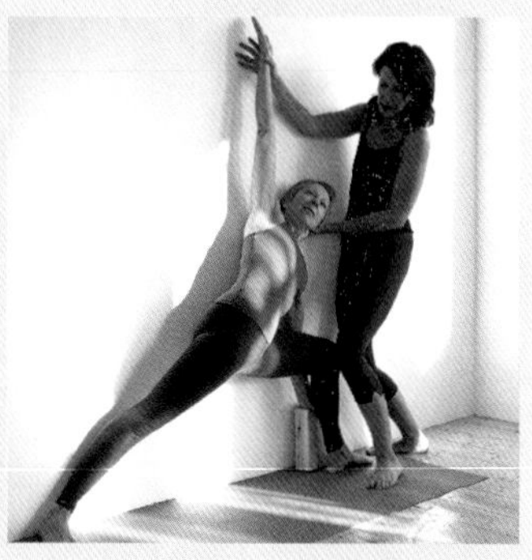

Modification

- Use a wooden block under the left hand to open the chest more.
- Do the posture with the back against the wall to improve the alignment.
- This posture can be done at right angles to the wall, with the back foot against the wall for support.

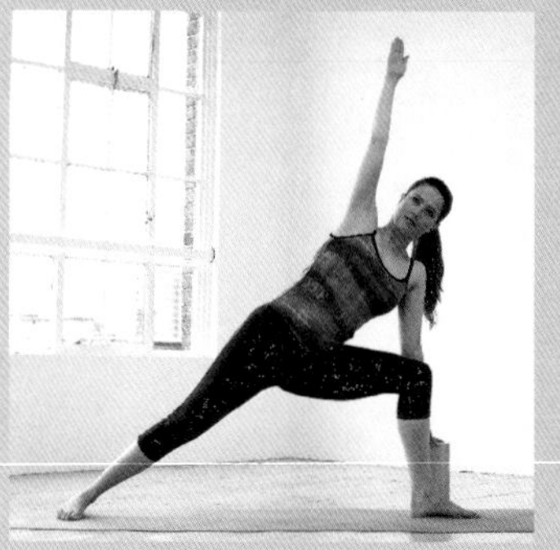

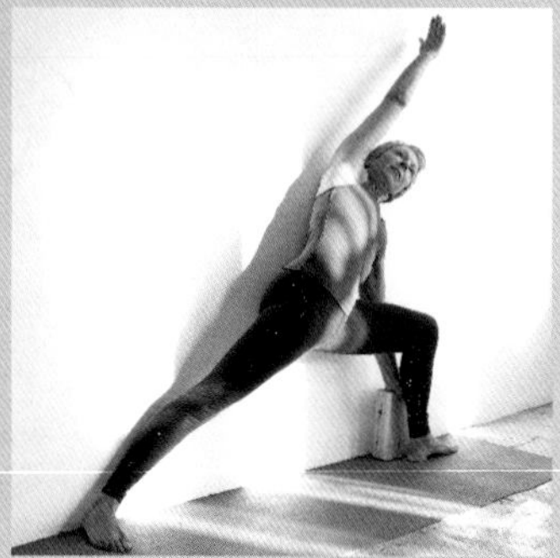

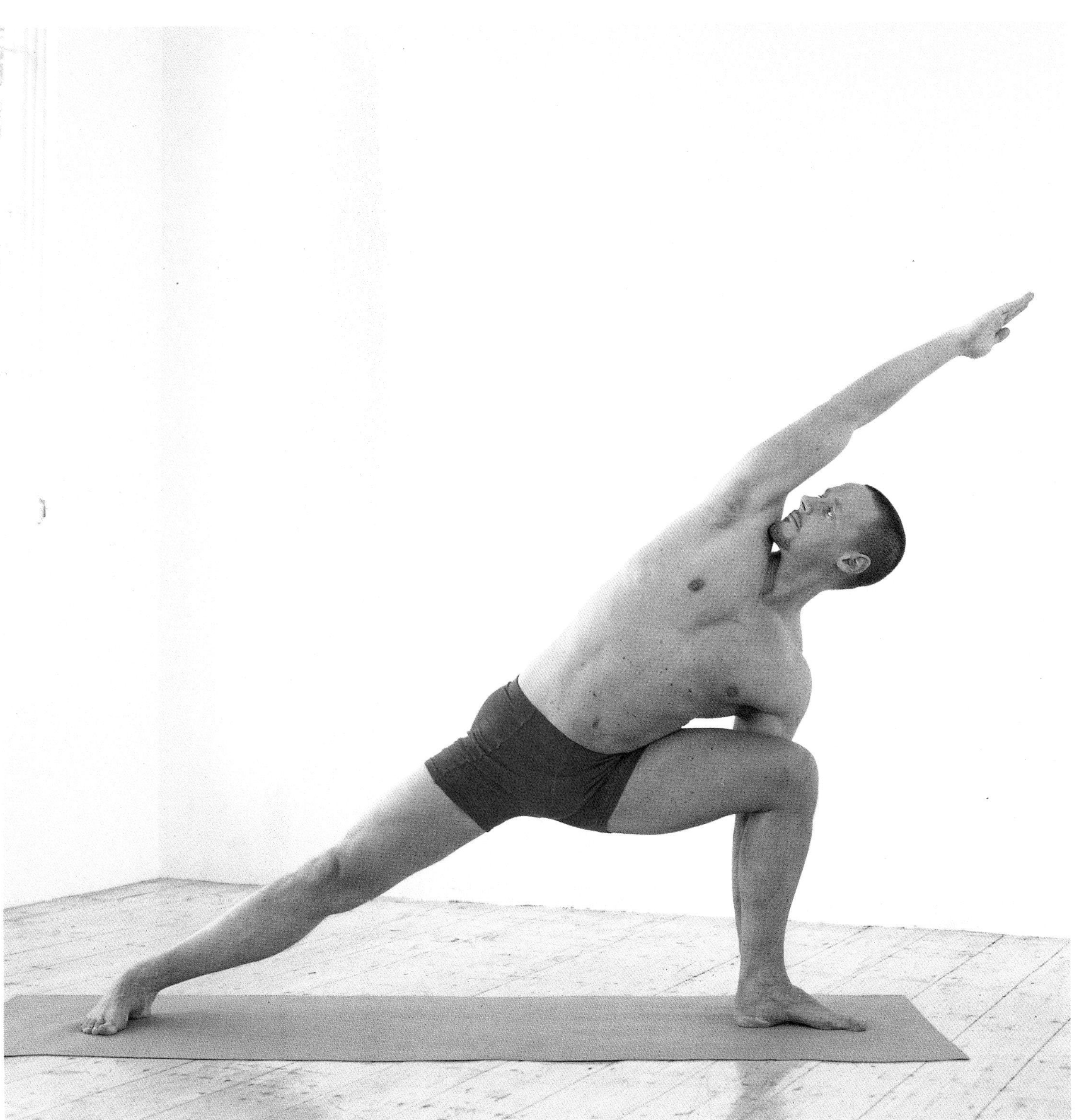

4 Turn the right arm towards the head and extend this arm over the head with the palm facing the floor. Turn the head to look towards the ceiling.

Fully extend the right leg and arm and turn the navel towards the ceiling.

Breathe normally and stay for 30–40 seconds. Inhale and come up, turn both feet forwards, rest hands on hips and then repeat the posture on the right side.

After finishing both sides, come back to Tadasana in the centre of your mat.

Virabhadrasana II | WARRIOR POSE II

This pose strengthens the legs, brings flexibility to the spinal muscles and tones the abdominal muscles. Although this is called the second posture it is practised first as it is less challenging.

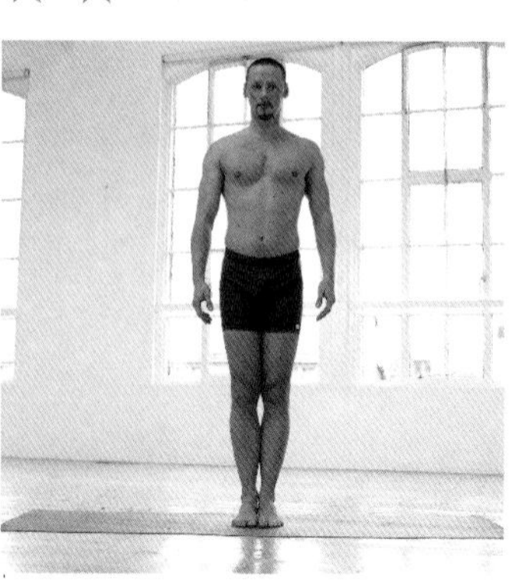

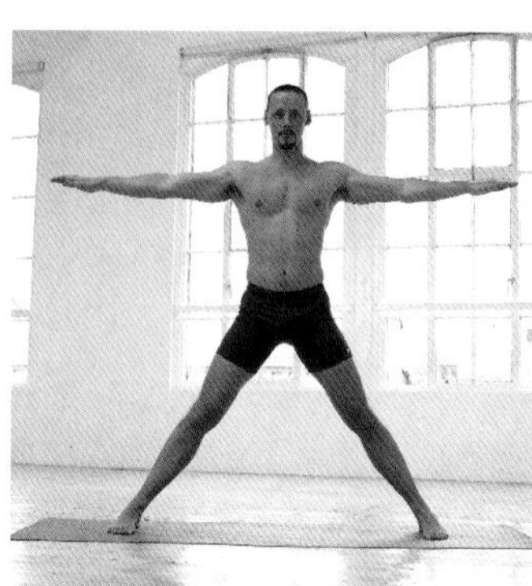

1 Stand in Tadasana.

2 Inhale deeply, jump or step your feet 1–1.2m/3–4ft apart and extend the arms out to the side, palms facing the floor.

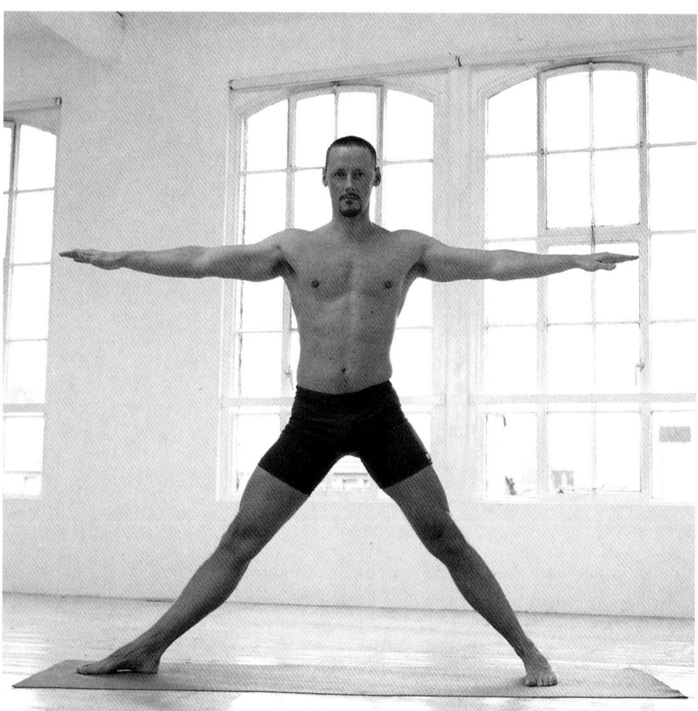

3 Turn the right foot out and the left foot in 15 degrees.

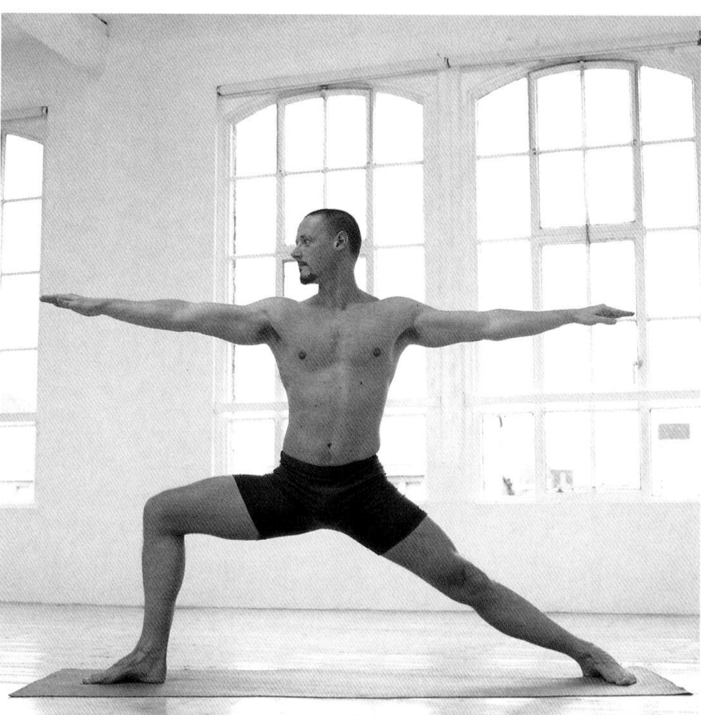

4 Extend the trunk up from the hips and, as you exhale, bend the right leg to 90 degrees, keeping the left leg firm and straight. Extend the arms strongly to the right and left with the palms facing the floor, stretch the trunk upwards, open the chest, turn the head and look along the right arm.

Extend the left arm more to the left so that the trunk doesn't lean towards the right. The crown of the head should be extending straight up towards the ceiling.

Open the chest, relax the face and breathe normally. Hold for 30–40 seconds, inhale and come up. Turn the feet forwards and repeat on the other side.

After completing both sides, come back into Tadasana.

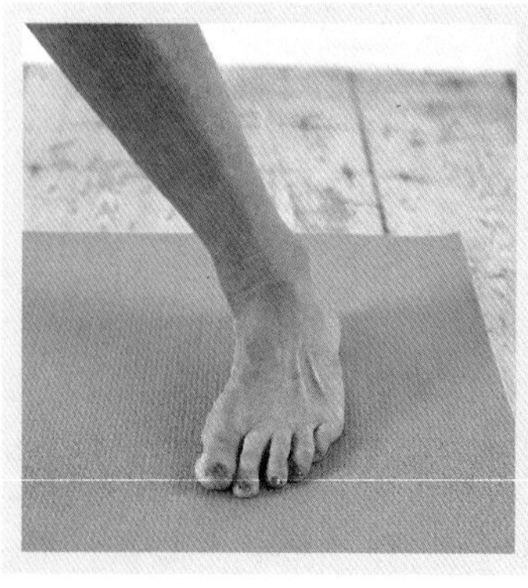

Focus

- Make sure that the back foot is turned in 15 degrees.
- Firmly press the outer edge and the heel of the back foot into the floor to create strength and stability in the back leg.

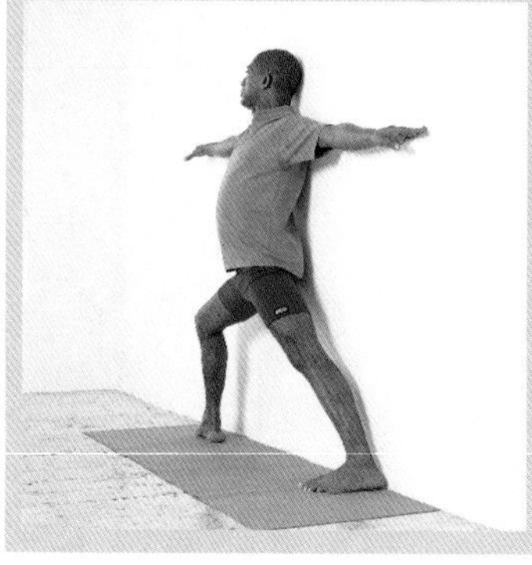

Modification

- Lean the back of the body against the wall for better alignment.
- Alternatively, place the back heel against the wall, with the fingertips of the back hand touching the wall.

Virabhadrasana I | WARRIOR POSE I

This is a challenging pose in which the chest is well expanded, which in turn improves breathing. It also helps with stiffness in the shoulders, back and neck.

★ ★ ★

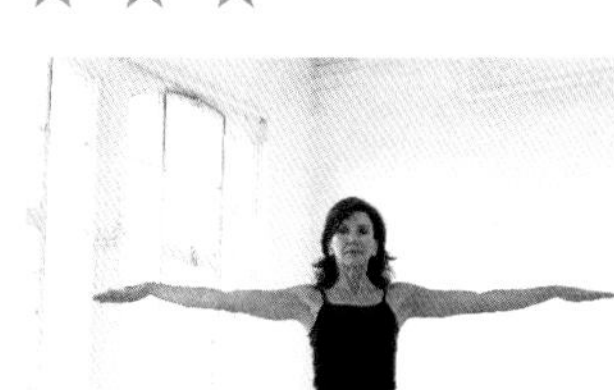

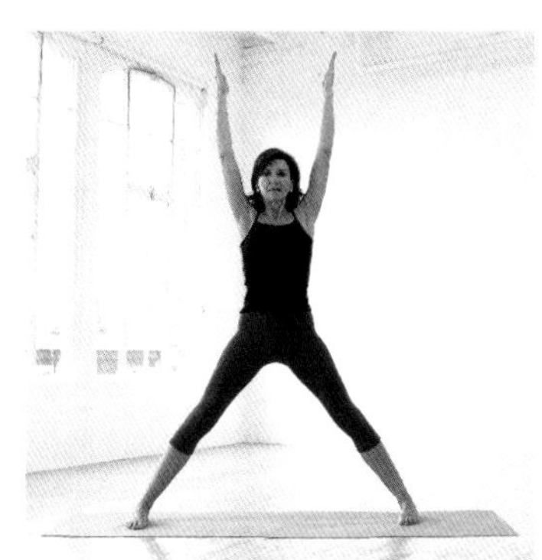

1 Stand in Tadasana, inhale deeply, jump or step the feet 1–1.2m/3–4ft apart and raise the arms to shoulder level.

2 Turn the palms upwards and extend the arms towards the ceiling, keeping the elbows straight and the palms facing one another. If your lower back aches when taking the arms up, then keep your hands on your hips.

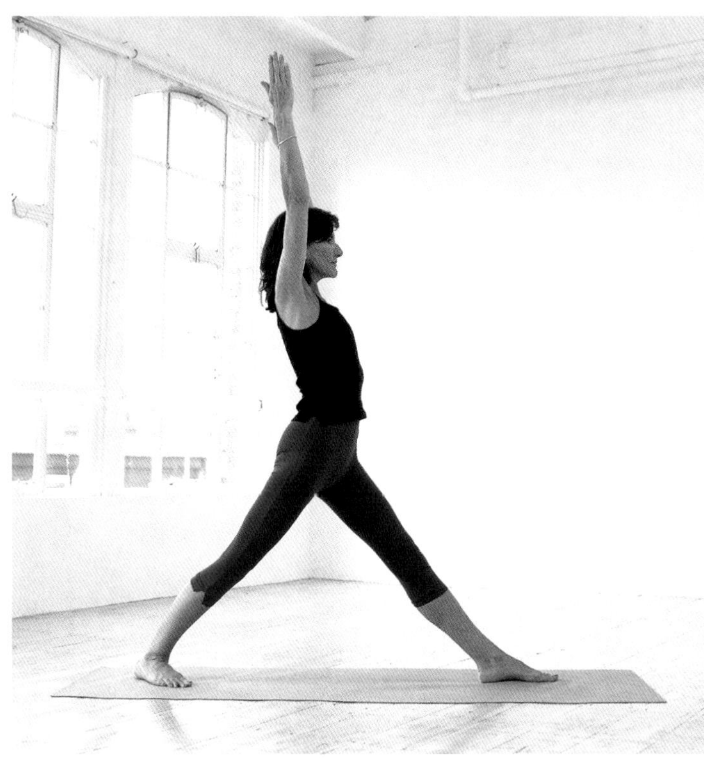

3 Turn the right foot and leg in deeply, about 40 degrees, and the left foot out 90 degrees. Simultaneously turn the hips, trunk and shoulders to the left.

Both sides of the trunk should be parallel – so bring the right hip forwards, while taking the left hip slightly back, to keep them even.

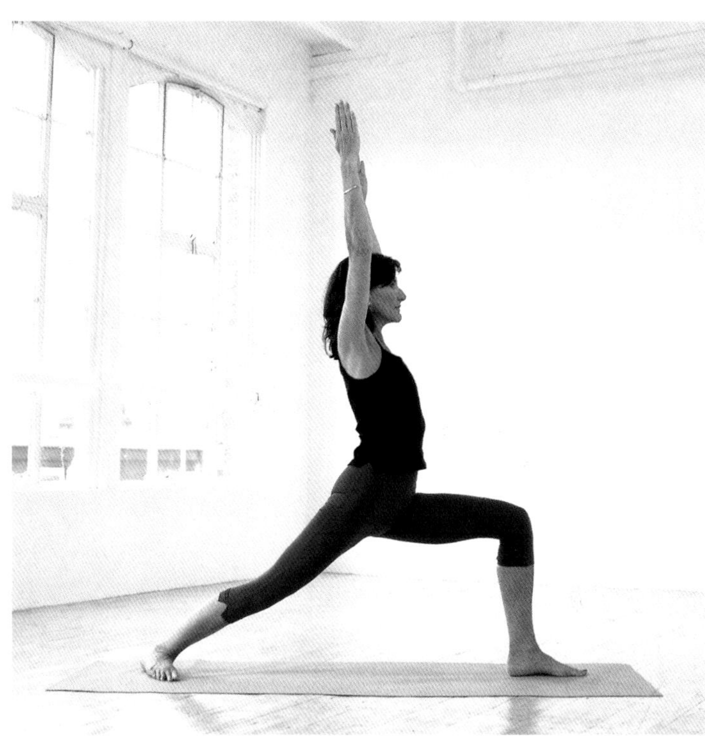

4 Exhale and bend the left leg to form a 90-degree angle. Extend the trunk upwards, as if it were being lifted out of the hips. Move the shoulder blades into the body to open the chest. Extend the chin towards the ceiling and look up. Maintain the full extension on the back leg and keep the hips, shoulders and trunk rotating to the left. Hold for 20–30 seconds, inhale, come up and lower the arms. Repeat on the other side, coming back to Tadasana.

Focus

• Don't strain or hold the breath in this posture. Breath is energy, so breathe evenly.

• If the lower back is uncomfortable in this pose, do it with the hands on the hips.

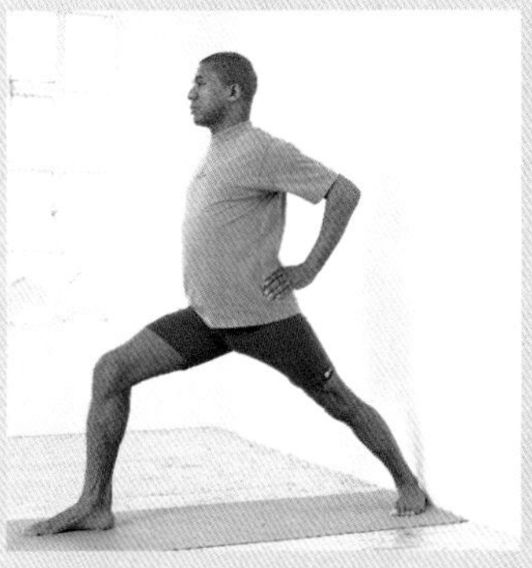

Modification

• If difficulty is experienced in turning the back foot inwards 15 degrees, either work with the back heel against a wall, or support the back heel with a foam block used as a raise.

Ardha Chandrasana | HALF MOON POSE

This pose strengthens the legs and helps improve balance. Regular practice will improve concentration and co-ordination. Because of the strong extension of the spine, it helps correct alignment and makes the back supple.

★ ★ ★

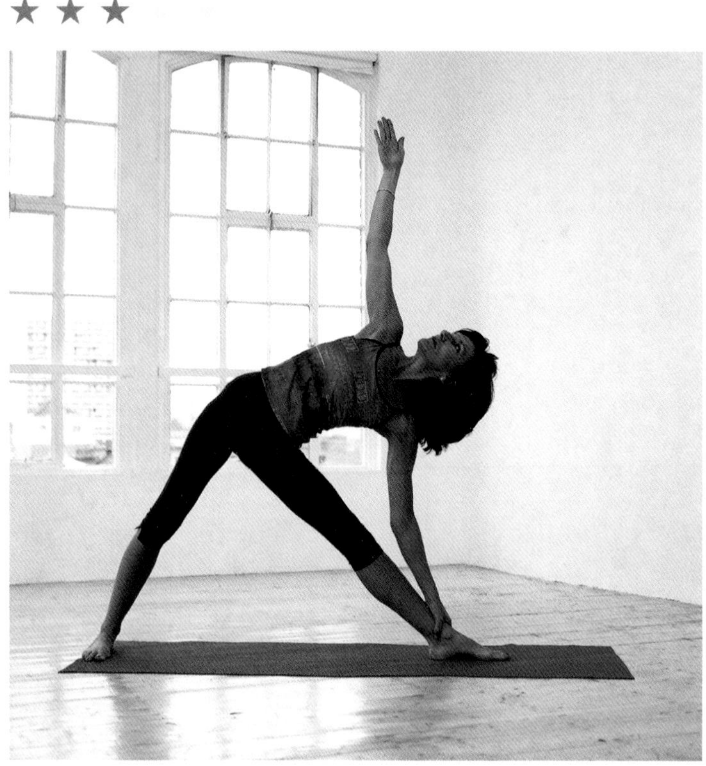

1 Start in Tadasana, then move into the full pose for Utthita Trikonasana.

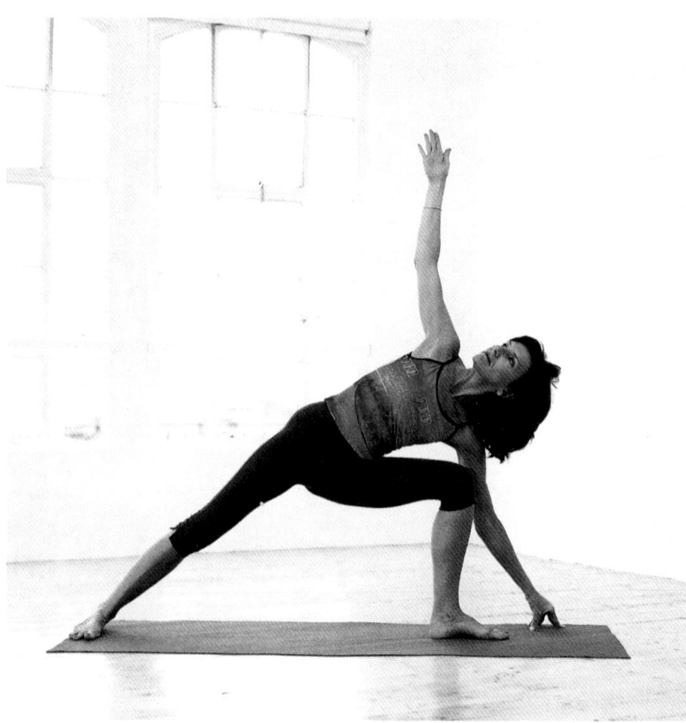

2 Bend the left knee and place the left hand about 30cm/1ft beyond the outer edge of the left foot. Bring the weight of the body on to this foot, using the hand to maintain balance.

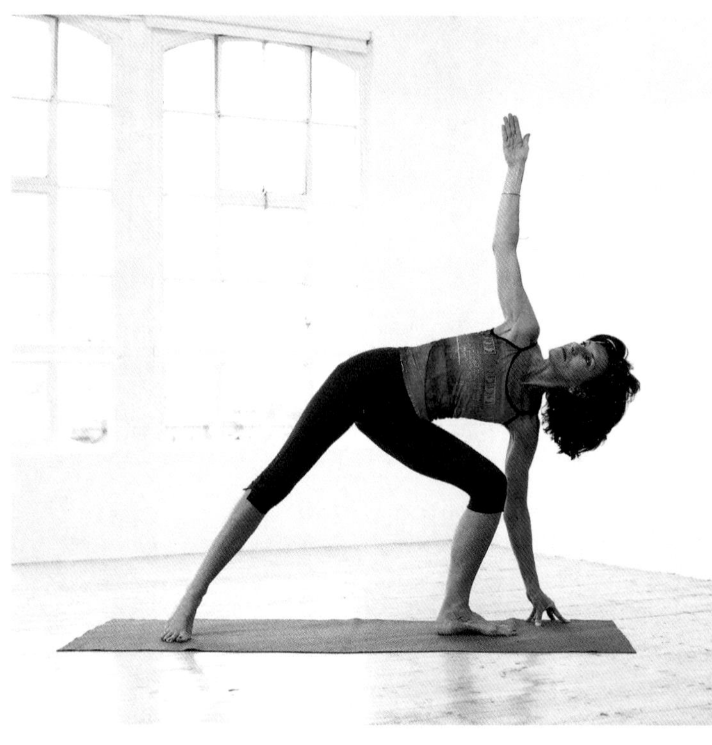

3 Exhale and draw the right foot slightly in towards the left leg. Straighten the left leg and the right leg will lift up.

Focus

- Keep the top hip (the one facing the ceiling) directly above the bottom hip (of the standing leg).
- If the neck is stiff, look ahead, not towards the top hand and the ceiling.

Modification

- If balancing is difficult, do the posture with the back of the body against the wall.
- Use a wooden block as support for the left hand.
- Alternatively, rest the foot of the lifted leg on a ledge or stool, using blocks to achieve the correct height.

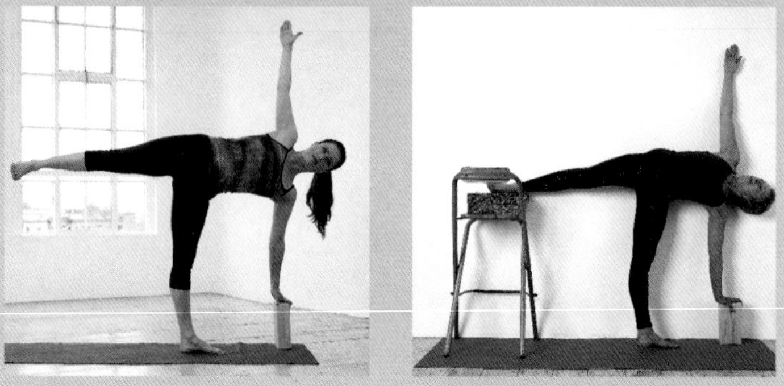

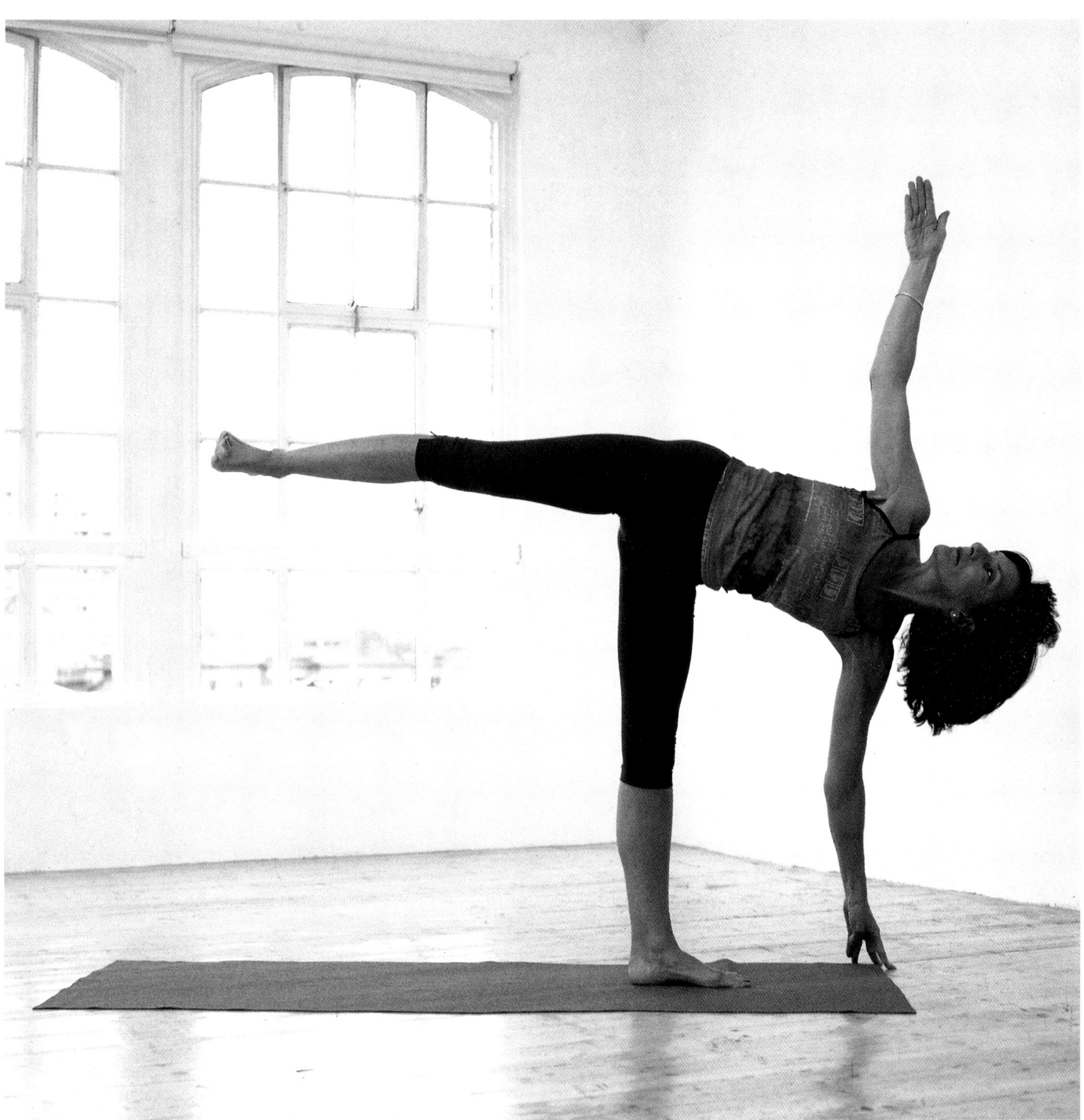

4 Raise and extend the right leg – keeping it parallel to the floor. Keep the left leg firm and pulled up and ensure that it is perpendicular to the floor.

If you are confident with the balance, extend the right arm up towards the ceiling, keeping it in line with the left arm.

Slowly turn the head to look at the right hand and open the chest, lifting the ribs upwards by twisting the waist.

Hold for 20–30 seconds, breathing normally, then come up and repeat on the second side. After finishing both sides, come back to Tadasana.

Utthita Hasta Padangusthasana I & II | EXTENDED LEG RAISES

This pose tones the muscles of the lower spine and strengthens the legs. It is done by standing on one leg, extending the other leg, to the front or the side, and catching the big toe with the fingers.

★ ★

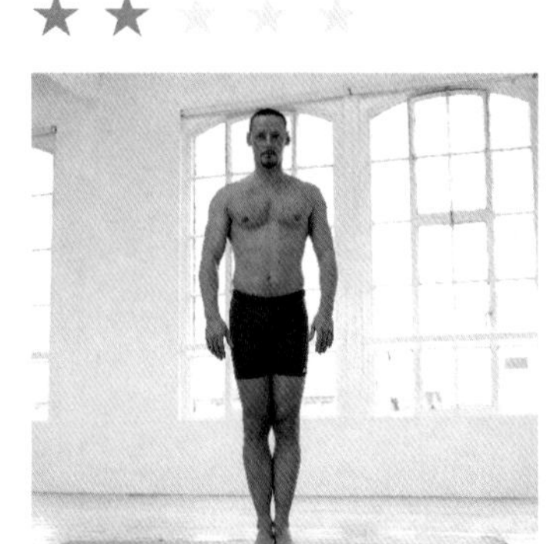

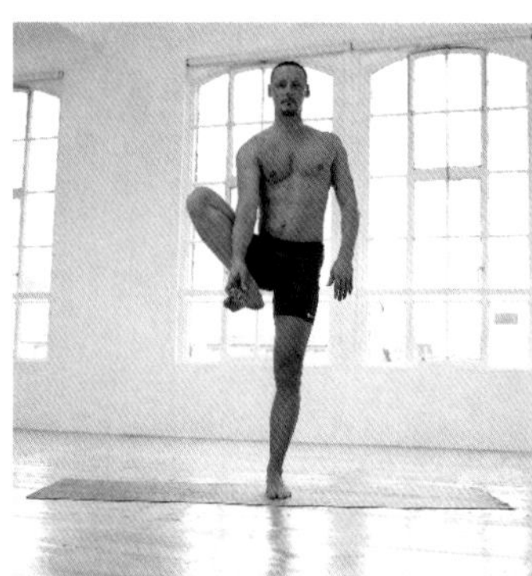

1 Stand in Tadasdana.

2 Bend the right knee and clutch the big toe with the first and second finger of the right hand.

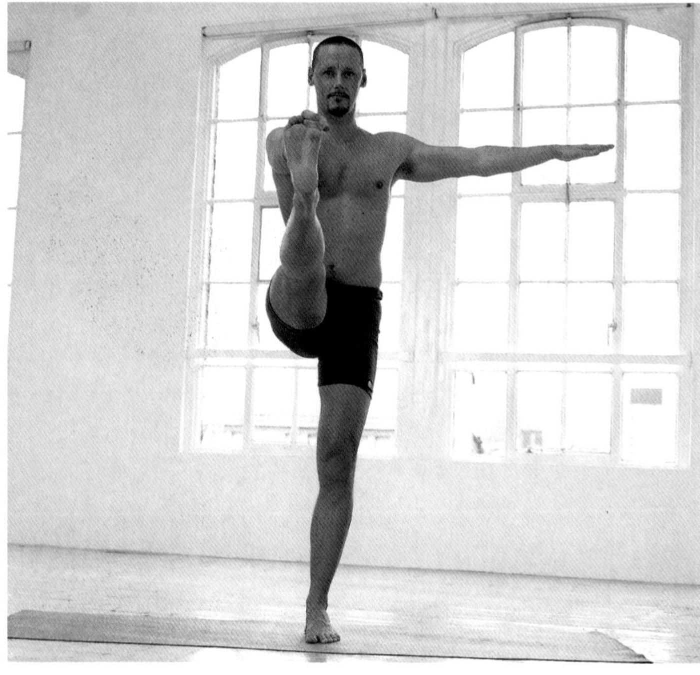

3 Utthita Hasta Padangusthasana I – Straighten the right leg forwards. Keep the knee of the extended leg pointing upwards, and the standing leg vertical.

Focus

• As the right leg is raised and straightened, ensure that the left foot (on the floor) does not turn out. Keep the toes on this foot pointing forwards.

• Keep the trunk upright, not leaning towards the raised leg. If this happens, support the lifted foot on a ledge.

• Balancing poses improve concentration and poise.

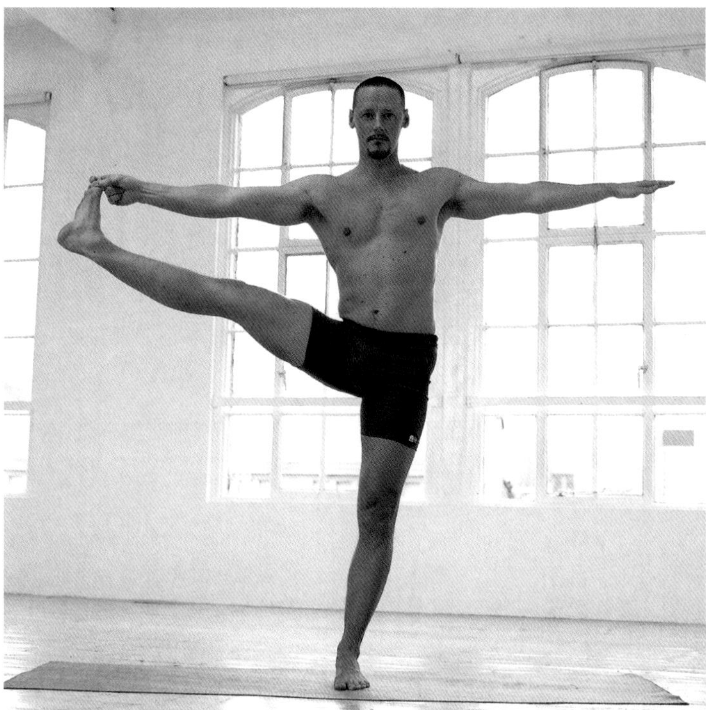

4 Utthita Hasta Padangusthasansa II – Sideways Extended Leg Raise – keep the left foot pointing forwards and bend the right knee to the side. Hold the big toe with the fingers of the right hand. Stretch the right leg out to the side. Ensure that the right knee faces the ceiling. Straighten the right arm. Extend the spine upwards. Stretch the left arm out to the side. Look ahead, breathing normally and stay for 20–30 seconds. Stretch the trunk up, open the chest, moving the shoulder blades into the back, and keep the left leg firm and straight.

Modification

• Initially holding the toes may prove to be too challenging, especially if you have tight hamstrings, so using a strap around the foot or resting the foot on a chair is recommended.

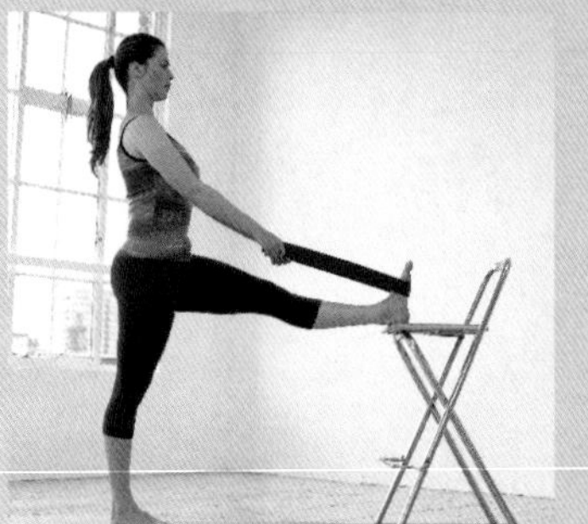

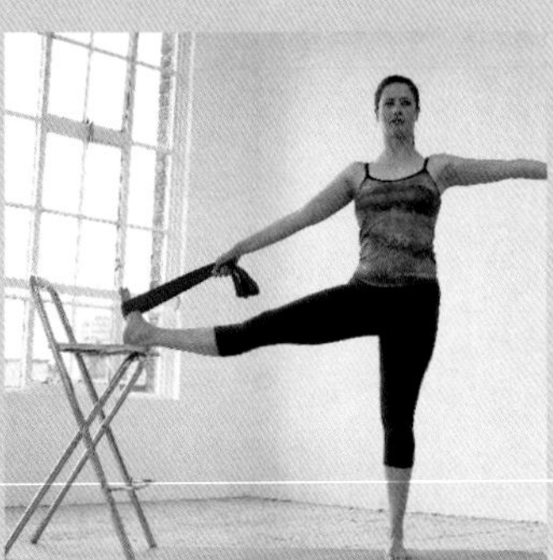

Virabhadrasana III | WARRIOR POSE III

This posture is an intensified continuation of Virabhadrasana I. It tones the abdominal organs, strengthens the legs, makes the spine more flexible and improves balance. It gives the practitioner agility in both body and mind.

★★★★

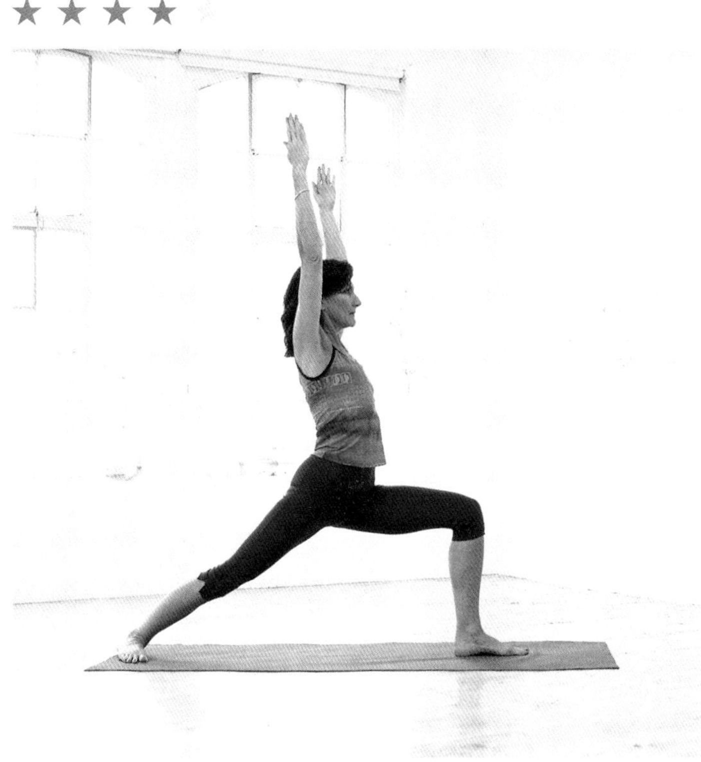

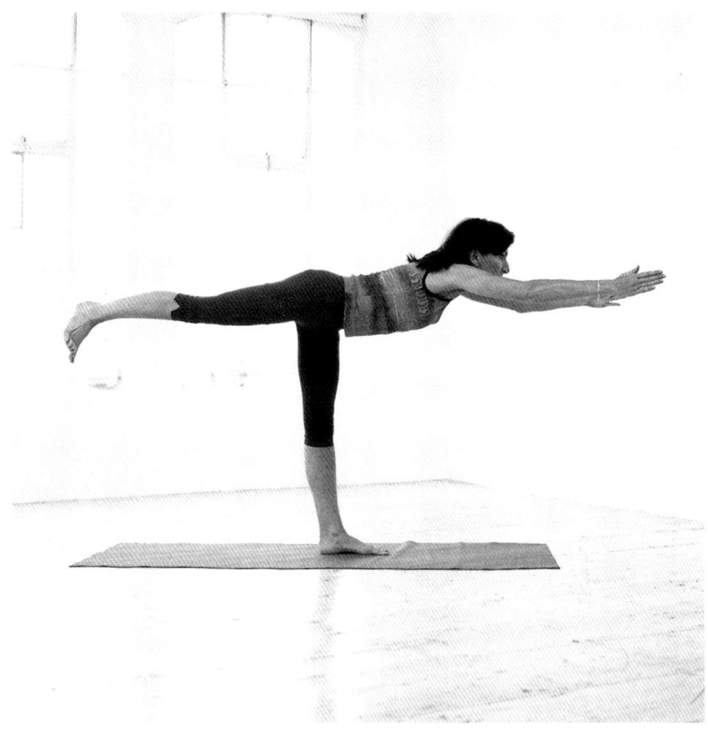

1 Follow the instructions for Virabhadrasana I.

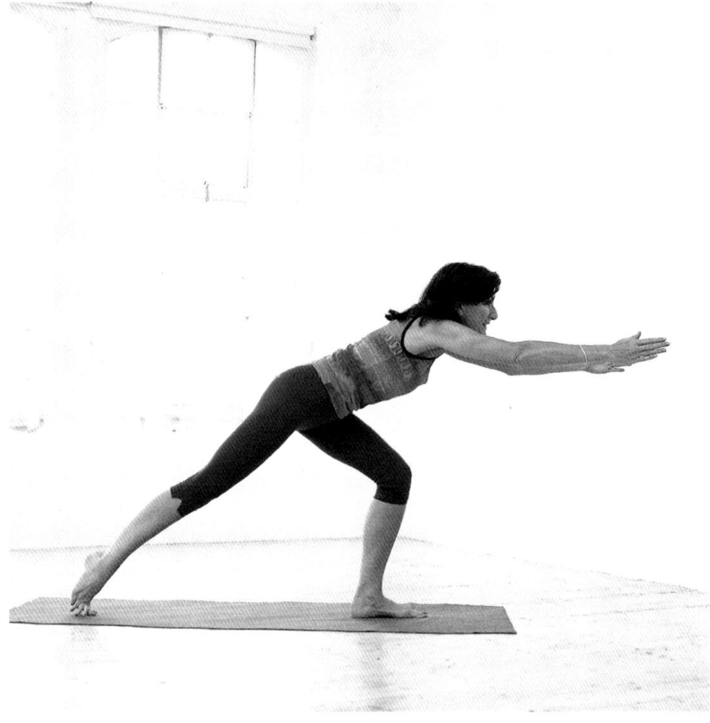

2 Exhale and extend the trunk and arms forwards over the left thigh.

Keep the hips level by pulling the right hip forwards if necessary.

3 Extend the trunk more, straighten the left leg and lift the right leg up so that it is parallel to the floor. With the right leg, trunk, head and arms parallel to the floor, extend the fingertips away from the head and extend the right inner heel away from the head. Hold this position for 20–30 seconds.

Come down by bending the left leg, lowering the right foot to the floor and raising the trunk up – this is Virabhadrasana I. Repeat on the other side, and then come back to Tadasana.

If the lower back is painful, support the lifted leg on a ledge and the hands on a chair. Do not strain or compress the back of the neck.

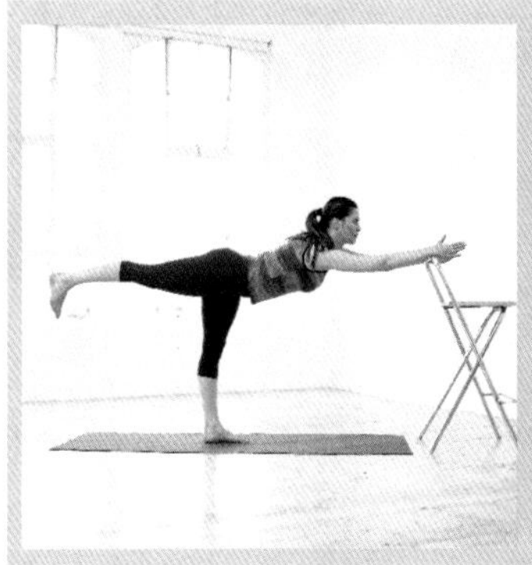

Modification

- The fingertips of the extended hands can press into the wall, or rest on a chair or ledge to extend the spine more.
- The hips must be level and the raised leg straight.

Parivrtta Trikonasana | REVERSE TRIANGLE POSE

This pose increases the flow of blood to the lower back region and therefore improves the flexibility of the spine. It also strengthens the legs and hips and invigorates the abdominal organs.

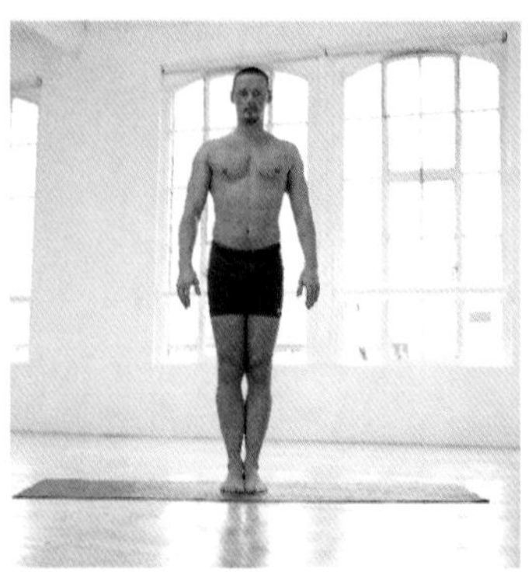

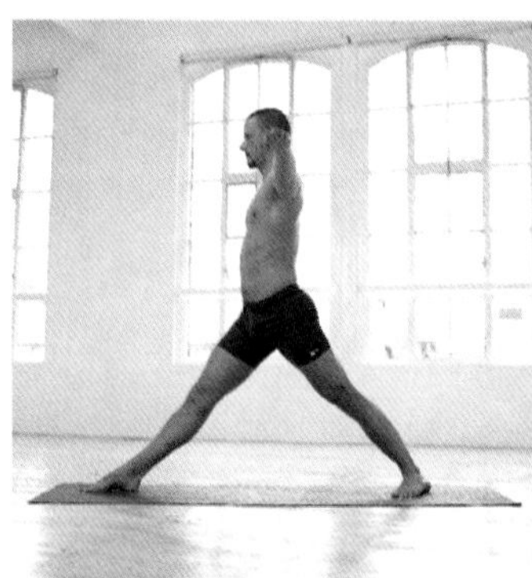

1 Stand in Tadasana, inhale and spread feet and arms apart.

2 Turn the right foot out 90 degrees and the left foot in 45 degrees. Exhale and rotate the trunk and head to the right.

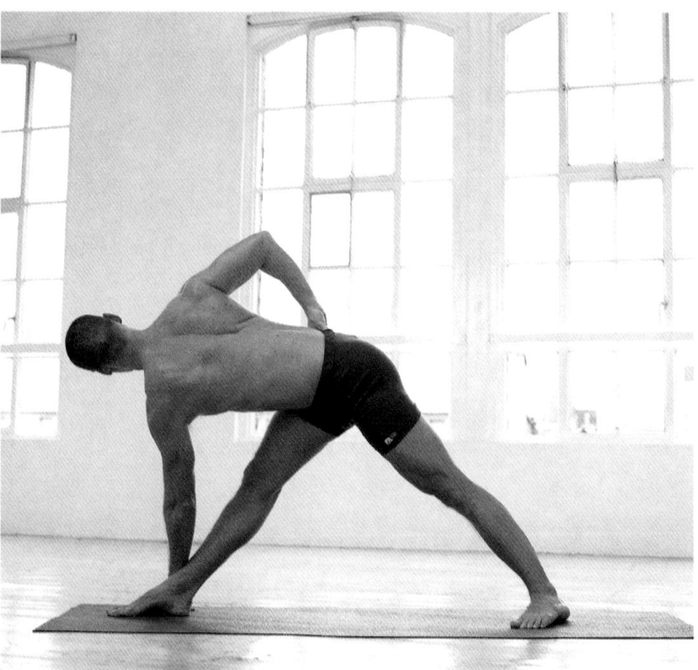

3 Extend the left arm over the right leg and place the fingertips of the left hand on the outside of the right foot.

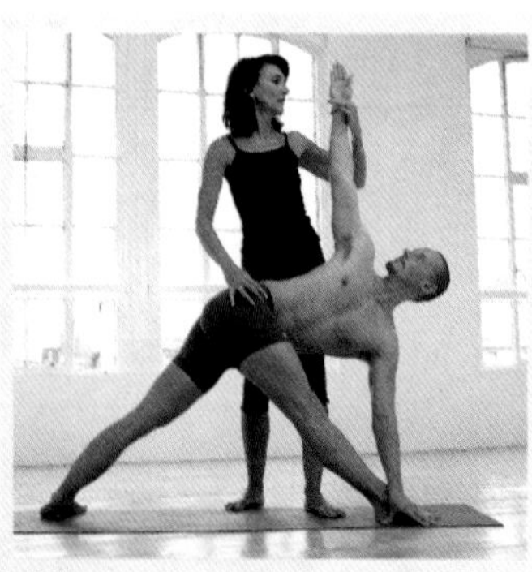

Focus

- Keep the right hip pointing upwards, so it does not collapse down into the body.
- Keep the head in line with the tailbone when looking up, maintaining a straightness in the spine.

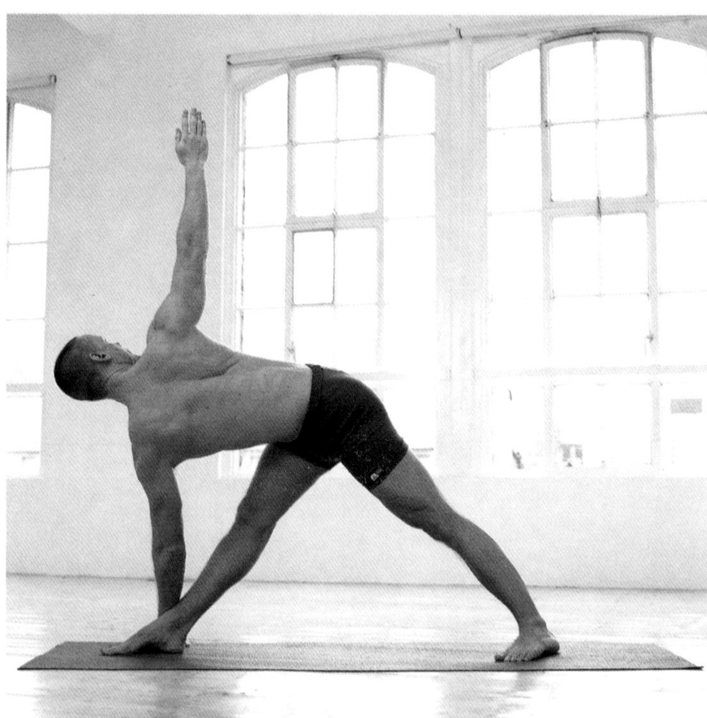

4 Turn the trunk towards the right and extend the right arm strongly upwards in line with the right shoulder. Extend the spine and open the chest. Keep the head in alignment with the tailbone. Hold for 30–40 seconds. Inhale, rotate the trunk back to its original position and come up. Repeat on the other side and then come back to Tadasana.

Modification

- Less-flexible students can do this posture with the back against the wall.
- Use a wooden block under the right hand to get more extension in the spine and to allow the chest to turn towards the ceiling.
- Do the posture with the back foot against the wall.
- Put a foam block under the right heel to allow the chest to rotate farther.

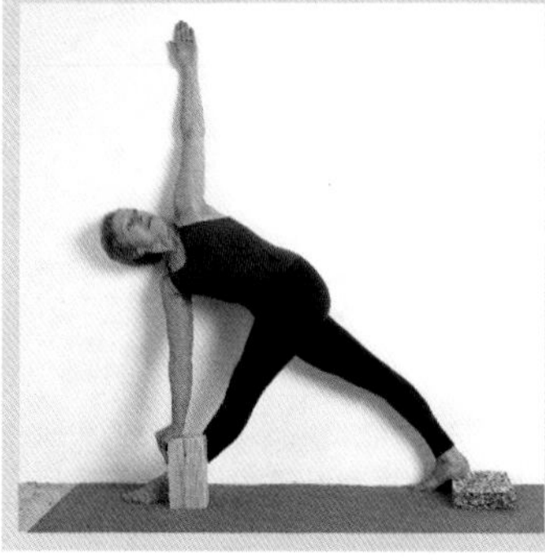

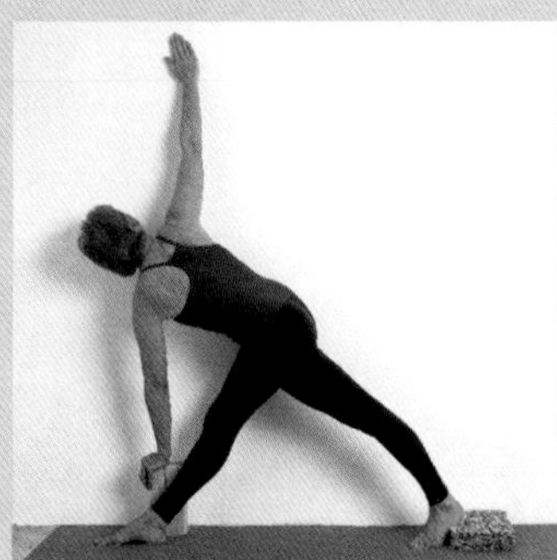

Parivrtta Parsvakonasana | REVOLVING LATERAL ANGLE POSE

This posture is a more intense version of Parivrtta Trikonasana and therefore the effects are greater. The abdominal organs are more constricted, thus aiding digestion and helping to eliminate toxins from the colon.

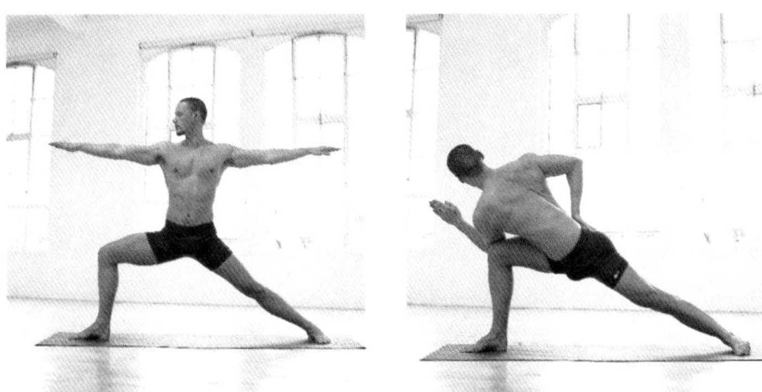

1 Begin in Virabhadrasana II, then bend the right leg, extending the arms out to the side and keeping the palms facing the floor.

2 Rotate the trunk, pelvis, abdomen and chest towards the bent right leg. Take the left side of the trunk over the right thigh, bend the left elbow and hook it over the right thigh.

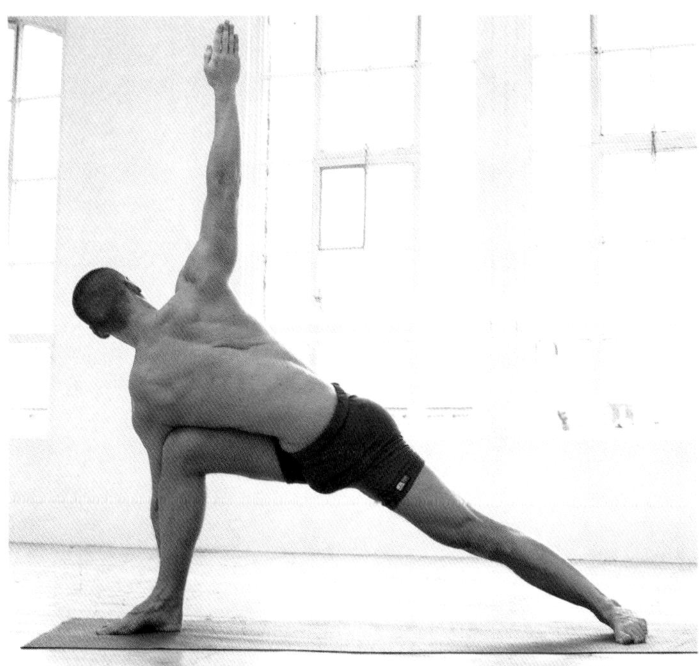

3 Rotate the trunk and chest more, and place the fingertips of the left hand on the floor on the outside of the right foot. Extend the right arm up towards the ceiling.

Focus

- Throughout this posture, make sure the back (left) leg is straight.
- Keep the right shin perpendicular to the floor.

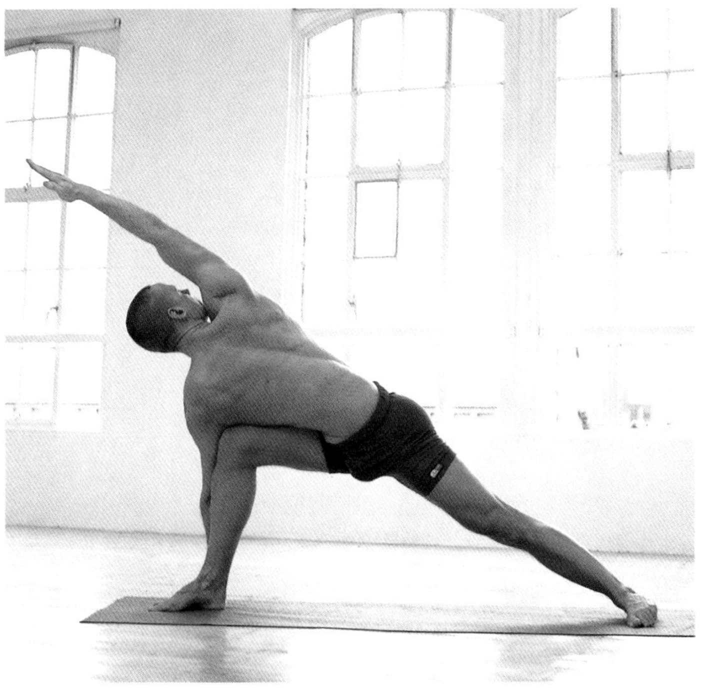

4 Turn the right palm towards the head, extending the arm over the head in line with the ear. Keep the left leg strong and straight. Turn the chest towards the ceiling more, and, if possible, look up.

Hold for 20–30 seconds, then inhale, lift the left hand from the floor, raise the trunk, and come up. Repeat on the other side, and then come back to Tadasana.

Modification

- Work parallel to the wall, supporting the lower hand on a block and the back heel on a raise.
- Work with the back heel against the wall. The heel is lifted on the wall while the toes are on the floor.
- This is a strenuous postition, so if it is too much, try keeping the top hand resting on the waist.
- Assistance in stretching the arm fully can help.

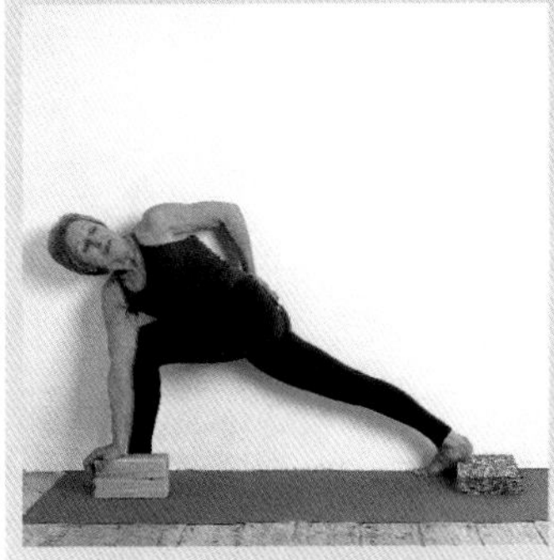

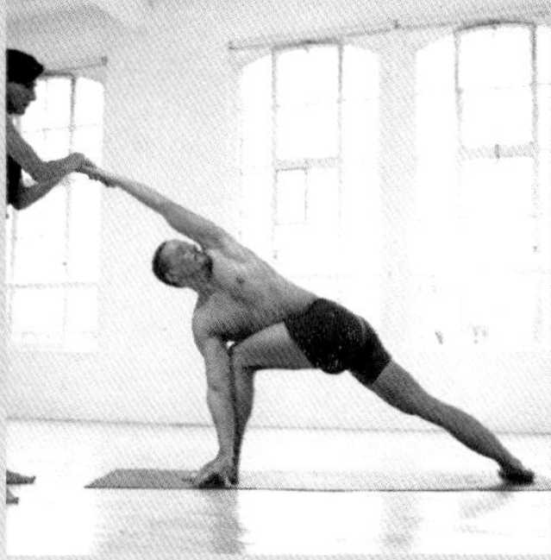

Parsvottanasana | INTENSE SIDE CHEST STRETCH

This pose helps to maintain mobility in the neck, shoulders, arms, elbows and wrists. It improves flexibility in the spine and hips and, once the head is down, it calms the brain. The abdominal organs are strengthened and digestion improves.

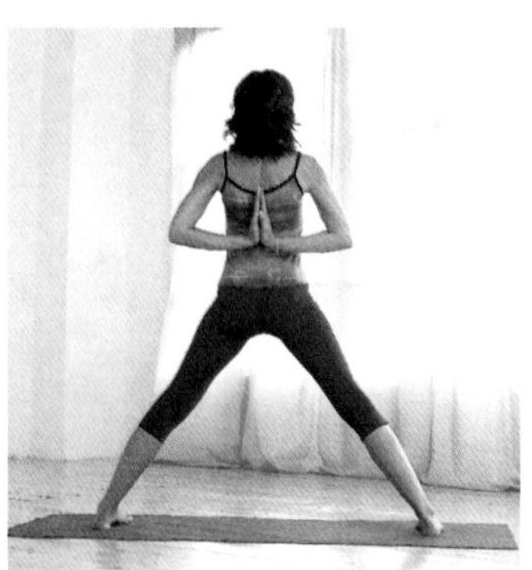

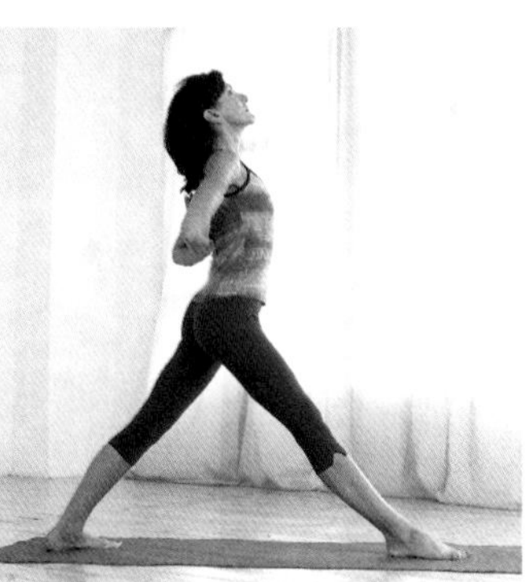

1 Stand in Tadasana, and join the hands behind in Namaskar. Inhale and jump or step the feet 1–1.2m/3–4ft apart.

2 Turn the right foot out 90 degrees and the left foot in 45 degrees. Turn the hips, trunk and shoulders to the right.

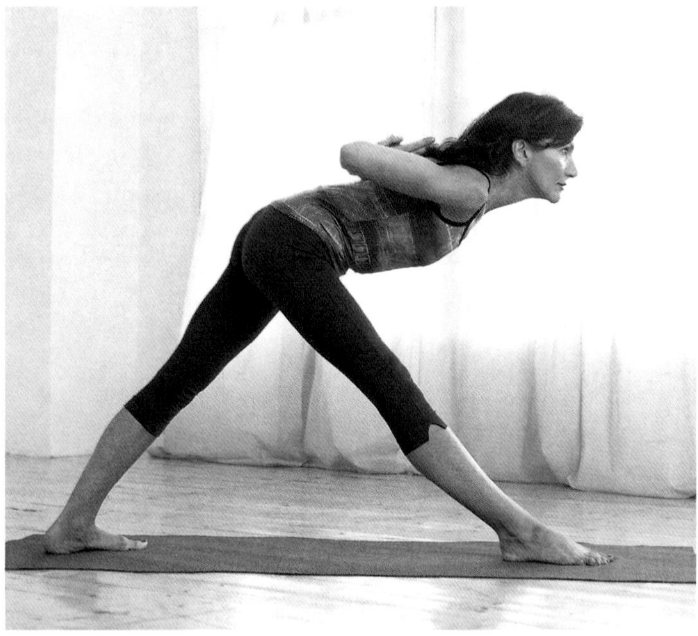

3 Extend the spine forwards. Lift the chin towards the ceiling and look up to make the back concave.

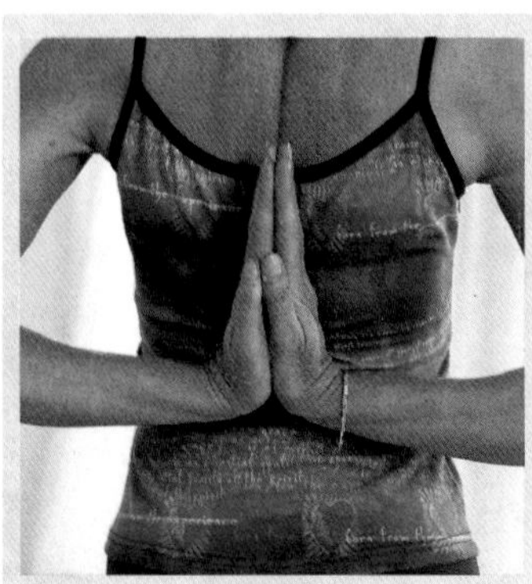

Focus

• Keep the palms flat together behind the back. This will increase flexibility in the wrists and shoulders. If the hands cannot go into Namaskar, however, hold the elbows behind the back.

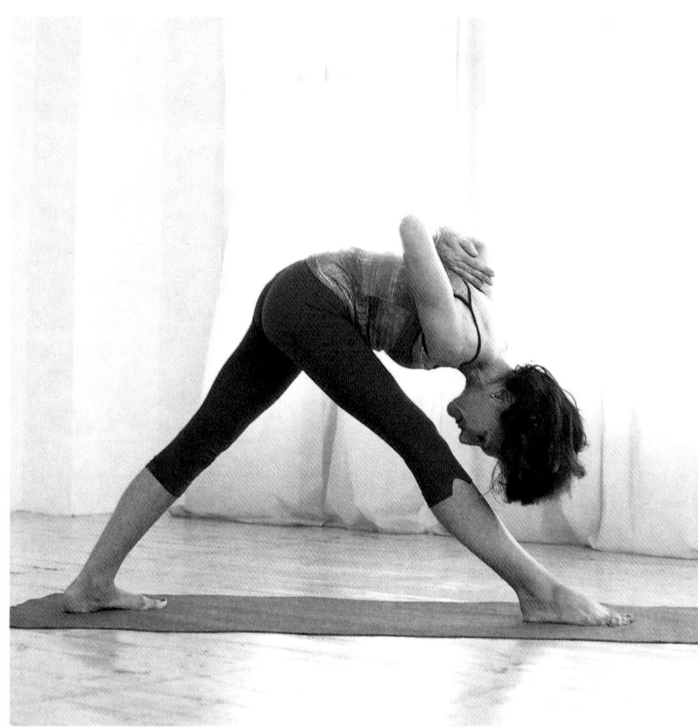

4 Exhale and extend the trunk over the right leg, taking the head towards the right foot. Keep both legs poker straight, the hips level and the weight evenly distributed between both feet. Hold for 30–40 seconds, raise the trunk, turn the feet forwards, release the hands and repeat on the other side. Come back to Tadasana.

Modification

• Until stability is learned, do the posture with the hands on the waist and, after coming forwards, place the hands on the floor on either side of the front foot.

• Don't allow all the weight to collapse on to the front leg. Press both feet equally into the floor.

• If the back is painful, place each hand on a wooden block after coming forwards, and then extend down.

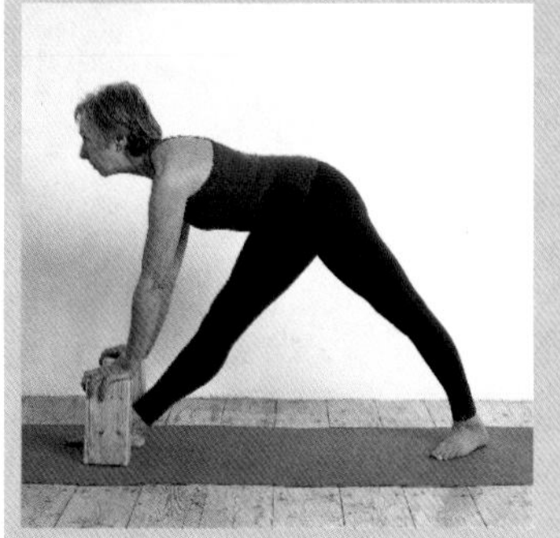

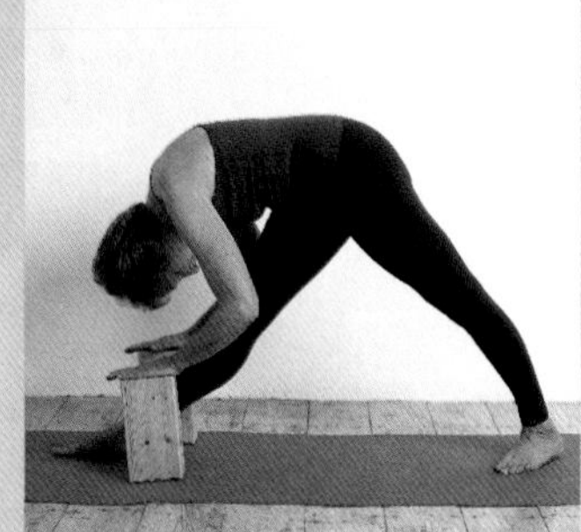

Prasarita Padottanasana | FORWARD EXTENSION LEGS WIDE APART

This pose is usually practised towards the end of the standing poses. Because the head is down, increased blood flows to the trunk and head, quietening the body and mind, and promoting a feeling of tranquillity and serenity.

★ ★ ★

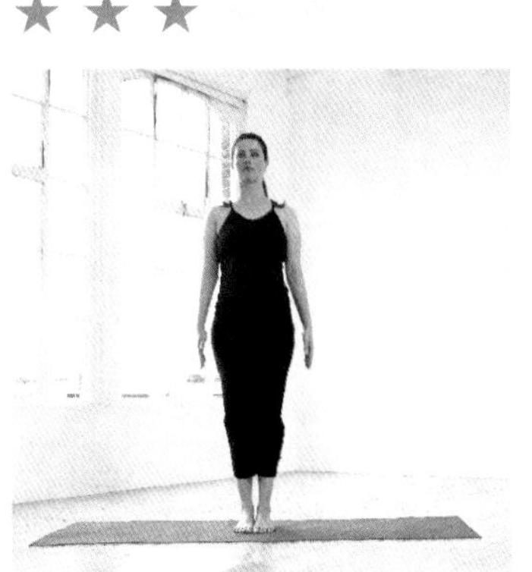

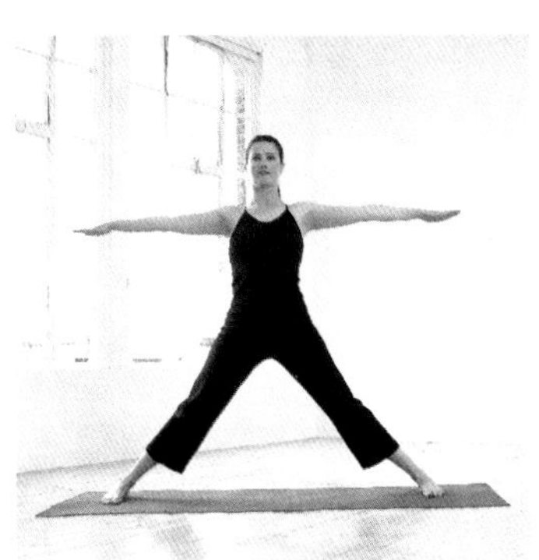

1 Stand in Tadasana.

2 Inhale and jump or step the feet 1.2–1.5m/4–5ft apart. Make sure the toes of each foot are level and the feet are parallel.

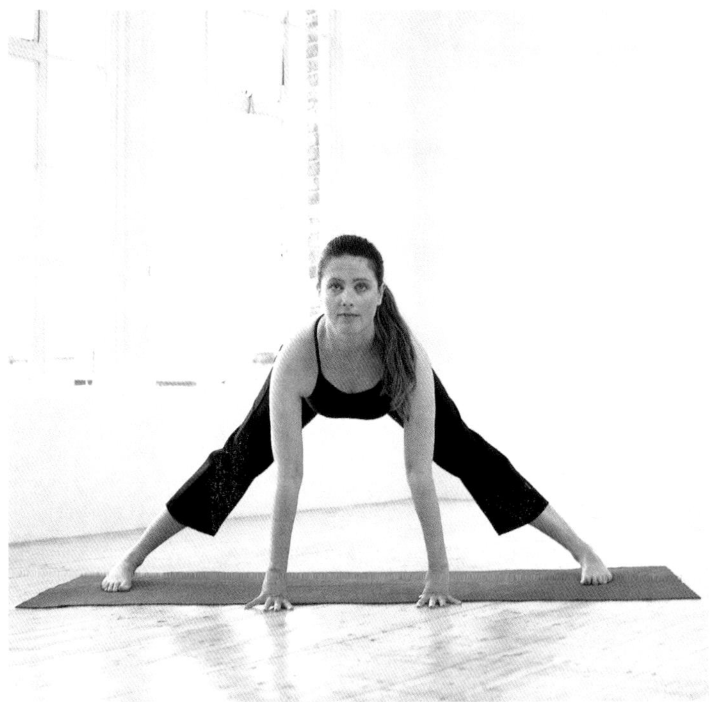

3 Straighten the legs by pulling up the knees and thigh muscles. Exhale and extend the trunk forwards from the hips, stretching the spine.

Place the fingertips on the floor, shoulder-width apart, directly under the shoulders.

Straighten the arms, stretch the legs and extend the trunk forwards, making the back concave and extending the front of the body from the pubis to the chin. Look up.

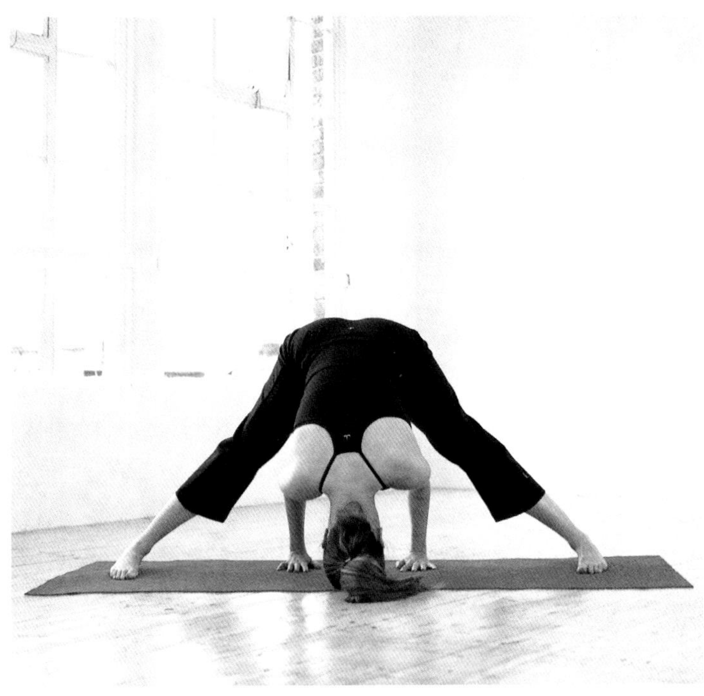

4 Bend the elbows back, extend the trunk to the floor and place the crown of the head on the floor. Lift the shoulders to release the head nearer to the floor, breathe normally and hold for 20–30 seconds. Inhale, lift the head and trunk and make the back concave. Place the hands on the hips and come back to Tadasana.

Focus

- Move the inner thigh muscles away from each other, i.e. inner thighs move towards outer thighs.
- Press the outer edges of both feet into the floor without letting the outer ankle bones bulge down.
- Even though the trunk moves forwards and then down, keep both legs stretching up towards the ceiling.
- This pose stretches the hamstring muscles.

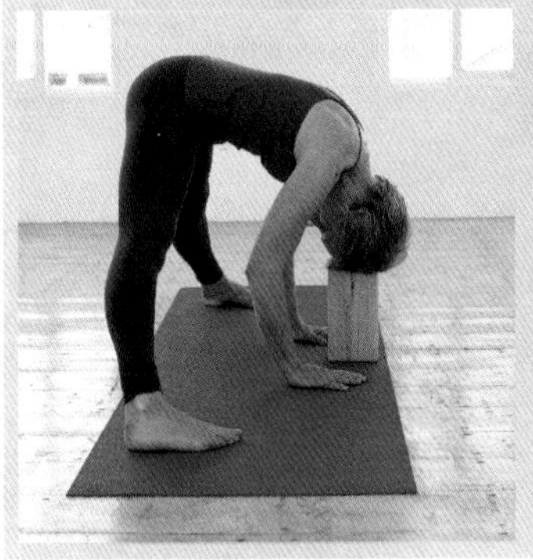

Modification

- If the hands don't reach the floor, support each hand with a wooden block.
- If the head doesn't reach the floor, support the crown of the head with foam or wooden blocks.

Uttanasana I | FORWARD EXTENSION

In this pose the spine is given an intense stretch. The abdominal organs are toned and, because the head is down, the increased flow of blood soothes the brain cells. It also relieves fatigue.

★ ★

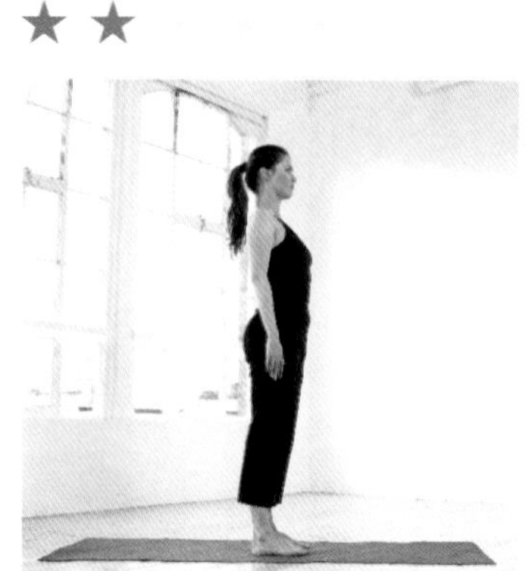

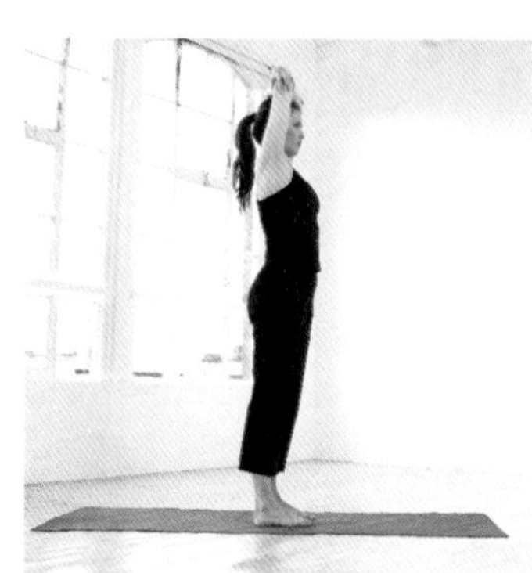

1 Stand in Tadasana with the feet 30cm/1ft apart. The inner edges of the feet should be parallel to one another and the toes level. Keep the legs and knees straight.

2 Fold the arms, catching the left elbow with the right hand and the right elbow with the left hand. Inhale and extend the folded arms above the head in line with the ears. Lift and extend the entire body upwards.

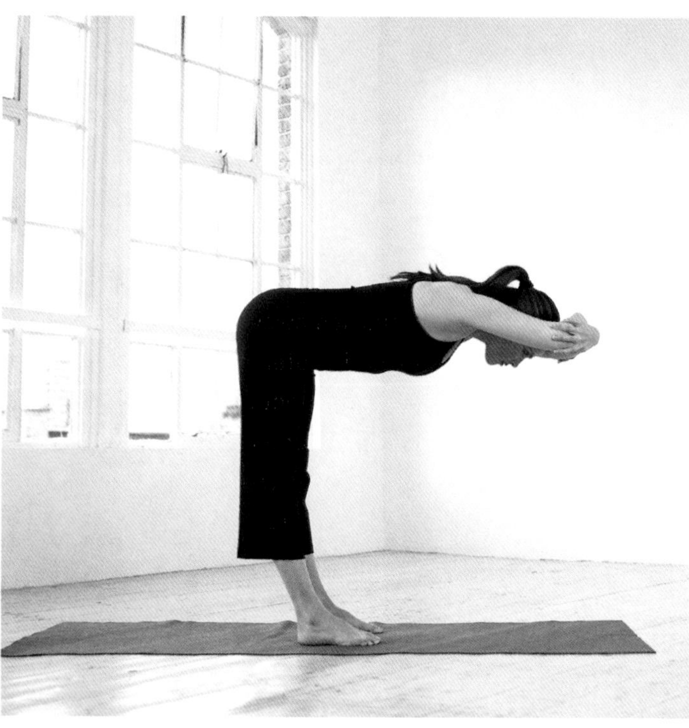

3 Exhale and extend the trunk forwards.

Focus

• This is a relaxing forward bend, although the legs remain strong, knees lifted. Allow gravity to do the rest of the work for you.

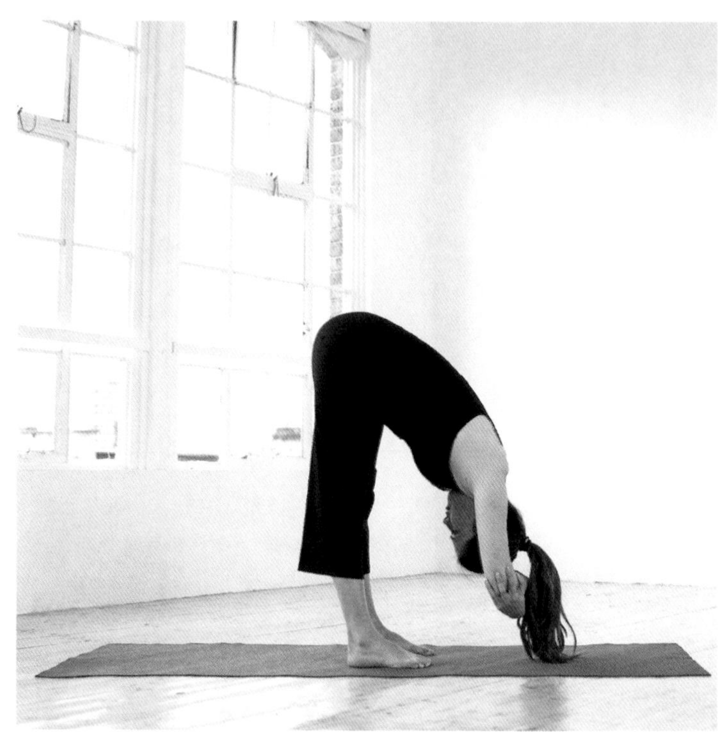

4 Extend the trunk down to the floor, keeping the legs straight, and extend the trunk and arms nearer to the floor. Inhale, lift the trunk, release the elbows and come back to Tadasana.

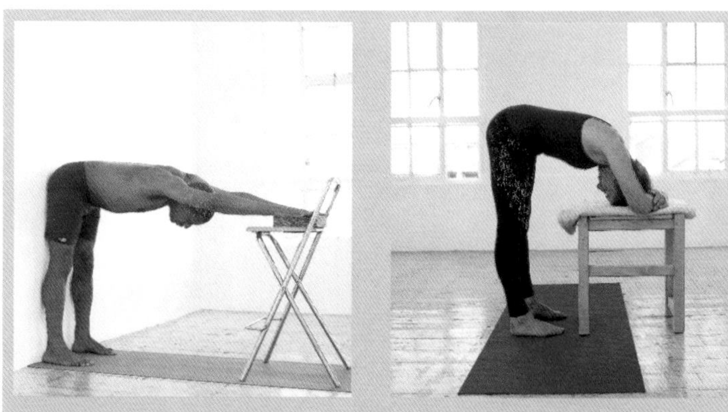

Modification

• For students with a stiff or painful back and tight hamstring muscles, do supported Uttanasana I – put the hands onto a support at hip level, and extend the spine forwards. An alternative is to rest the head on a support, such as a Halasana stool softened with a blanket.

• If the back is uncomfortable in the final posture, take the feet wider apart and turn the toes slightly inwards.

• Keep the legs extending strongly upwards to elongate the spine and to protect the lower back.

Padangusthasana | FINGER TO TOE POSE

This posture strengthens the legs, makes the spine more flexible and also activates and tones the abdominal organs which improves digestion. Students who cannot catch their toes can hold their ankles.

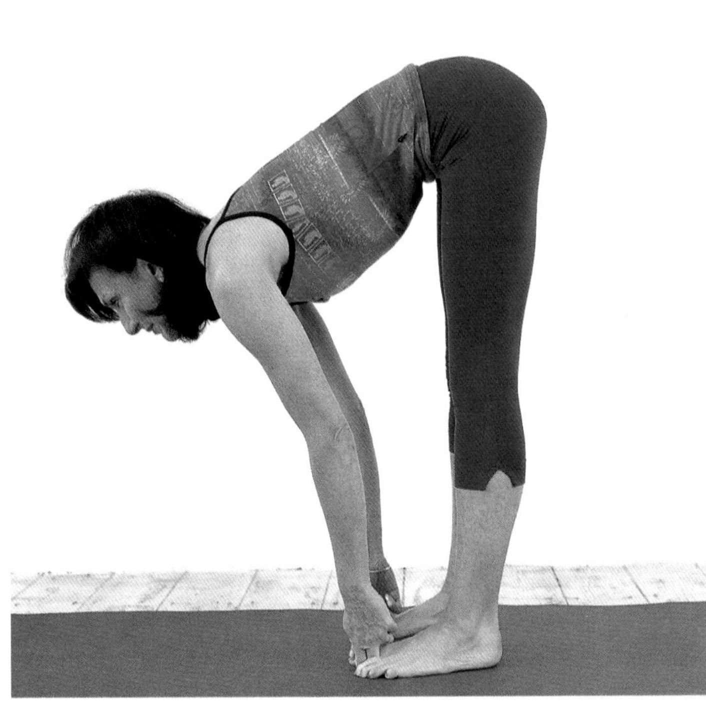

1 Stand in Tadasana with the feet 30cm/1ft apart. Bend the trunk forwards and down, then catch the big toes with the thumbs, index and middle fingers. Stretch the legs up and extend the trunk forwards. Straighten the arms, inhale, make the back concave, lift the chest and look up.

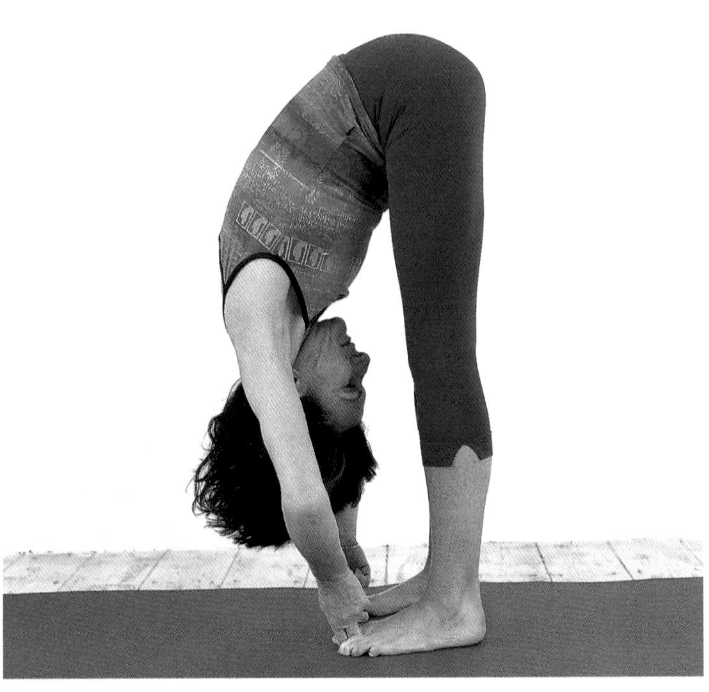

2 Exhale, bend the elbows out and extend the trunk down.

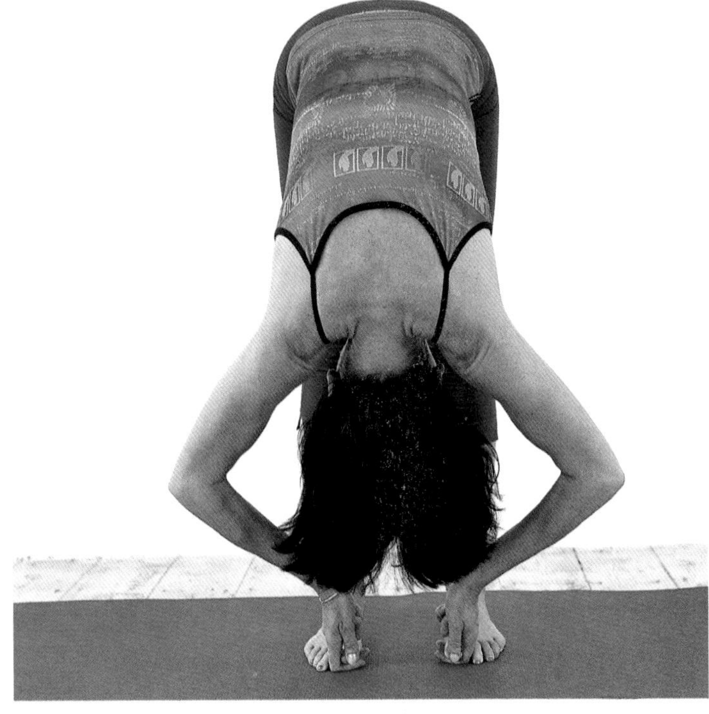

3 On the next exhalation, bend down farther by pulling on the toes, and take the head towards the feet.

Hold for 20–30 seconds, inhale and come up into Tadasana.

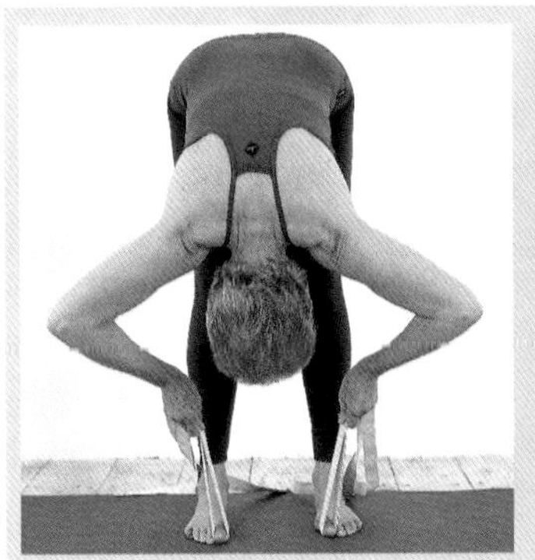

Modification

- If you are unable to reach the feet, use two straps wrapped around the toes, or rest the hands on blocks.
- If the back hurts, take the feet slightly wider apart and turn the toes inwards.

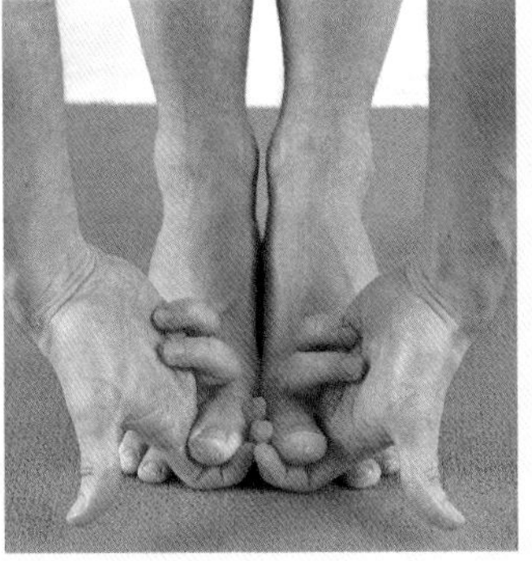

Focus

- Use the first two fingers on each hand to wrap firmly around the big toe so you can use the leverage to pull your top half down. Move further into the posture with each exhalation.

Garudasana | EAGLE POSE

This is a balancing posture that keeps both ankles and shoulders flexible and is recommended for preventing cramps in the calf muscles. Concentration and balance are also improved.

★ ★

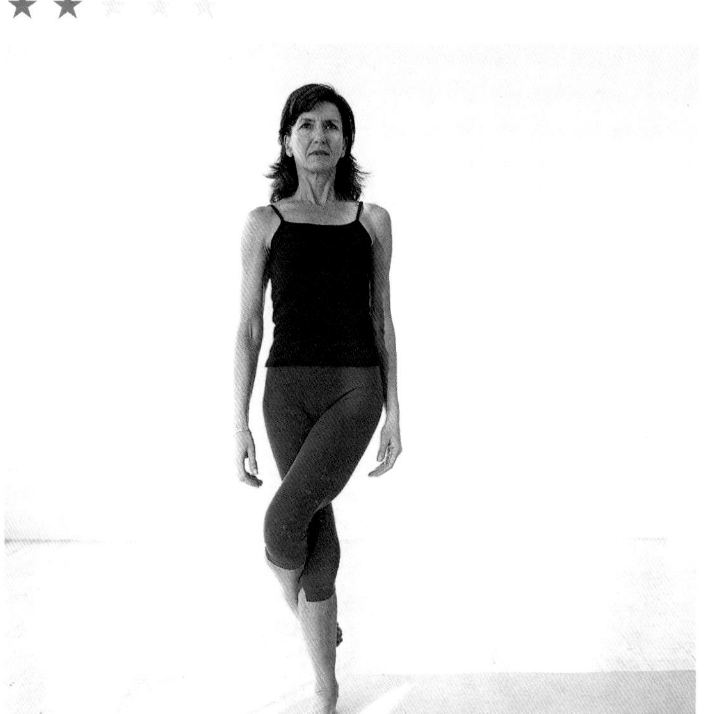

1 Stand in Tadasana. Exhale and slightly bend the right knee and cross the left thigh and knee over the right thigh. Take the left shin behind the right calf, and hook the left foot behind the right calf muscle.

Balance on the right foot, spreading out the foot, with the weight evenly distributed between the toes and heel. Ensure that both hips are level and face forwards. If the knees are painful, practise the pose with the legs in Tadasana and intertwine the arms only.

When first learning this posture, it is necessary to separate out the hand and foot movements, but eventually these will become one flowing movement.

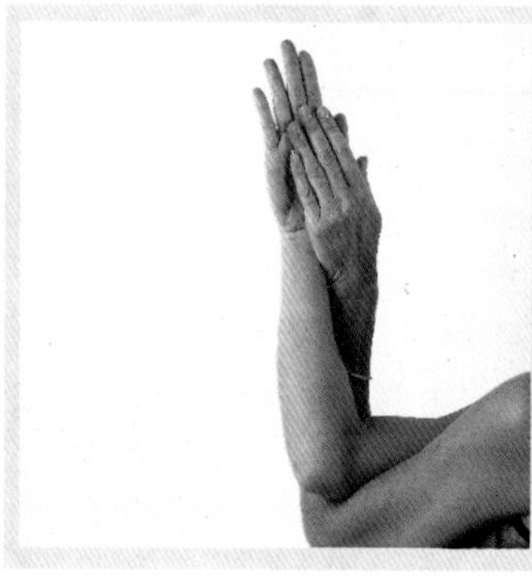

Focus

- Cross the right arm over the left, and touch palms.
- If you find it hard to balance, it may help to keep the eyes still, focusing on an object or a spot in the distance in front of you.

2 Bend the elbows and lift them to shoulder level with the thumbs towards the face. Cross the right elbow over the left, intertwining the forearms, placing the palms together.

Hold for 15–20 seconds, release the arms and legs, come back to Tadasana and repeat on the other side, i.e. crossing right thigh over left and left elbow over right.

Modification

- To help with balance, do the posture with the back against the wall.
- To practise the leg work only, push the fingertips against a wall to hold you upright.
- In full posture, keep both knees facing forwards and extend the trunk upwards.

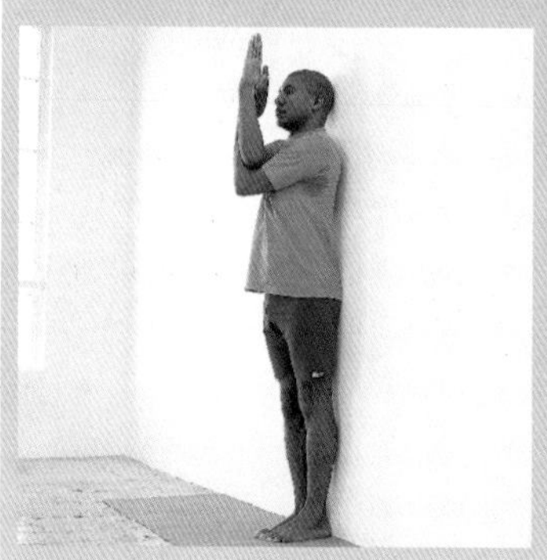

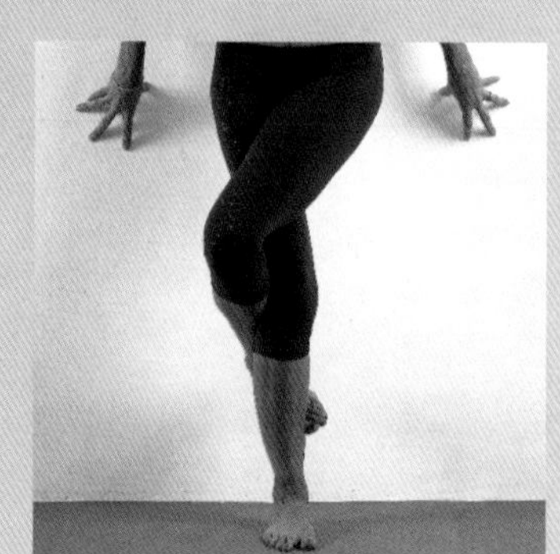

Utkatasana | FIERCE POSE

This pose is like sitting on an imaginary chair. It relieves stiffness in the shoulders, makes the ankles more flexible and strengthens the leg muscles. The abdominal organs and the spine are toned and the chest is fully expanded.

★ ★

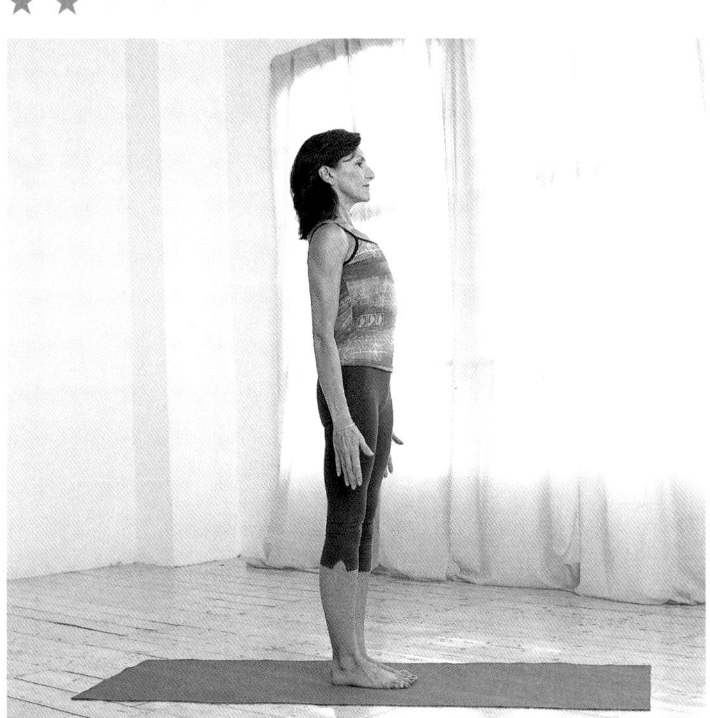

1 Stand in Tadasana – feet together, chest lifted, shoulders relaxed and down.

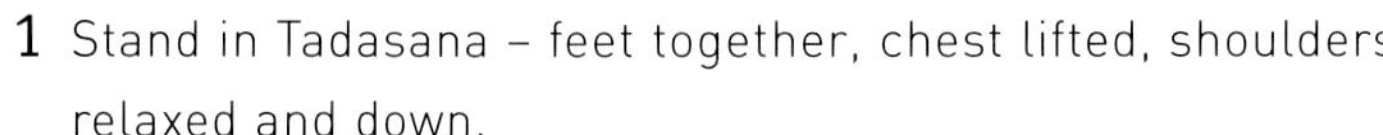

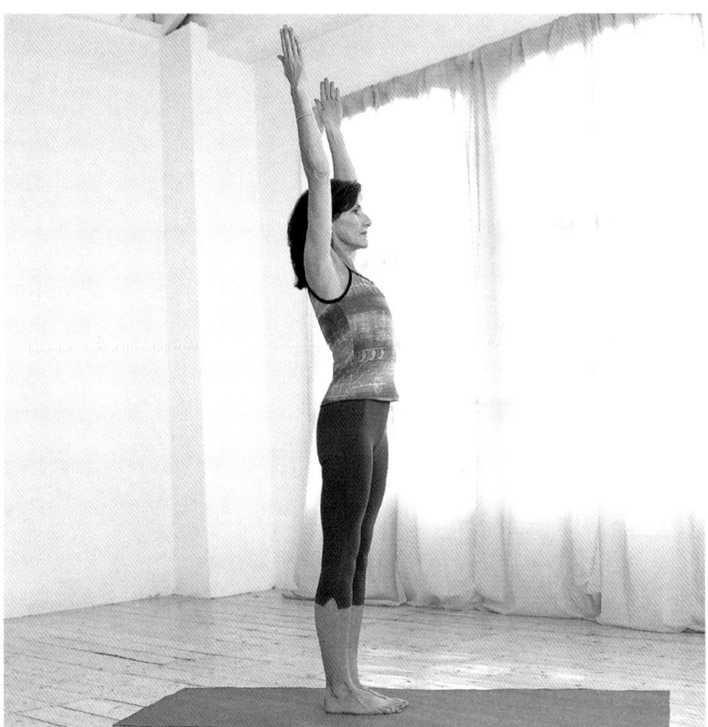

2 Inhale and extend the arms up towards the ceiling with the palms facing one another. Straighten the elbows and extend the palms and fingers up.

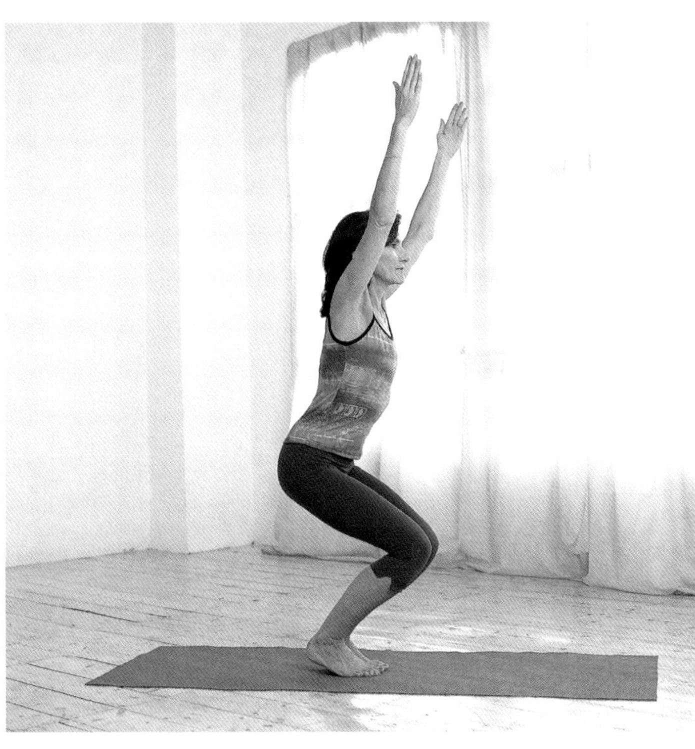

3 Exhale, bend the knees and lower the trunk down – as if you were going to sit on a chair.

Bend strongly in the ankle joints, press the heels down, bend in the knees, bend in the hips and stretch the arms strongly up. Keep the chest as far back as possible. If the elbows are straight, then join the palms.

Focus

- Bend more at the ankle and knee joints.
- Move the thighs down towards the floor while lifting the hips and trunk away from the legs.
- Although the trunk leans forwards, try to draw it back towards the vertical.

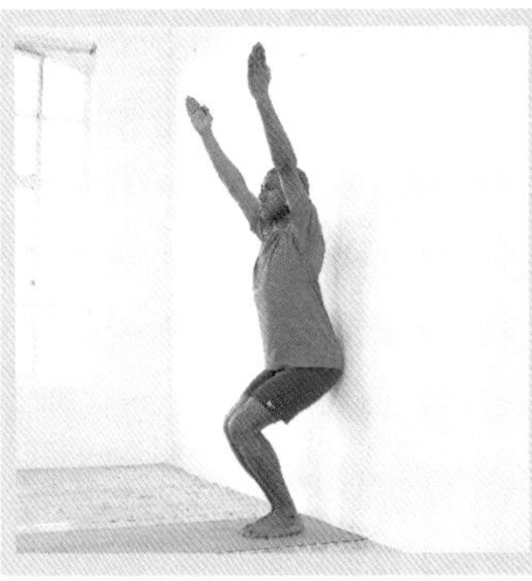

Modification

- It may be easier, at first, to rest against the wall to help with balance. Regular practice will help with stiff shoulders and ankles, strengthening the legs and activating the spine.

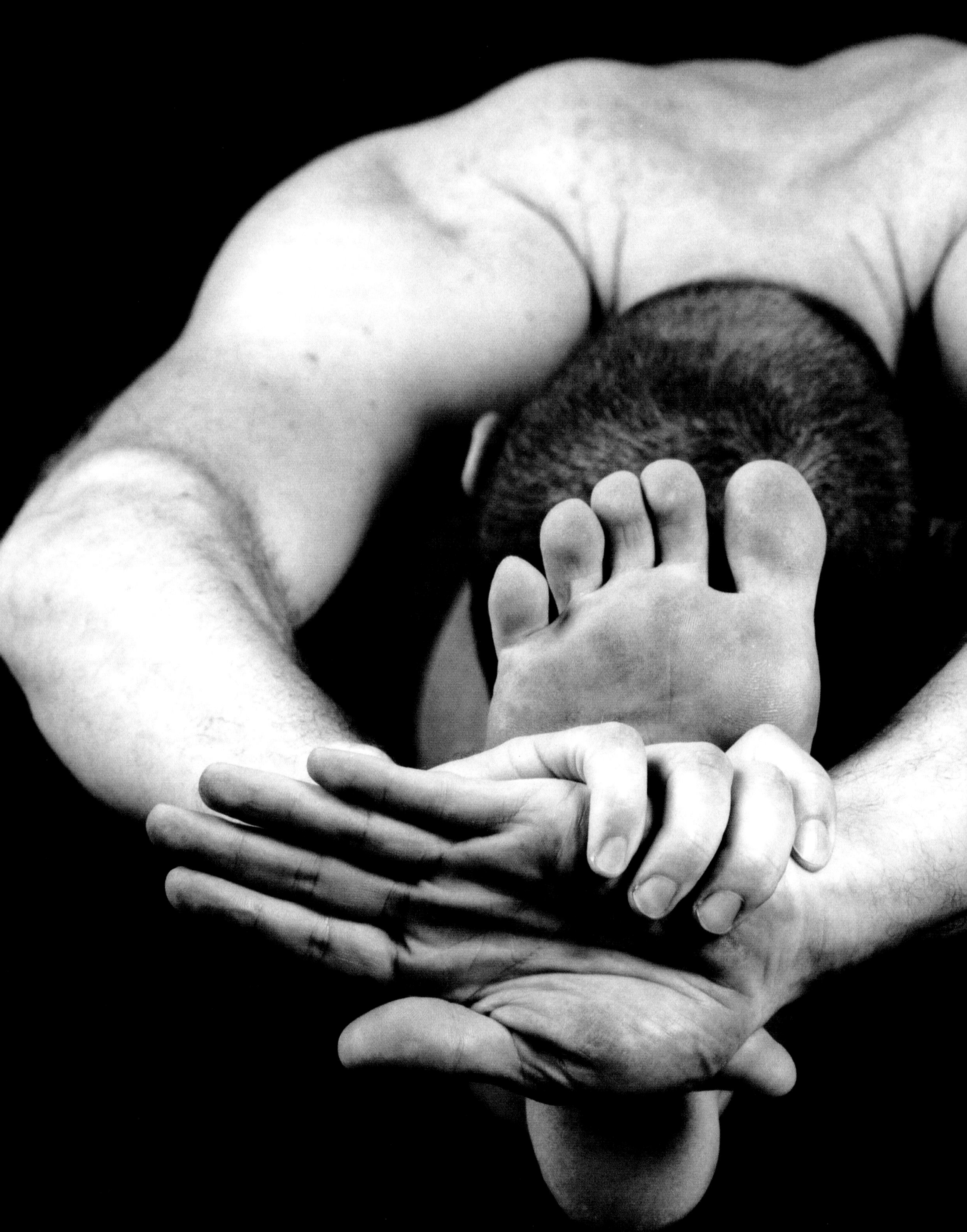

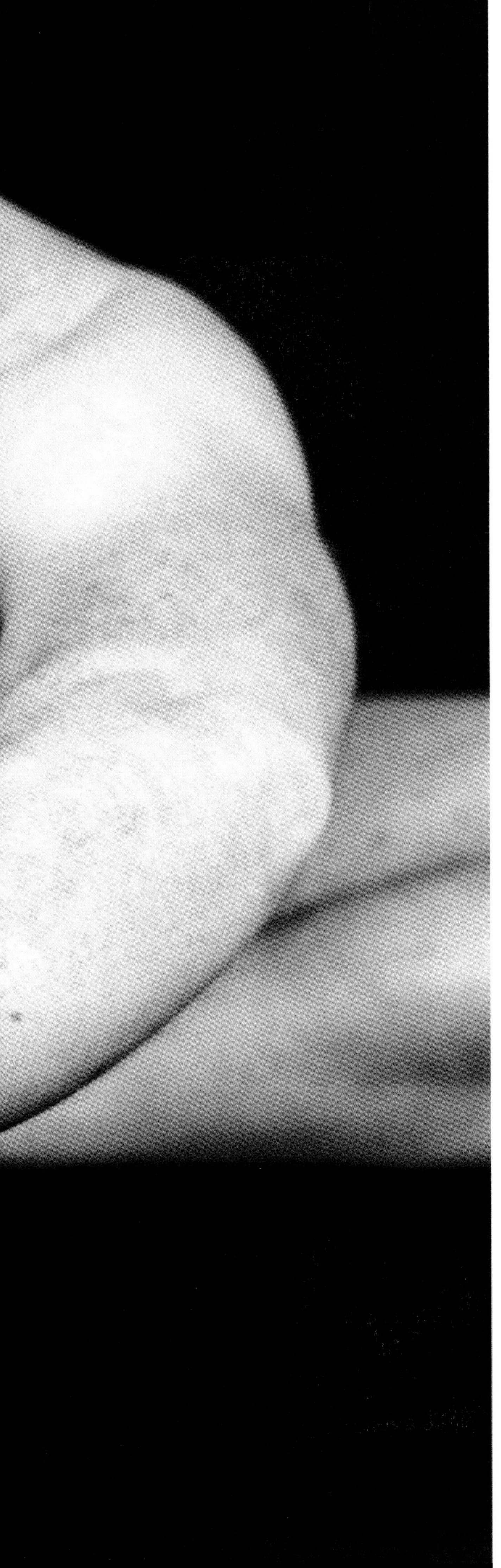

Seated Asanas

All seated postures improve flexibility to the hips, knees and ankles. They reduce tension in the diaphragm and throat, making breathing smoother and easier. They keep the spine firm, pacify the brain and stretch the muscles of the heart.

Sukhasana | SIMPLE CROSS LEGS

This posture keeps the knees and ankles flexible and nourishes the abdominal organs by encouraging blood circulation in the lower back and the abdomen. Since the spine is erect in this pose, the mind stays alert and attentive.

★

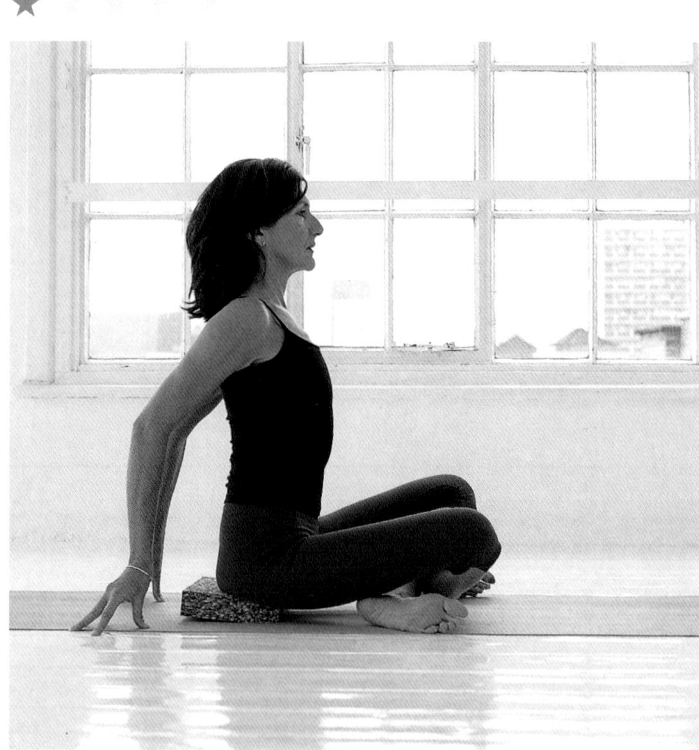

1 Sit on a foam block and cross the legs – place the left foot under the right thigh. Press the fingertips into the floor in order to lift the trunk.

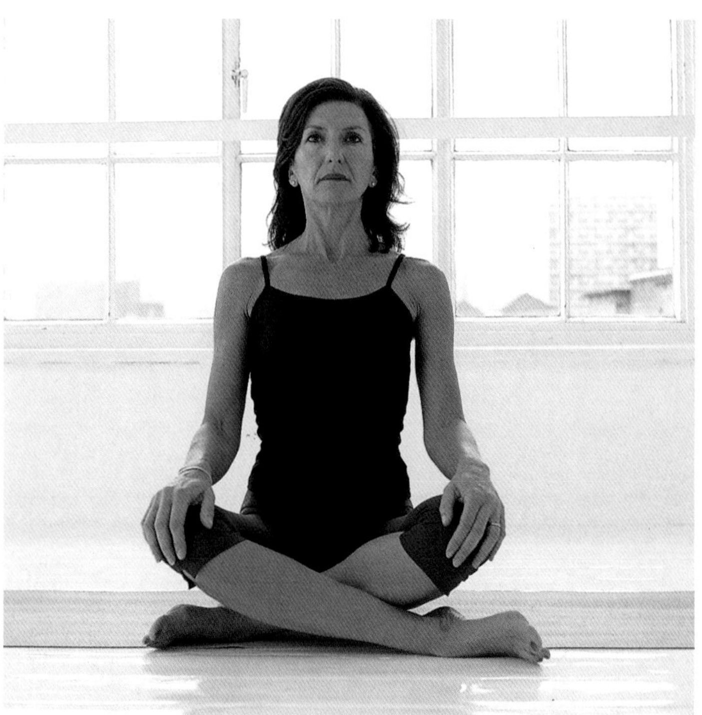

2 Extend the spine up, take the shoulders back and open the chest. Maintain the extension of the spine and put the hands on the knees.

3 Hold for 30–60 seconds. Change the cross-over of the legs – so that the other shin-bone is in front – and repeat, extending the spine and then placing the hands on the knees again.

Soften the groin area so that the knees release down towards the floor. Note which shin-bone is in front. Cross at the shins, not the ankles, and ensure the shin-bones cross in line with the centre of the body.

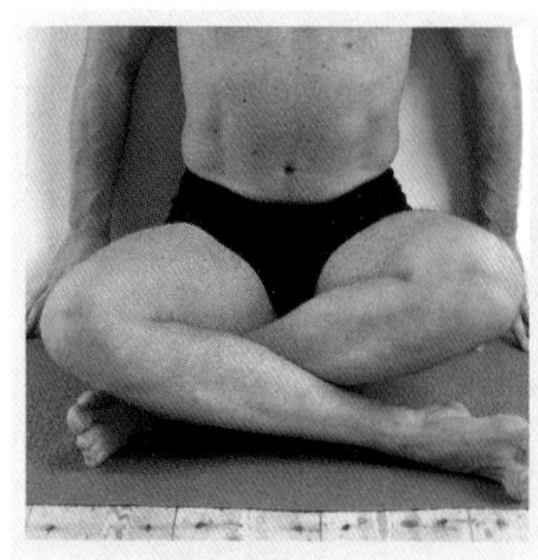

Focus

- Sukhasana can be done with the back against the wall, extending the spine up the wall.
- Broaden the base of the posture by spreading the buttocks to the sides.

Virasana | HERO POSE

This pose stretches the tops of the feet, ankles and knees. It helps to relieve leg cramps and is a good remedy for indigestion. Because of the position of the feet, it helps to correct flat feet and reduces discomfort in the legs.

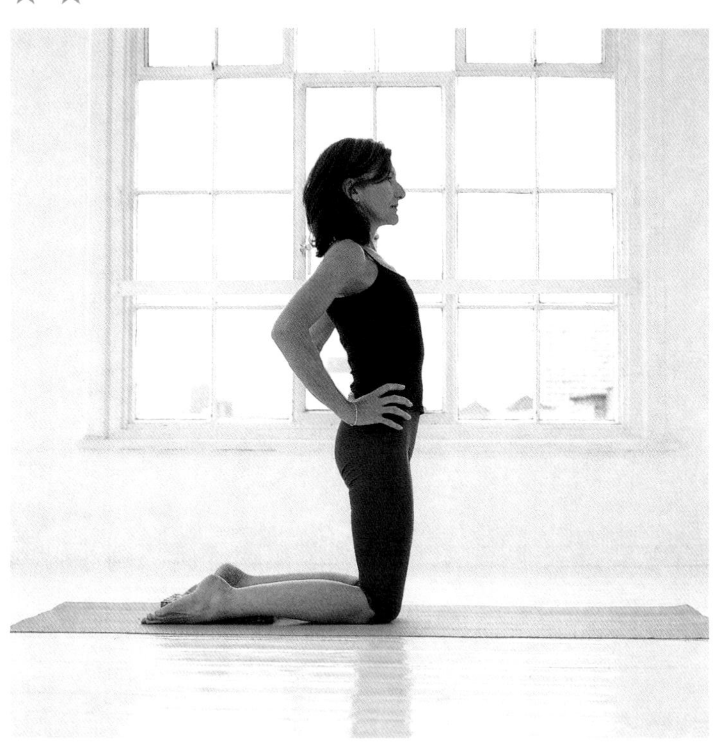

1 Kneel on a blanket or yoga mat with the knees together, the feet hip-width apart and the toes pointing straight back behind you.

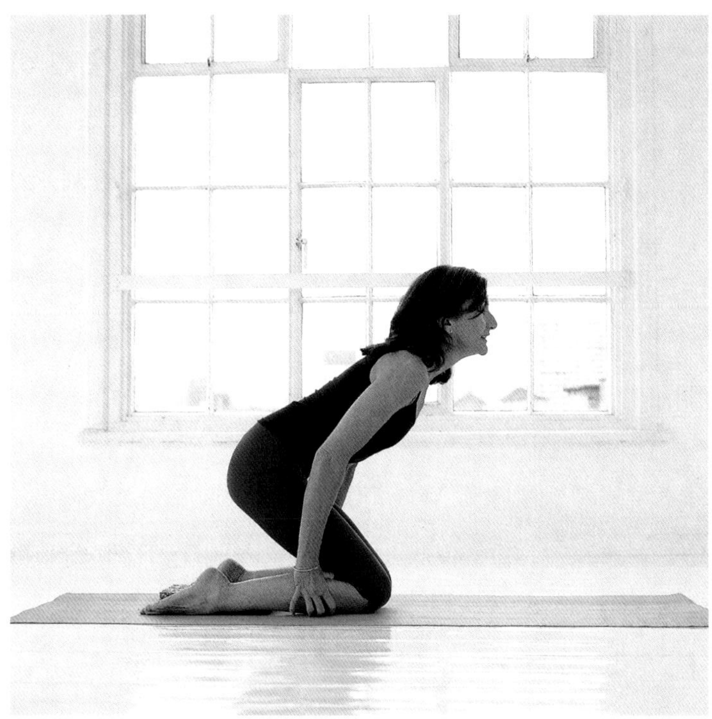

2 Sit between the feet, using the fingers to move the calf muscles away. If you cannot reach the floor comfortably, use a foam block or rolled-up blanket to raise you up.

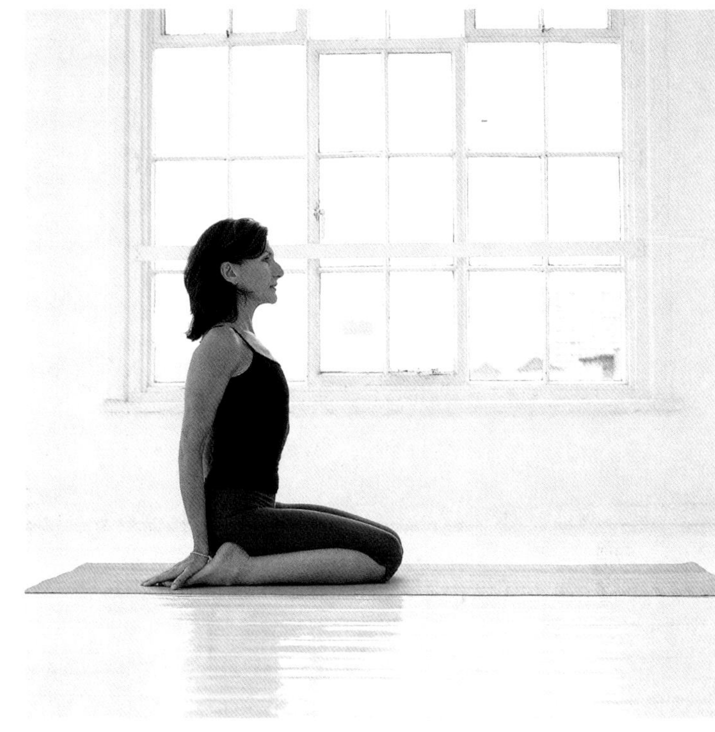

3 Put the palms of the hands on the soles of the feet (fingers pointing towards the toes) and stretch the trunk up. Take the shoulder blades into the body, lift the chest and extend the spine up.

Hold for 1–2 minutes, come out of the pose and straighten the legs.

Modification

- Sit on the edge of a foam block, or two, using as much support as is needed to alleviate knee pain.
- If the tops of the feet are painful, put them on a rolled-up blanket.
- If the knees are uncomfortable, put a rolled-up blanket between the calf and back thigh muscles.

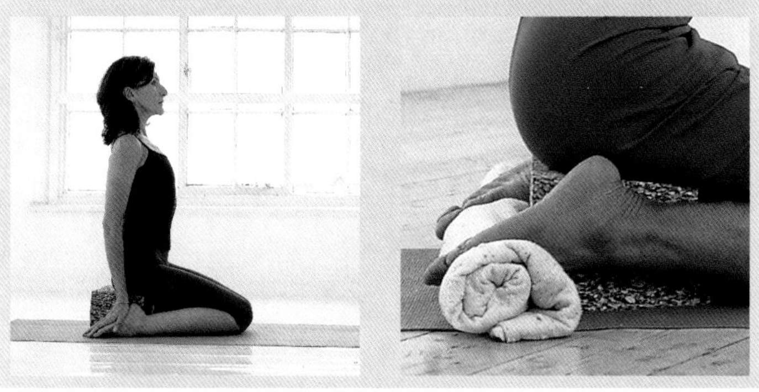

Virasana with Parvatasana | HERO POSE WITH EXTENDED ARMS

This pose can also be done sitting in Sukhasana. Parvatasana creates movement in the shoulder joints and develops the muscles of the chest. When the arms are raised, the abdominal organs are drawn in and the chest lifts and opens.

★ ★

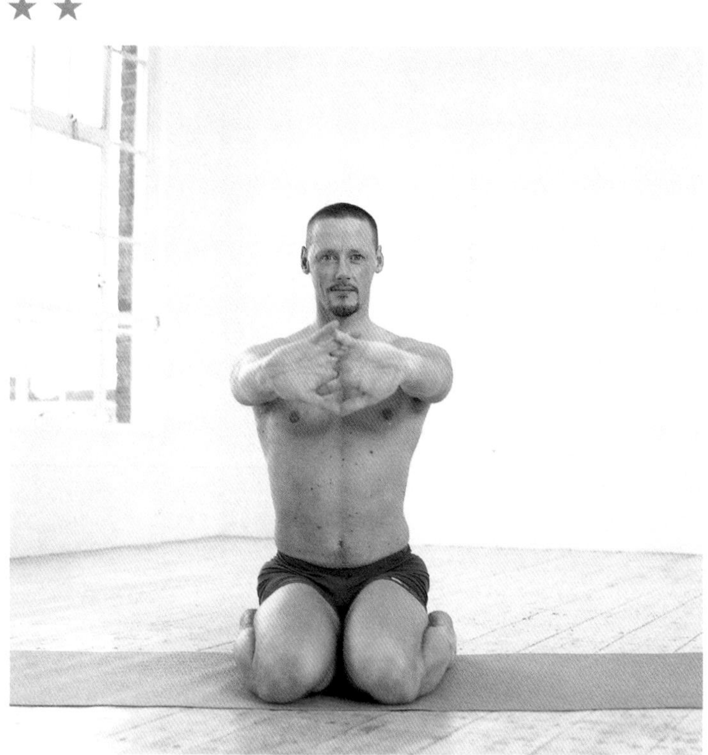

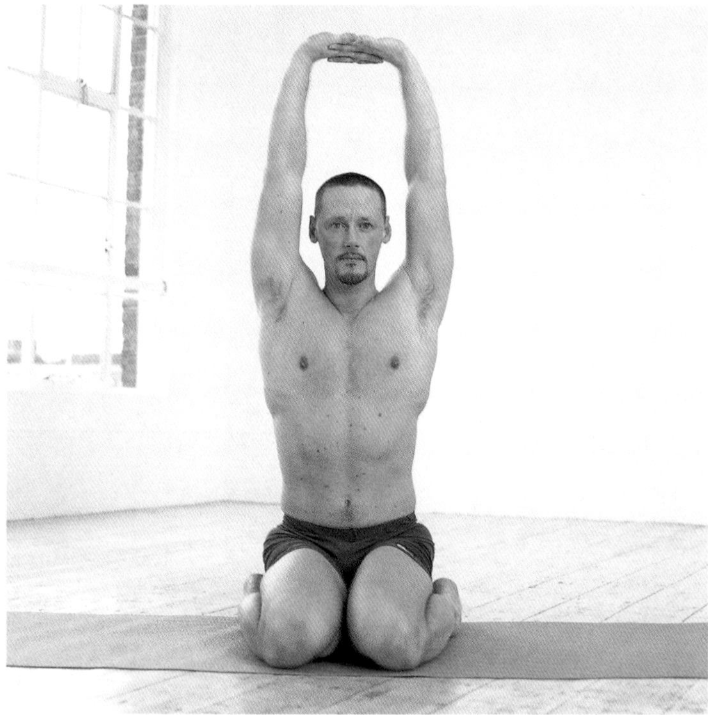

1 Sit in Virasana and interlock the fingers with the right index finger over the left.

Turn the palms away from you, stretch the arms forwards and straighten the elbows.

2 Extend the arms up with the elbows straight. The upper arms are in line with the ears and the palms are facing the ceiling.

Don't overarch in the lower back – extend the trunk and arms strongly upwards. Hold for 30–60 seconds, lower the arms, change the interlock of the fingers (i.e. left index finger over right) and repeat.

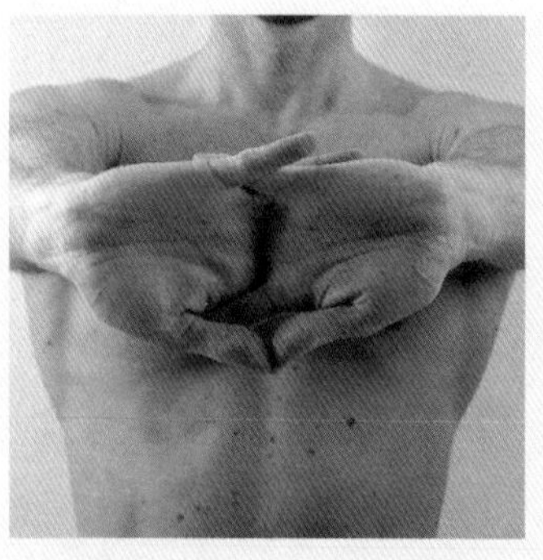

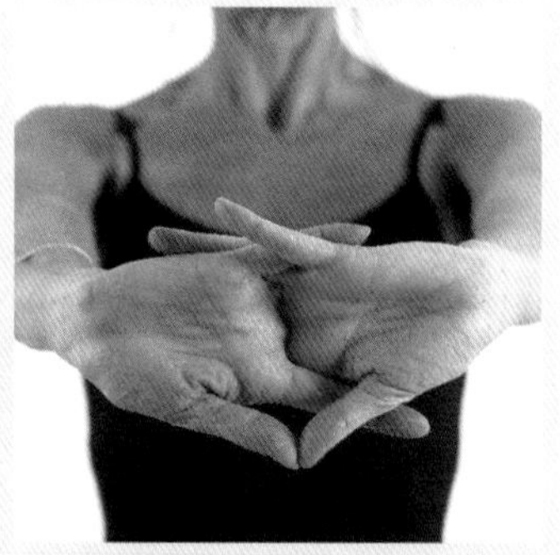

Focus

- Clasp the hands at the root of the fingers and, when extending the arms up, don't allow the fingers to slide apart.
- Change the interlock of the fingers half-way through this pose.

Modification

- If there is difficulty clasping the hands together due to stiffness in the shoulders, then use a strap. Practising this pose will help to relieve the problem.
- If the tops of the feet are painful, put them on a rolled-up blanket.

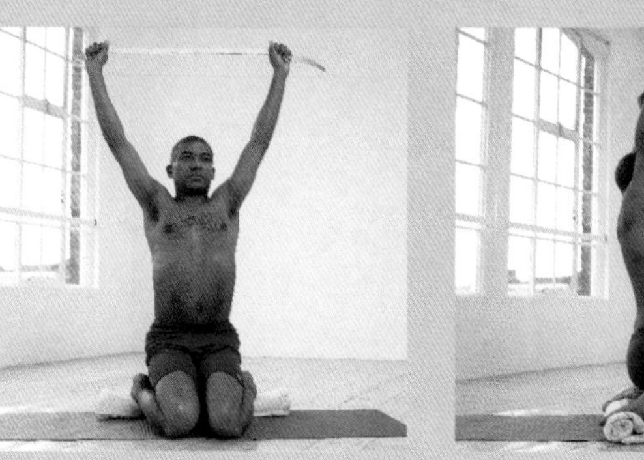

Adho Mukha Virasana | HERO POSE FORWARD BEND

This posture helps to soothe and calm the brain, as well as allowing the body to rest. It relieves fatigue and headaches, stretches and tones the spine and relieves back and neck pain.

1 Kneel on a blanket with the big toes together and the knees hip-width apart. Sit on the heels with the buttocks, and if they don't reach the heels, put a folded blanket on the heels.

Once the buttocks are down, extend the trunk forwards and put the forehead on the floor. Stretch both arms and the sides of the trunk forwards, and put the palms on the floor. Don't take the knees too far apart.

Focus

- The tailbone end of the spine must be supported on the heels. If this cannot be done, put a foam block between the buttocks and the heels.
- If the forehead cannot reach the floor, rest it on a foam block or a folded blanket.

Dandasana | STAFF POSE

This is the basic posture for seated poses and forward bends. It teaches how to sit up straight and extend the spine up.

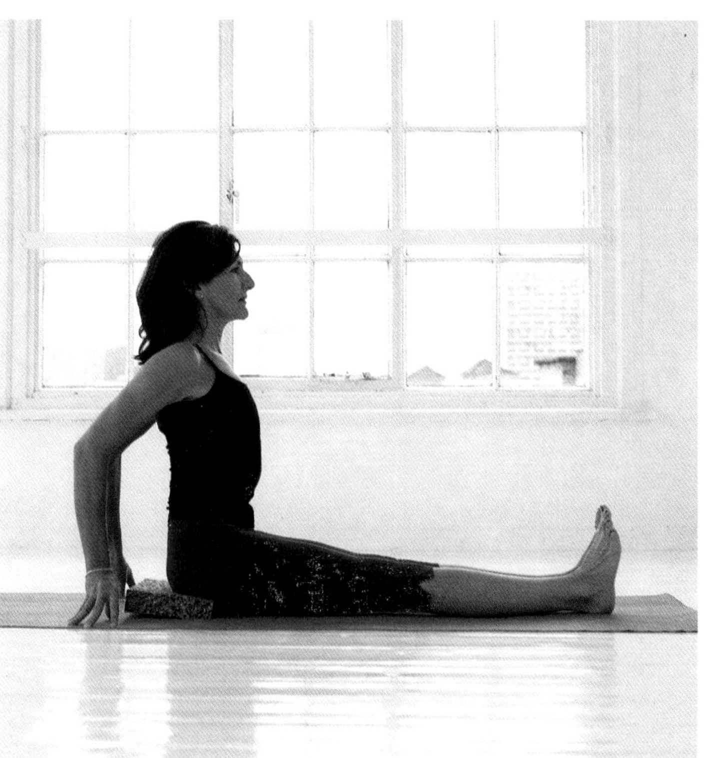

1 Sit on a raise with the legs stretched out in front. Keep the legs and feet together. Tighten the thigh muscles and knees and extend the heels forwards and extend the toes up towards the ceiling. Place the fingertips on the floor behind the hips, press into the floor and extend the trunk up. Don't overarch the lumbar spine. Roll the shoulders back, open the chest. Look straight ahead and relax the eyes. Move the shoulders away from the ears and the shoulder blades towards the front of the body.

Focus

- Balance the head on the spine centrally.
- Open the ribcage.
- Press the backs of the legs into the floor. Extend the inner heels away from the body, keeping feet upright.

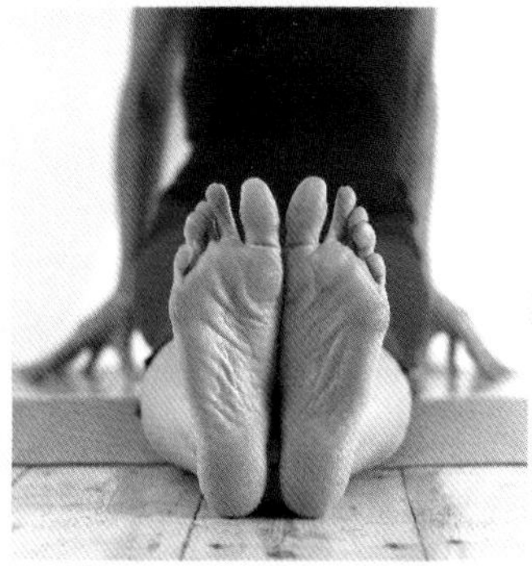

Gomukhasana (arms only) | HEAD OF COW POSE

Gomukhasana expands the chest and gives flexibility to the shoulders. As the spine extends strongly upwards, the shoulder joints become less restricted and the shoulder muscles are fully stretched. This pose also makes the wrists more flexible.

★★

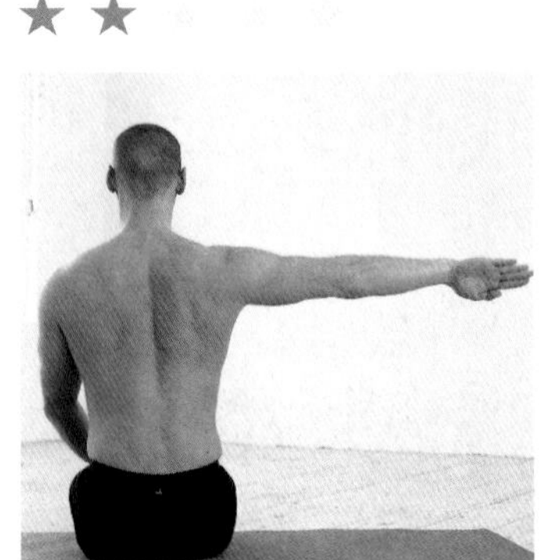

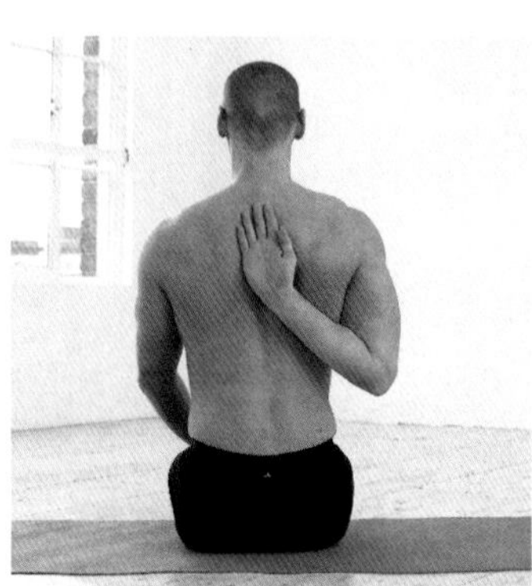

1 Sit in Sukhasana or Virasana and extend the right arm.

2 Bend the right arm behind the back and take the forearm up the back with the palm facing outwards.

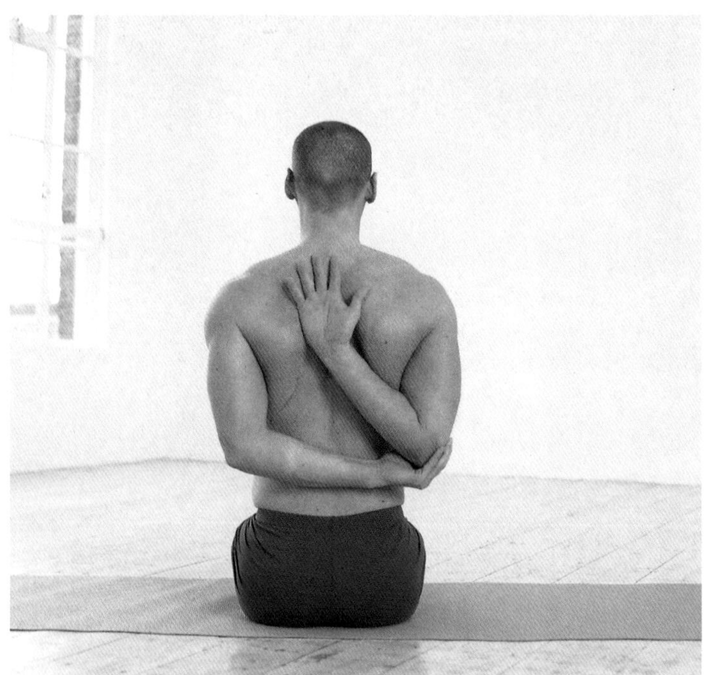

3 Use the left hand to bring the right elbow closer to the trunk, so that the right hand moves farther up the back.

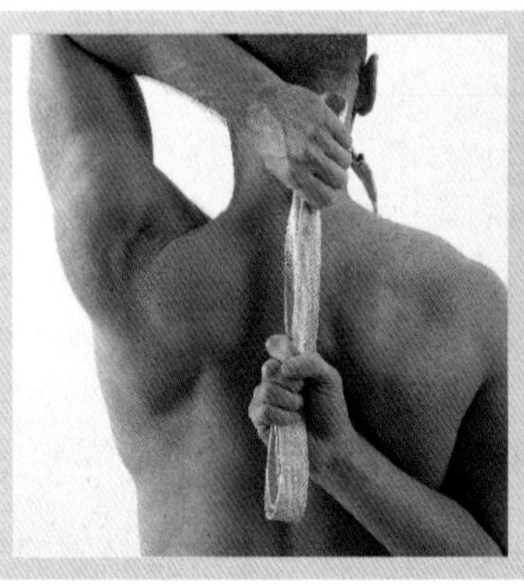

Modification

- Use a strap if the hands cannot grasp one another.
- Keep both sides of the trunk at an equal length and keep the head straight and the eyes level. Don't overarch the lower back.

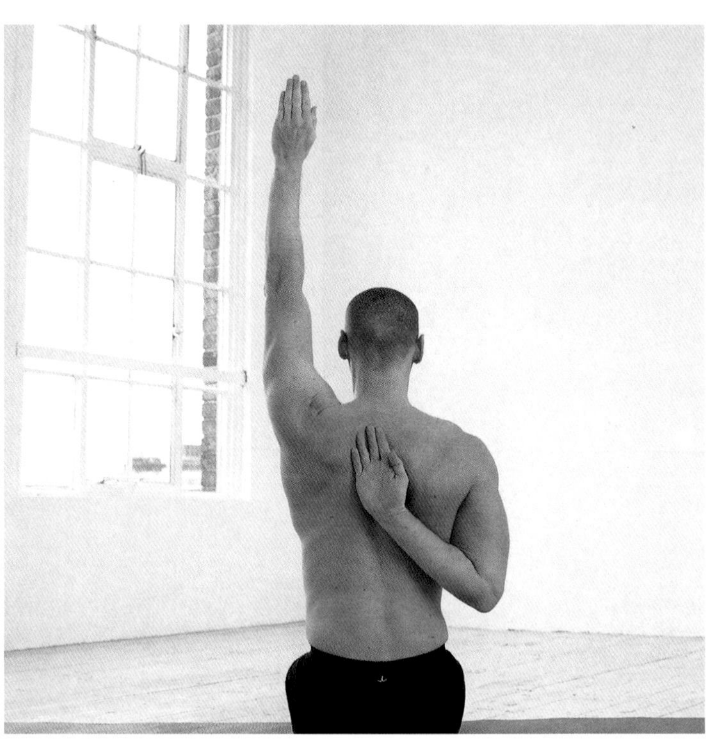

4 Extend the left arm up, turn the palm back, bend the elbow, put the palm of the hand below the nape of the neck and clasp the right hand.

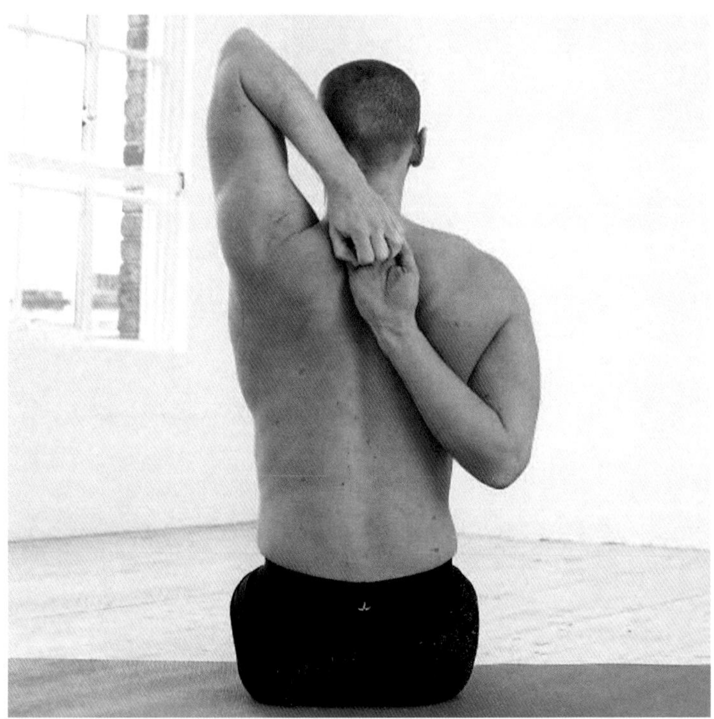

5 Roll the right shoulder back and stretch the left elbow towards the ceiling. Keep the trunk upright and look straight ahead. Hold for 30–60 seconds and repeat on the other side.

Baddhakonasana | COBBLER POSE

This pose keeps the knees and hips flexible. It stimulates the pelvis, abdomen and lower back and keeps the kidneys healthy. It strengthens the bladder and uterus and keeps the prostate healthy, and also helps to reduce sciatic pain.

★

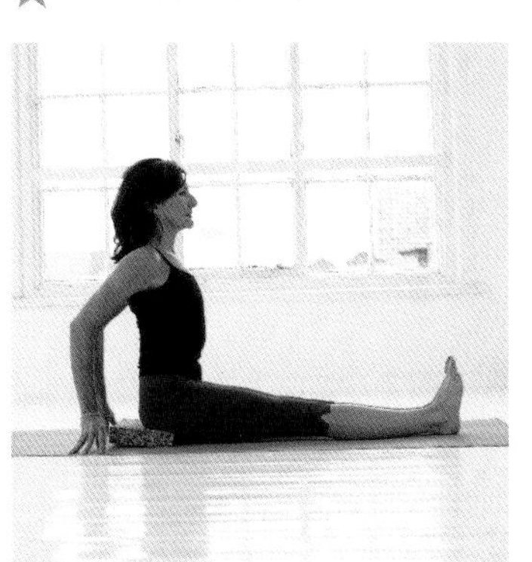

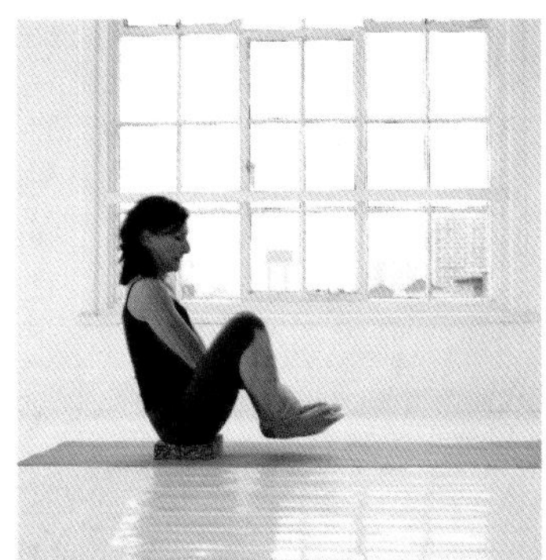

1 Sit in Dandasana on a folded blanket or foam block.

2 Taking the knees out to the side, bend the legs, and use the hands to bring the heels towards the groin.

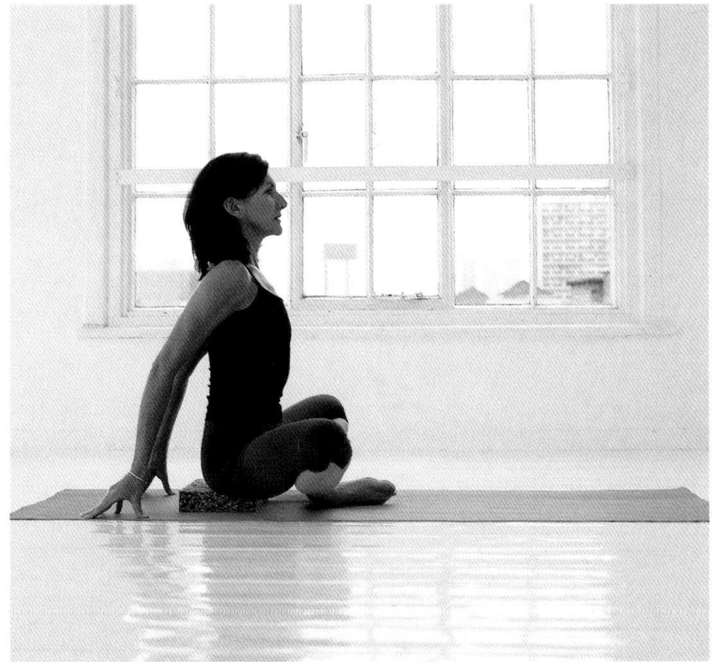

3 With the fingertips on the floor beside the hips, lift up the trunk, take the shoulders back and open the chest.

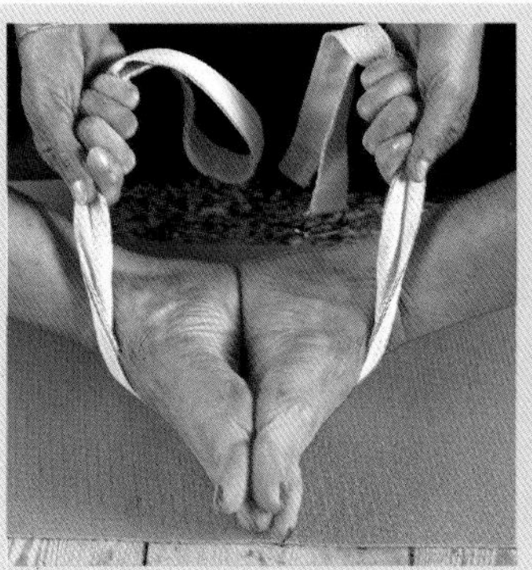

Modification

- If you cannot hold the ankles, use a strap.
- If it is difficult to sit up straight, sit with the back supported against a wall.
- Place a support under the knees to relieve the groin.

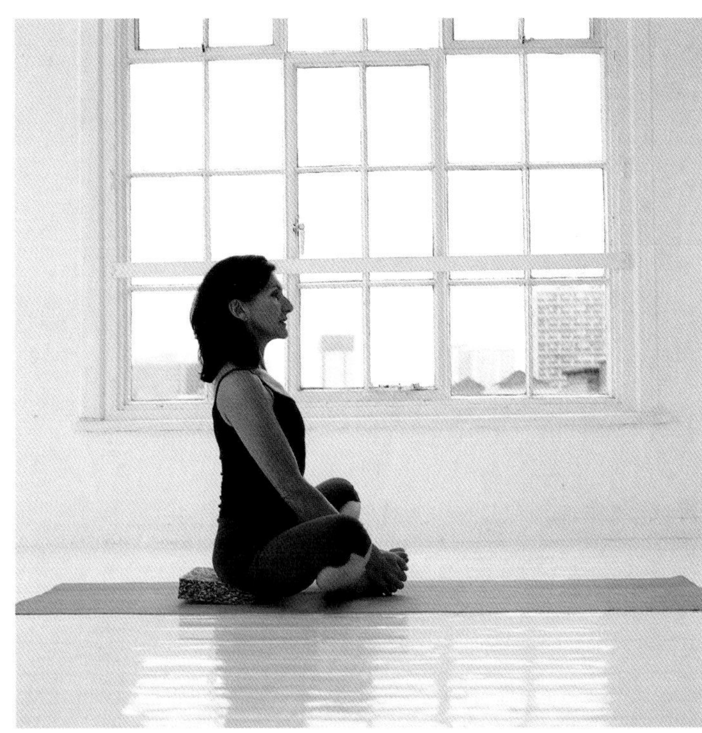

4 Keep the spine lifted, the chest open and hold the ankles, pressing the soles of the feet together.

Roll the shoulders back and down towards the floor, without overarching the lower back.

Hold for 30–60 seconds, release the ankles and come back to Dandasana.

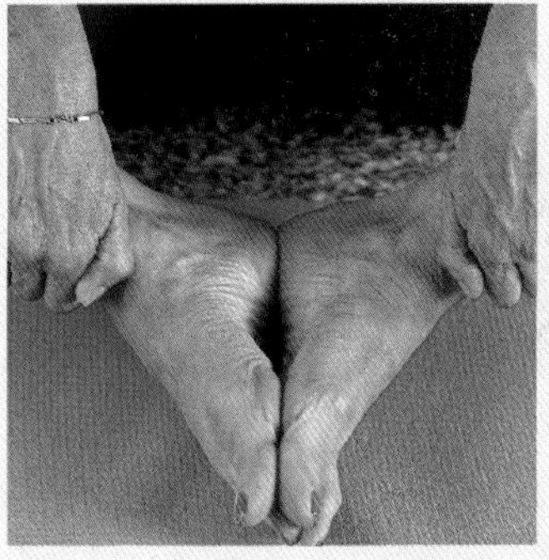

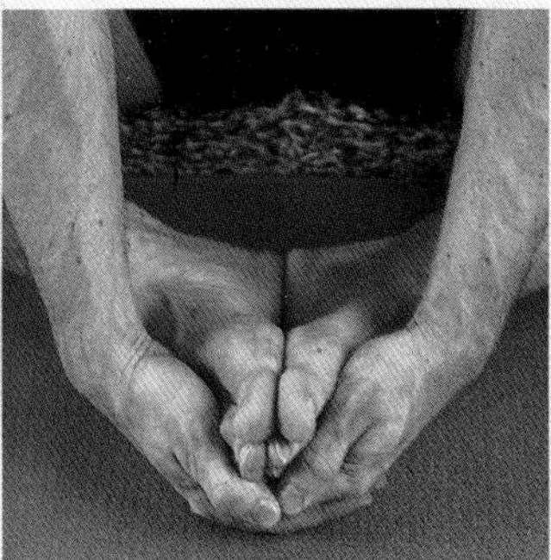

Focus

- Pull the feet in towards the groin as far as you can.
- In the final pose, hold the toes with the hands and lift from the base of the spine.

Upavistakonasana | SEATED ANGLE POSE

This posture stretches the hamstrings and helps blood circulate in the pelvic region, keeping it nourished. It strengthens the muscles that hold the bladder and uterus in position, relieves stiffness in the hip joints and reduces sciatica.

★ ★ ★

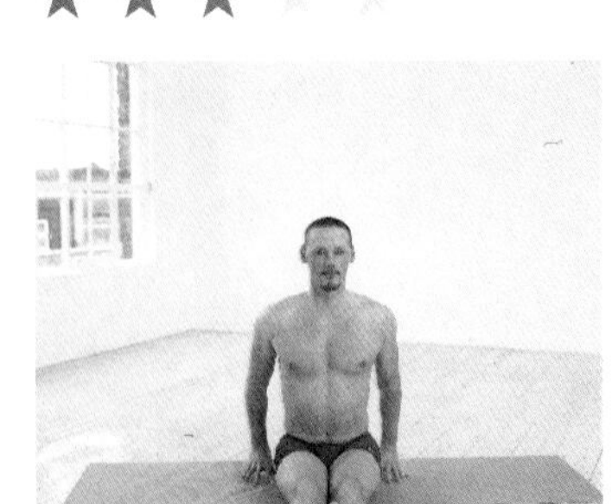

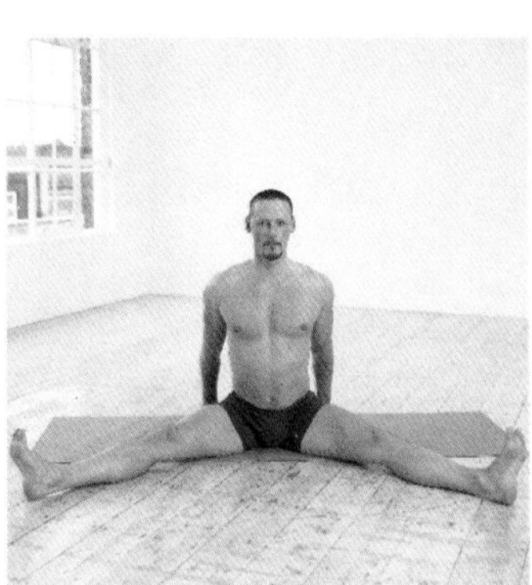

1 Sit in Dandasana on a blanket or mat with no support.

2 Take one leg out to the side, then the other, and widen the distance between the legs. Ensure that the centre of each knee, thigh and foot faces the ceiling. Put the fingertips on the floor behind the hips, press down and extend the spine and trunk up.

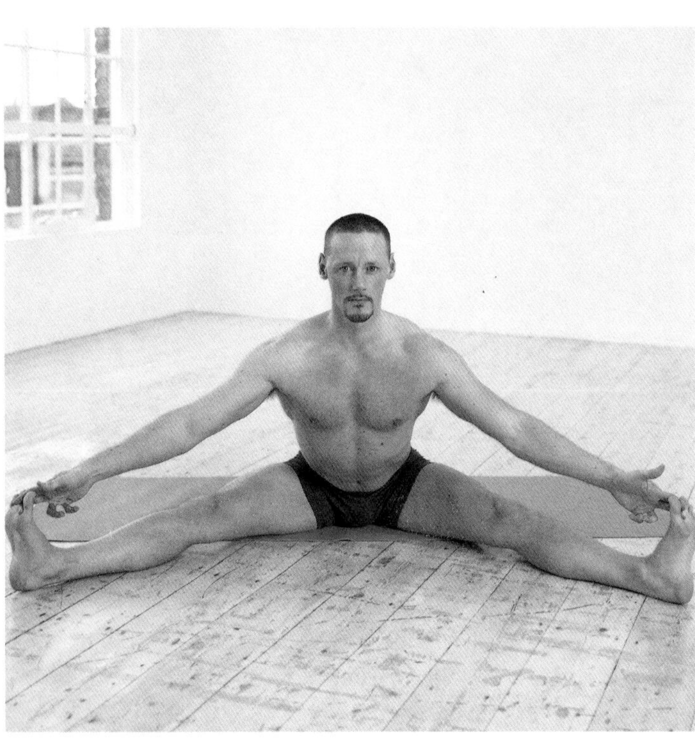

3 Keeping the spine erect, catch the big toes with the first two fingers and pull on them. Alternatively, put a strap around each foot. Hold the straps as close to the feet as possible.

Extend the spine, keeping the back concave and opening the chest. Look up.

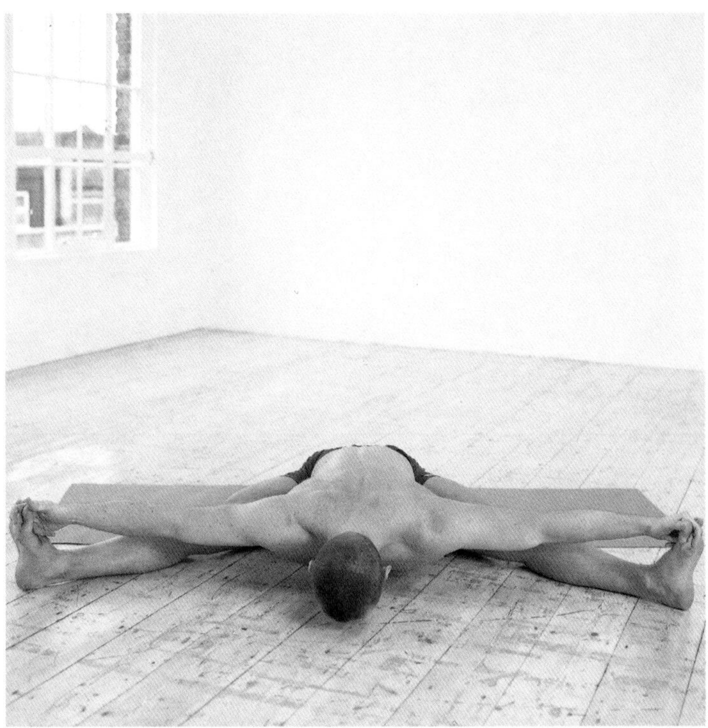

4 Exhale, bend forwards and, keeping the spine stretched, extend the trunk along the floor, trying to get the chest as close to the floor as possible, breathing normally.

Hold for 30–60 seconds and come back to Dandasana.

Modification
- Sit against the wall to support the back.
- Sit on a foam block positioned by the wall for further support.
- Hold the feet with straps if it is difficult to reach.

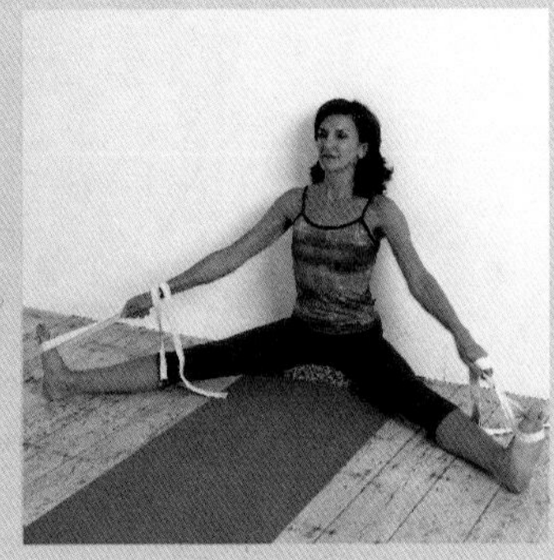

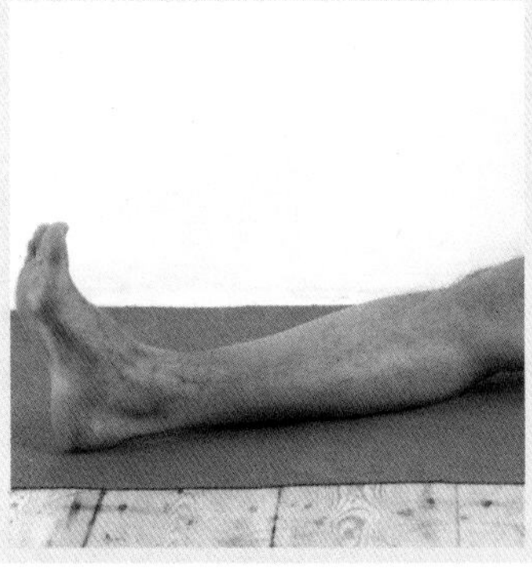

Focus
- Don't allow the feet to roll out. Keep the toes up.
- Extend the inner heels away from the body.
- Press the backs of the legs into the floor and keep the knees facing up.

Paripurna Navasana | BOAT POSE

This pose increases the circulation in the abdomen and tones the abdominal muscles. It improves digestion and relieves lower backache by strengthening the spinal muscles. It also stimulates the thyroid gland.

★ ★

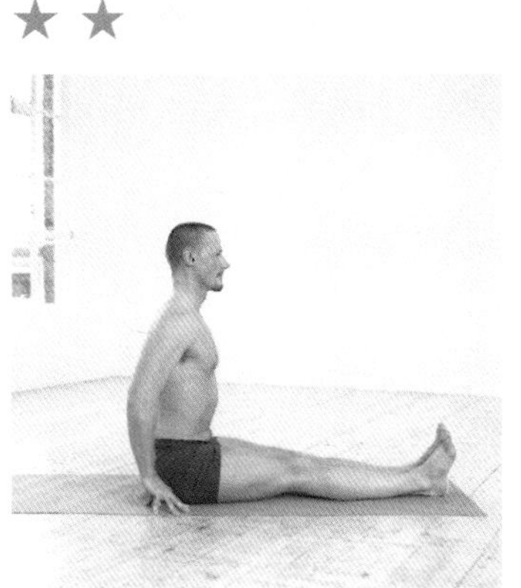

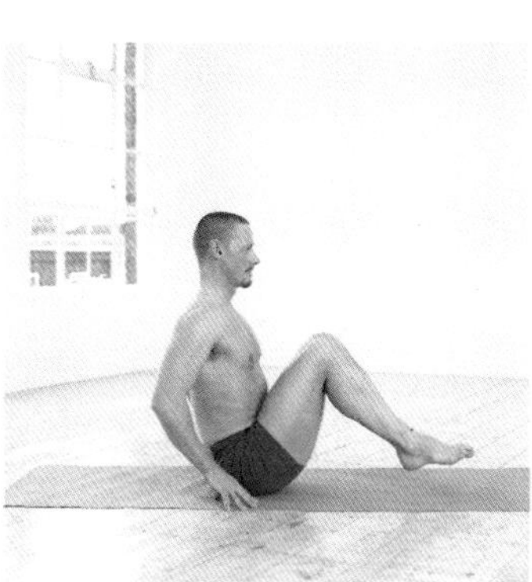

1 Sit in Dandasana on a blanket or mat with no support. Place the hands on the floor beside the hips.

2 Take the trunk slightly back, bend the knees and raise the bent legs, stretching them forwards.

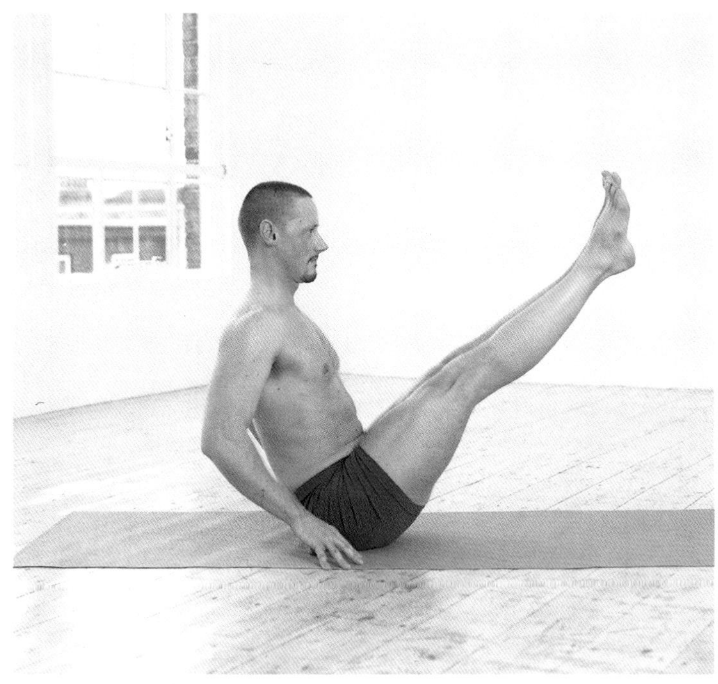

3 Keep both legs very straight (knees and thighs pulled up) and balance on the buttock bones. Raise the feet to 60 degrees, so that they are higher than the head.

Focus

- The abdominal and leg muscles are used to maintain the balance, not the back muscles.
- Don't collapse the lower back – move it into the body and upwards.
- Stretch the backs of the legs strongly.

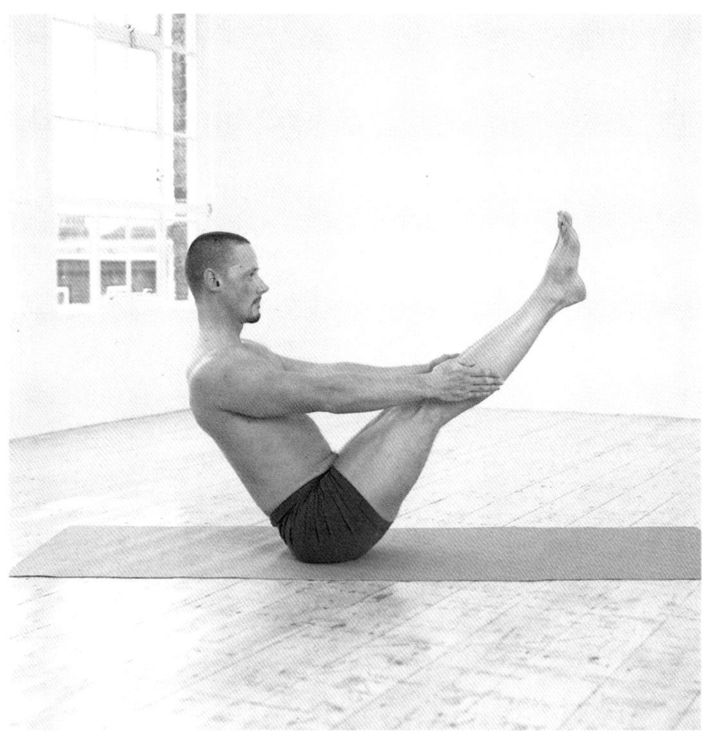

4 Stretch both arms forwards, keeping them parallel to the floor and palms facing one another.

Keep stretching the spine and take it into the body so that the trunk doesn't collapse and the chest remains open.

Look straight ahead and make sure there is no tension or strain in the head and neck. There is a tendency to hold the breath in this pose, which causes tension in the eyes, so breathe normally throughout.

Hold for 30–60 seconds, exhale and come back to Dandasana.

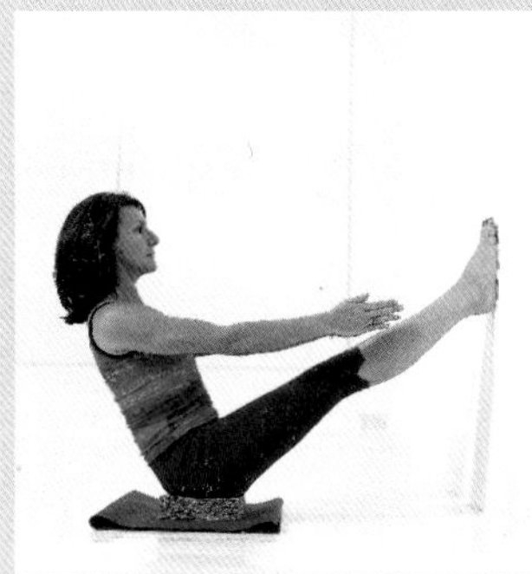

Modification

- If balancing on the buttock bones is difficult, keep the hands on the floor, or put the raised feet against the wall.
- If the back is painful, do the posture with bent knees.

Ardha Navasana | HALF BOAT POSE

The difference between this pose and Paripurna Navasana is the height to which the legs are lifted. Because the legs are lower in Ardha Navasana, it tones the liver, gall bladder and spleen. It also strengthens the spinal muscles.

★★

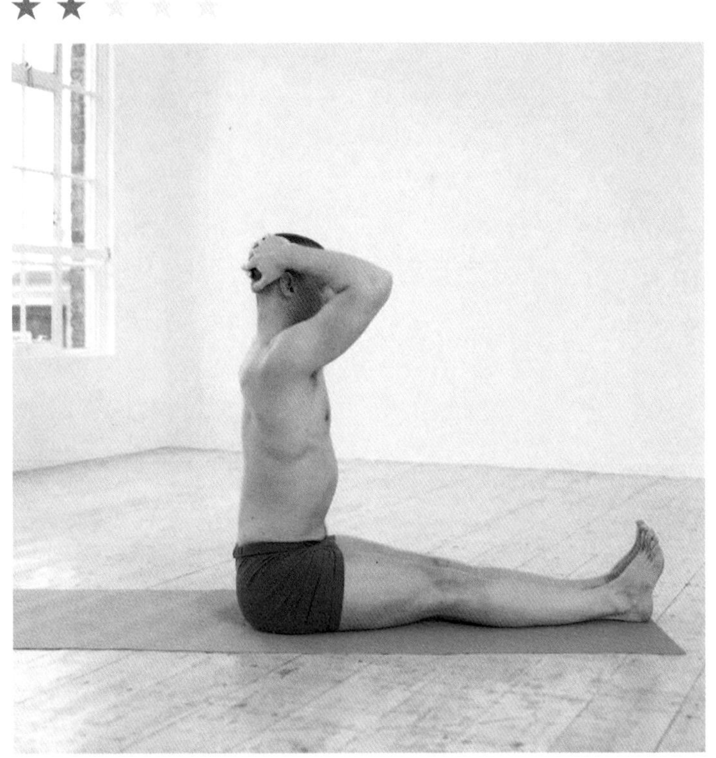

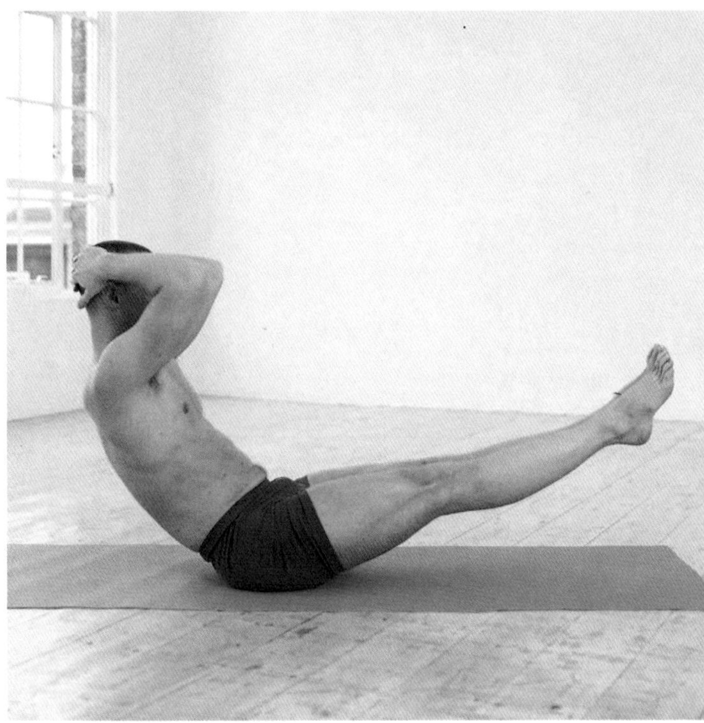

1 Sit in Dandasana on a blanket or mat with no support. Place the hands on the floor beside the hips.

Interlock the fingers and put the hands behind the head just above the neck. Bring the elbows slightly in so that the arms form a semi-circle.

2 Exhale, simultaneously taking the trunk slightly back and raising the legs from the floor to 30 degrees. Keep the knees and thighs pulled up, extend the backs of the legs towards the heels and keep the feet level with the head.

The body rests on the buttock bones and no part of the spine should touch the floor. Look towards the feet.

Breathe normally and keep the eyes soft. Don't strain the neck by pulling the head forwards with the clasped hands – the palms should touch the back of the head and the head should rest lightly on the palms.

Hold for 30–60 seconds, remembering to breathe normally.

Focus

- The difference between Paripurna Navasana and Ardha Navasana is that here the legs are raised to only 30 degrees, not to 60 degrees, and the body is not lowered.
- Interlock the fingers at the back of the head just above the neck.

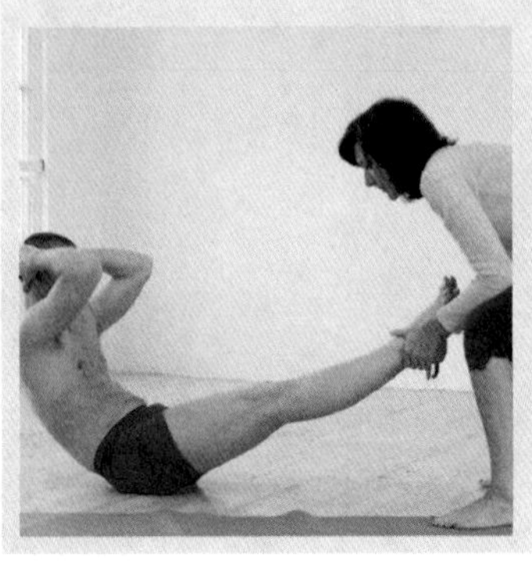

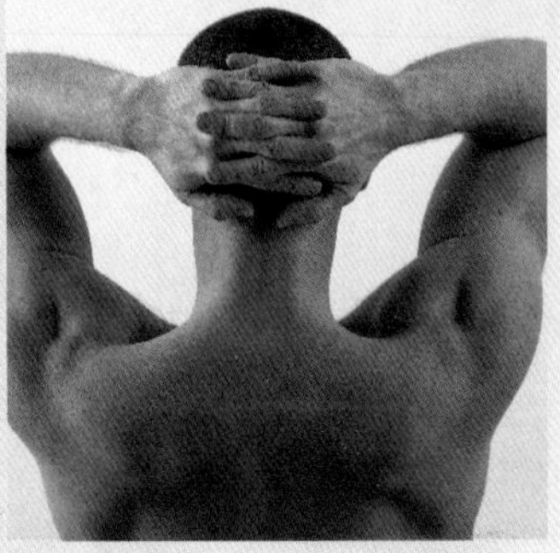

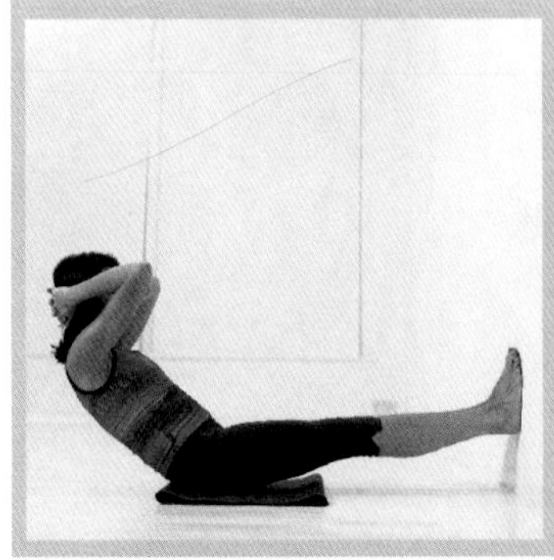

Modification

- If there is a problem with balance, position the raised feet flat against the wall.

To hold this position for any length of time requires very strong abdominal muscles, so help may be required.

Janusirsasana | HEAD TO KNEE POSE

Janusirsasana stimulates the digestive system, tones the abdominal muscles and brings the brain and heart into a restful state. Forward bends are beneficial for a good night's sleep.

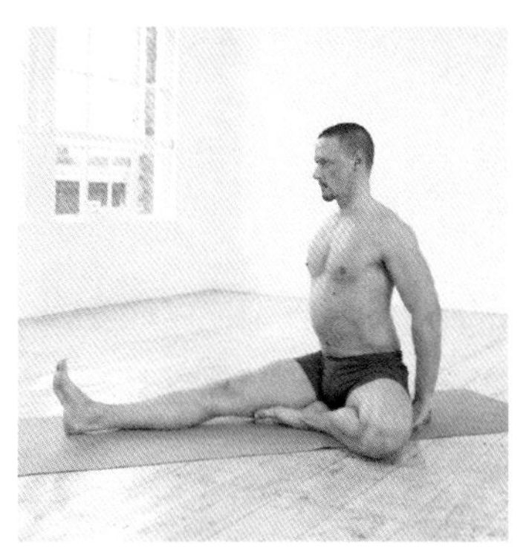

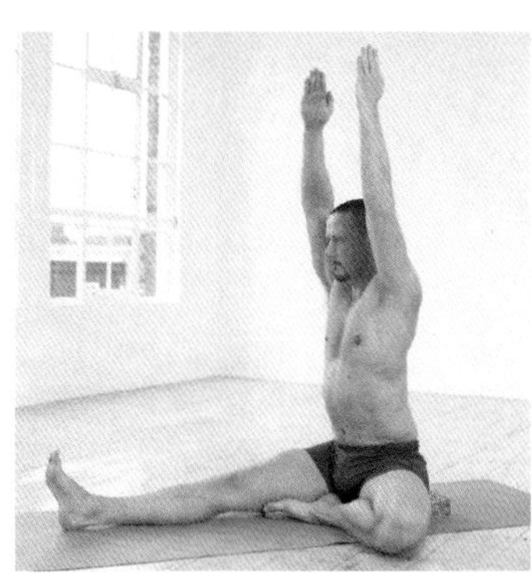

1 Sit in Dandasana on a support, bend the left knee to the side and place the left foot so that the big toe touches the inside of the right thigh.

2 Inhale and extend both arms straight up to the ceiling, moving the shoulder blades into the body. The upper arms are beside the ears. Stretch the spine upwards.

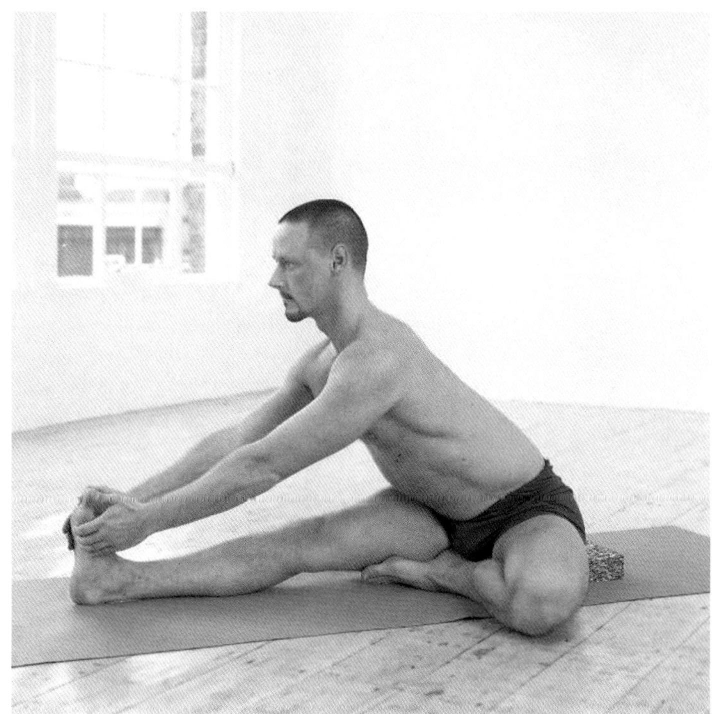

3 Exhale, bend forwards and catch the sides of the right foot with both hands. Make the spine concave and look up. If the lower back aches, do not proceed any further.

Focus

• Keep the right leg straight with the toes pointing up. Press the back of the right leg down on to the floor.

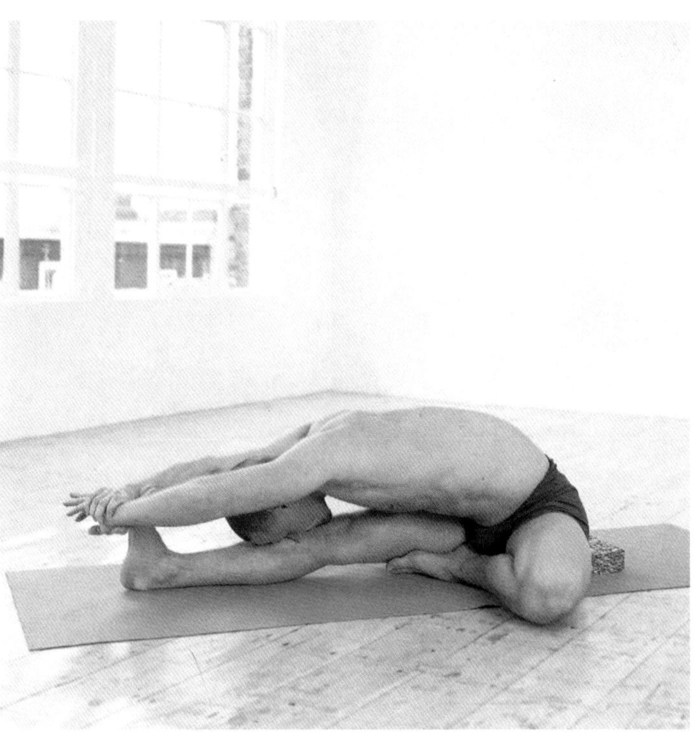

4 Exhale, widen the elbows out to the side, extend the trunk further forwards and take the head down.

Hold for 30–60 seconds, inhale, release the foot, come up and repeat on the other side.

Modification

• If you can't reach the right foot, use a strap around the foot, holding it in a "V" shape with both hands.

• If you are able to catch the foot, hold it around the sides of the foot, not the toes.

• If the lower back is painful, rest the forehead on a stool or bolster.

• Sit on a foam block and support the bent knee on a foam block if it is uncomfortable.

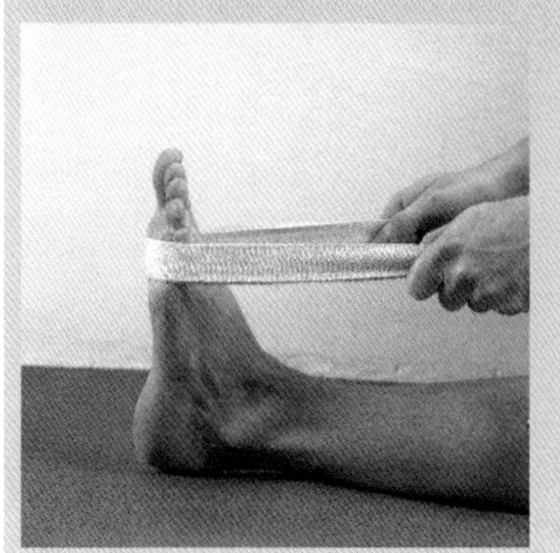

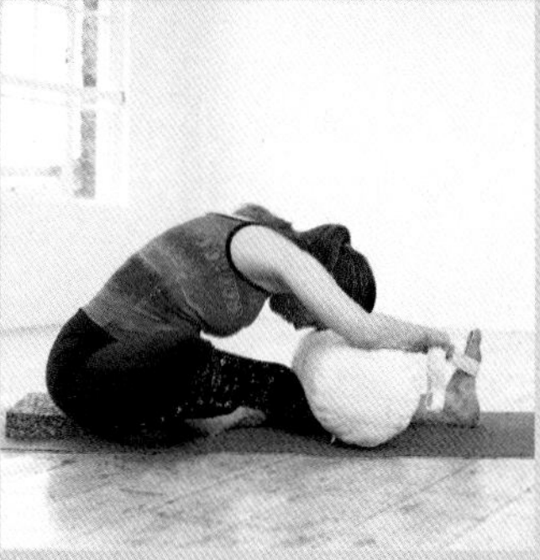

Trianga Mukhaikapada Pascimottanasana | FORWARD BEND WITH ONE LEG BENT BACK

This posture improves flexibility of the ankles and knees. It also helps to tone the abdominal muscles and organs.

★ ★

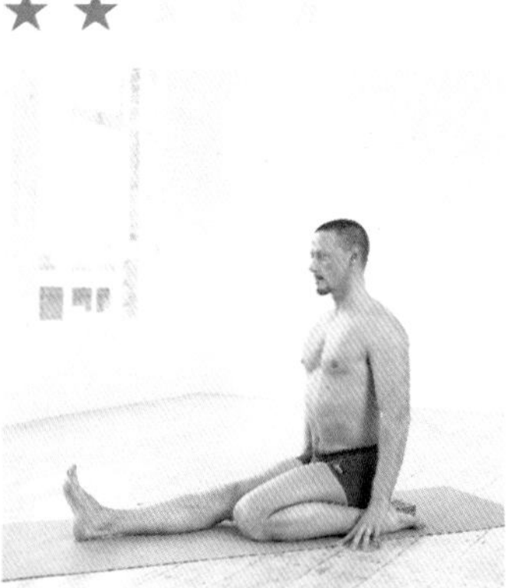

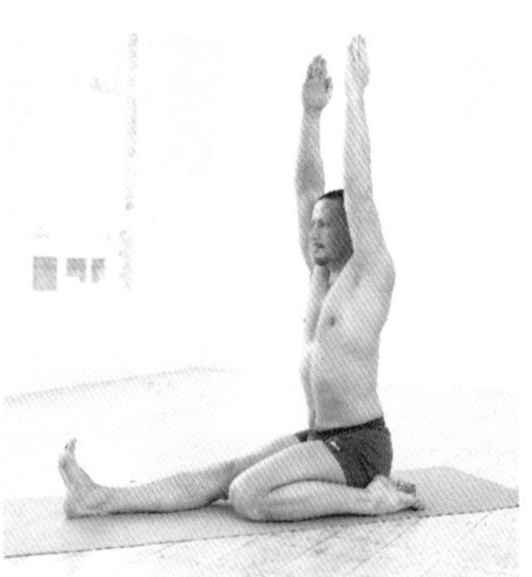

1 Sit in Dandasana on a support. Bend the left leg back and place the foot beside the left hip.

2 Inhale and extend the arms up, palms facing and upper arms beside the ears. Extend the spine and trunk.

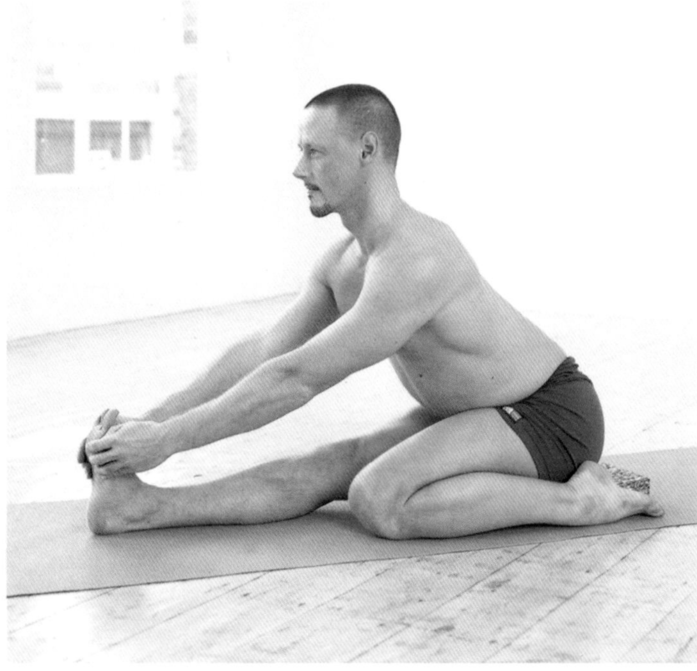

3 Exhale, extend the trunk forwards and clasp the right foot.

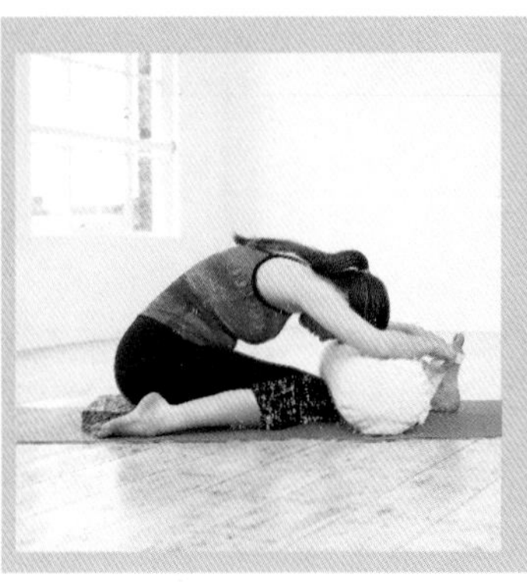

Modification

• An easy version is to rest the head on a bolster or rolled-up blanket.

• It may also help to sit on a raise – a folded blanket or a foam block are both good for this.

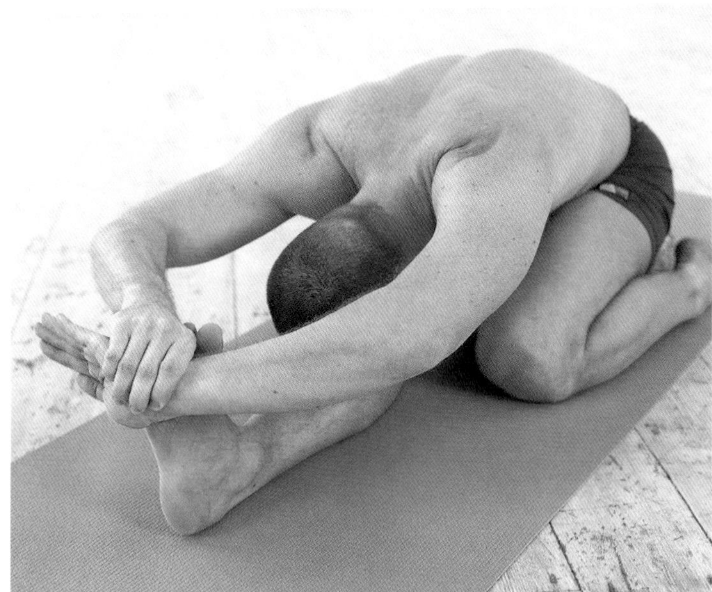

4 Inhale, lengthen the spine upwards, make the back concave and look up. Exhale, extend the trunk forwards, elongating the spine and taking the head towards the right leg. Widen the elbows out to the side.

Hold for 1–2 minutes, inhale, release the foot, raise the head and come up. Repeat on the other side.

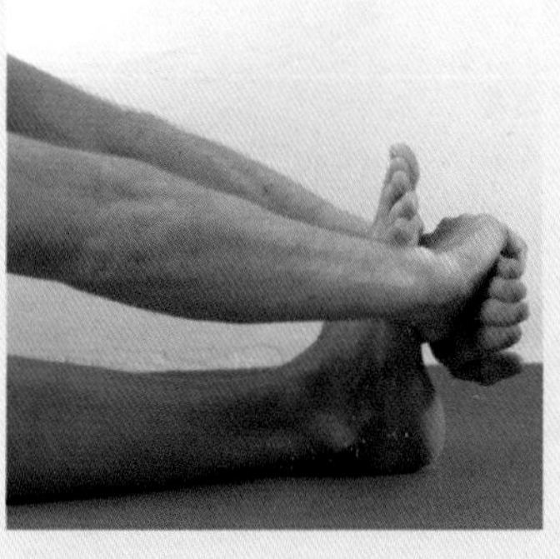

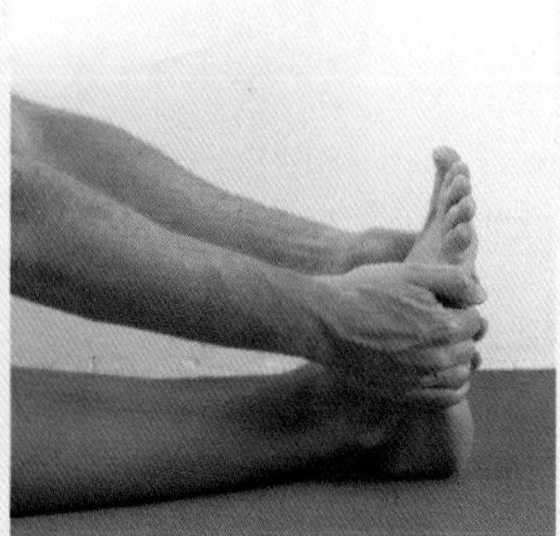

Focus

• Try to catch the hands around the foot. If you can't manage this at first, then use a strap, or clutch the foot on either side, but not the toes.

• Press both buttocks down towards the floor. Pull on the foot (or strap) to lengthen the spine and open the chest.

• Move the shoulders away from the ears and relax the neck and head.

Pascimottanasana | FULL FORWARD BEND

This posture tones and activates the abdominal organs, aids digestion and rejuvenates the spine. As the body is in a horizontal position in forward bend poses, there is less strain on the heart.

★★★

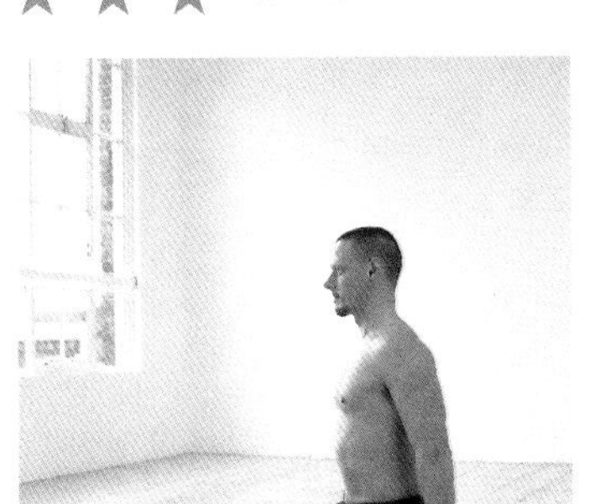

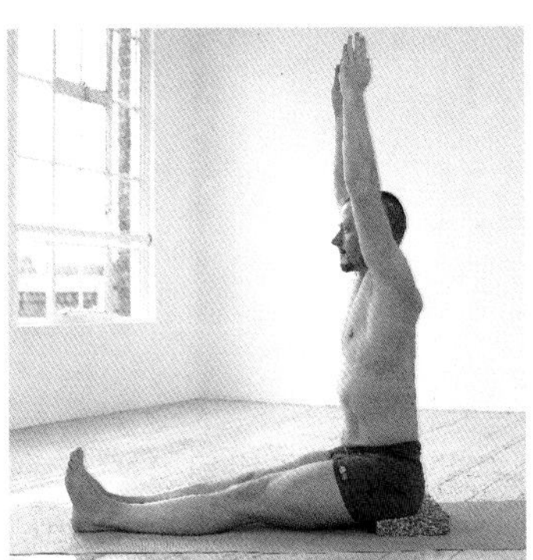

1 Sit in Dandasana on a support.

2 Inhale, extend the arms up (palms facing), keeping the upper arms besides the ears.

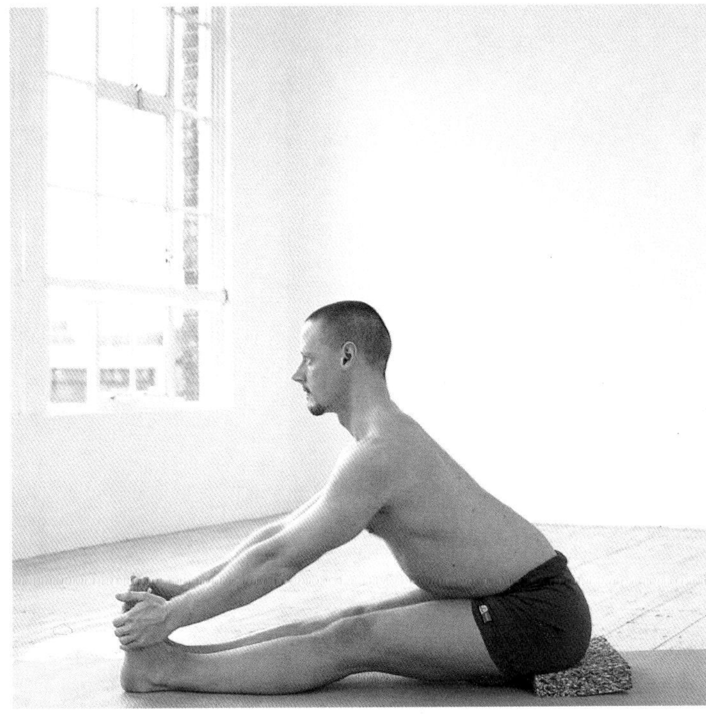

3 Exhale, extend the trunk forwards, clasp the sides of both feet with the hands (or use a strap). Inhale and extend forwards, make the back concave, lift the chest and look up.

Focus

- Press the back of the legs down into the floor to extend the spine more.
- Extend the inner heels away, with toes stretching towards the ceiling.
- Pull on the feet or the strap to lengthen the trunk.

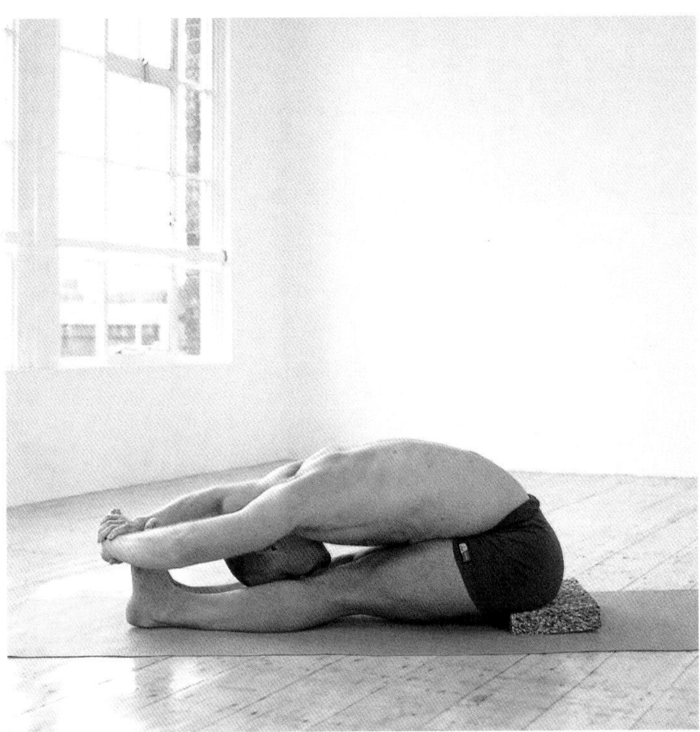

4 Exhale, continue extending the spine/trunk forwards over the legs and catch the hands around the foot (or reach further with the strap). Bend the elbows out to the side.

Fully extend the front of the body and the sides of the trunk. Take the head down. If the back aches, rest the head on a bolster or stool. Hold for 30–60 seconds, inhale and come up.

Modification

- If the backs of the knees are painful when pressed into the floor, place a rolled-up blanket under the knees.
- If the forehead cannot reach the floor, rest it on a foam block or a folded blanket.
- In cases of extreme stiffness, or pain in the back, rest the head on a stool covered with a blanket.

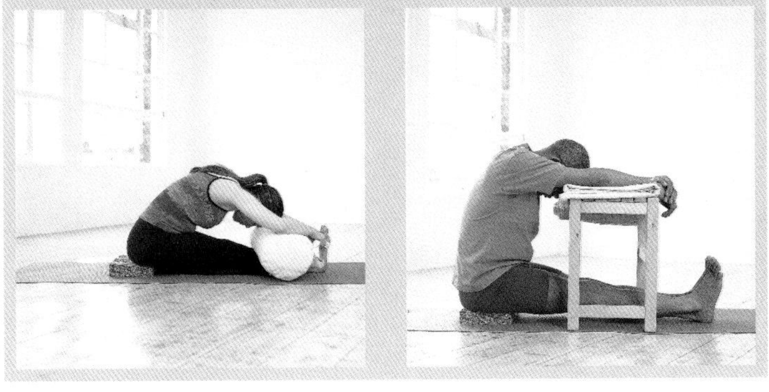

Malasana | GARLAND POSE

In this pose the arms hang from the neck like a garland. It relieves lower back pain and reduces stiffness in the knees and ankles. It also activates and nourishes the abdominal organs.

★ ★

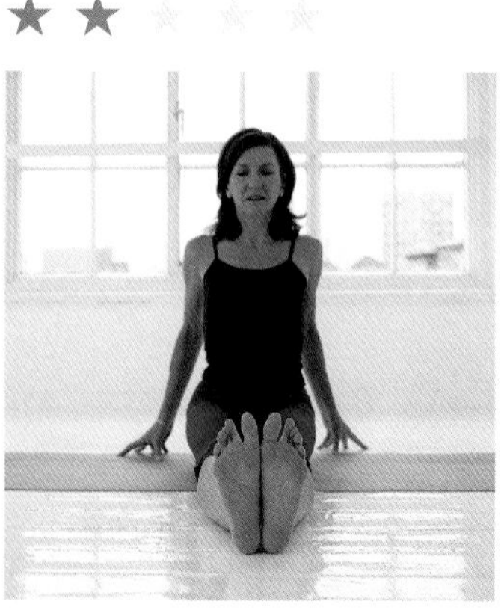

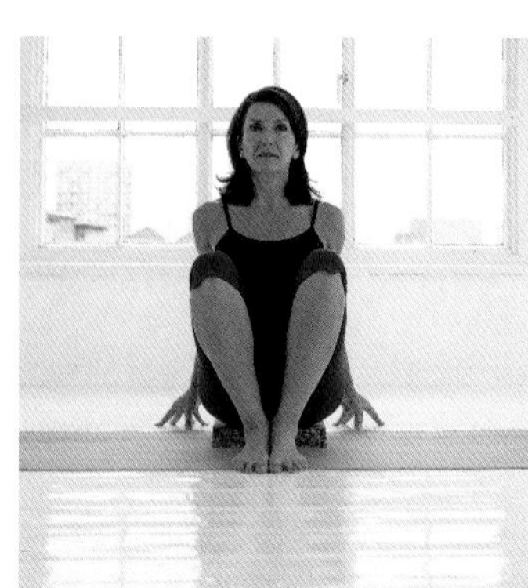

1 Sit in Dandasana on a support.

2 Bend the knees and come up into a squatting position.

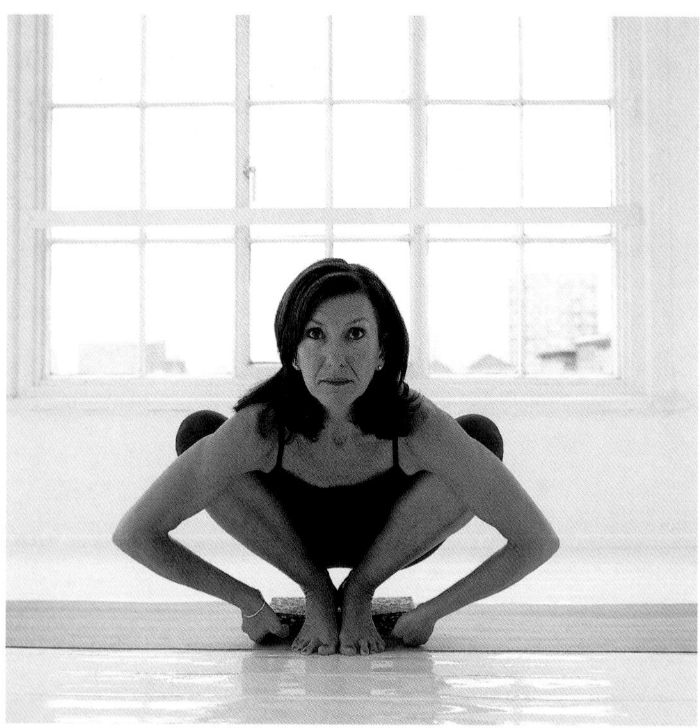

3 Keep the feet together and support the heels by pulling the support forwards underneath the heels. Separate the thighs and knees and extend the trunk forwards between the legs.

Focus

- If the heels come off the support, add another support. The heels must press on to something.
- The inner thighs lightly grip the sides of the trunk.
- Extend the spine and lengthen the side ribs.
- Round the back when taking the head down.

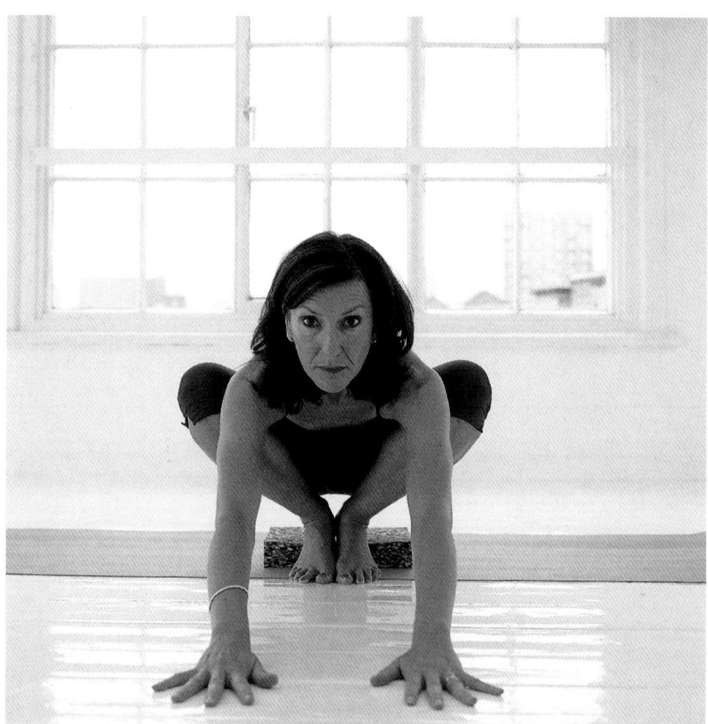

4 Stretch the arms forwards, pressing the palms into the floor, extend the spine towards the head and look up. Wrap the arms around the legs.

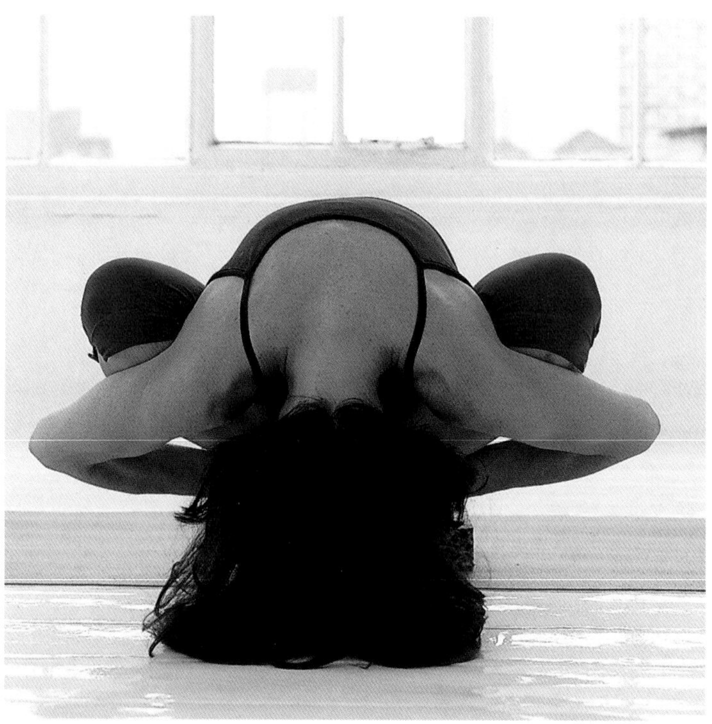

5 . Exhale, bend forwards and take the head down towards the floor. Hold the ankles with the hands. Hold for 30–60 seconds and then come up.

Padmasana | LOTUS

Exercise extreme caution when attempting this posture. If the knees are painful, stop immediately and practise Sukhasana as a preparation for Padmasana.

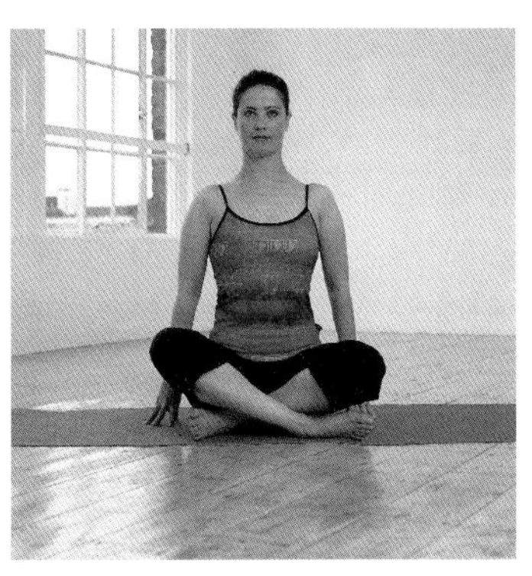

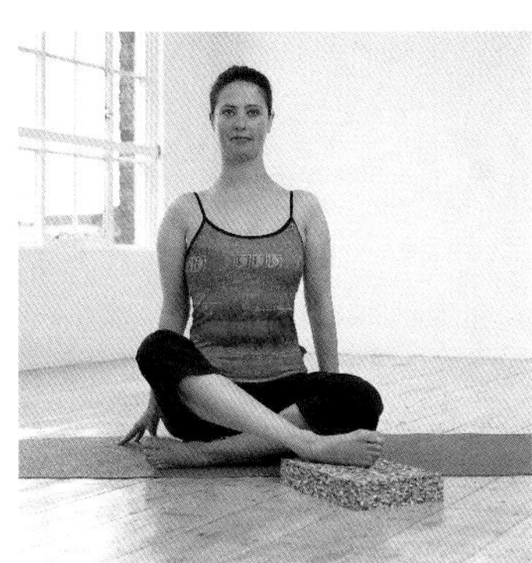

1 Sit in Sukhasana (simple cross legs), with the right shin-bone crossed in front.

2 Bring the right foot forwards, supporting it on a foam block if necessary.

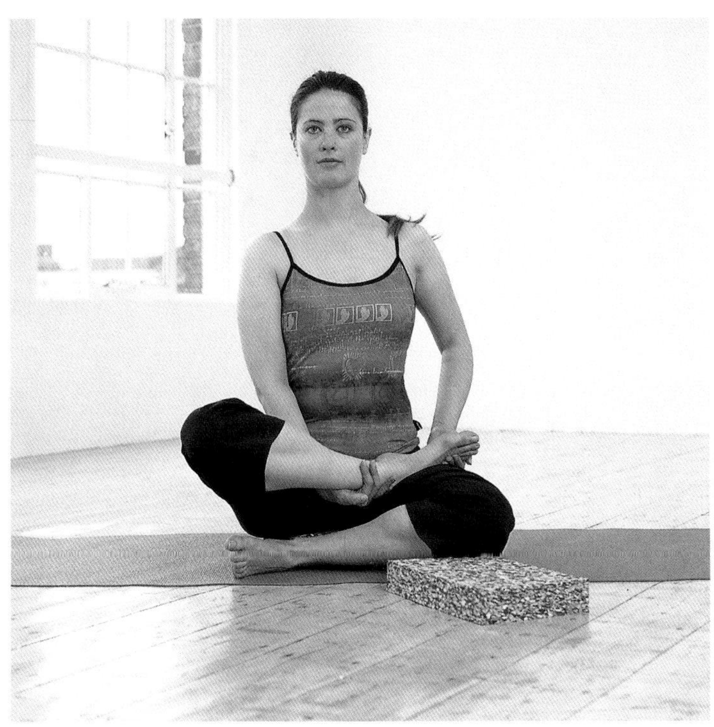

3 Carefully lift the right foot and place it as high up on the left thigh as possible.

Bring the left foot forwards and support it on a block on the other side.

Lift the left foot on to the right thigh. If there is pain in the knees, sit in half-Padmasana, i.e. first leg in Padmasana and second leg in Sukhasana.

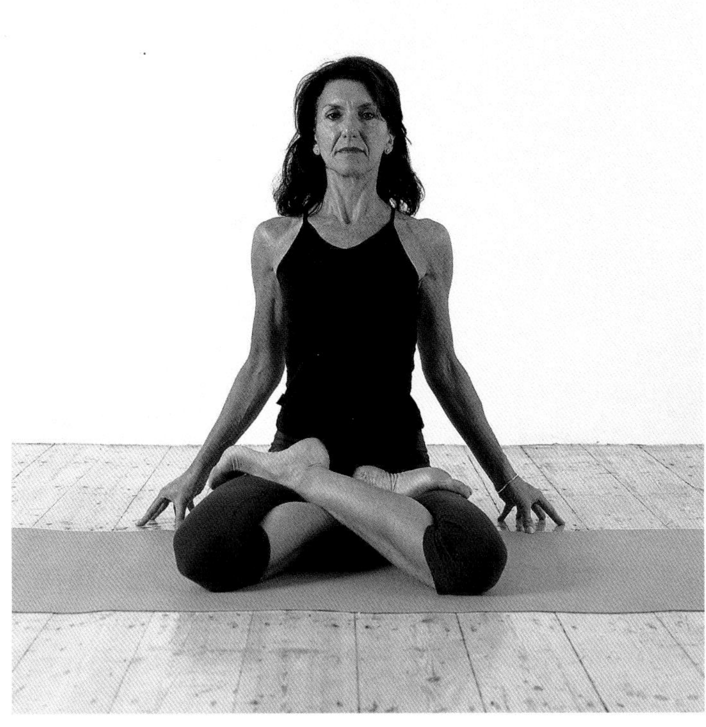

4 Press the fingertips into the floor beside the hips to extend the spine up. Continue to lift from the base of the spine upwards through the neck to the top of the head.

Hold for 30–60 seconds. Release the legs, and repeat with the left shin-bone crossed in front of the right.

Many people will find they lack the flexibility in the knees to do this posture at first, but after time suppleness will increase and the posture become comfortable. Changing the cross of the legs regularly means that they will develop evenly on both sides.

Focus

- When bending the knee, to avoid straining and to create space, use the fingers to draw the top of the calf muscle and the bottom of the back thigh muscle away from the back of the knee.
- For painful knees, place a strap at the back of the knee and pull on it as you take the leg into Padmasana.
- If the right knee doesn't reach the floor, support it on a foam block, then take the left leg into Padmasana.

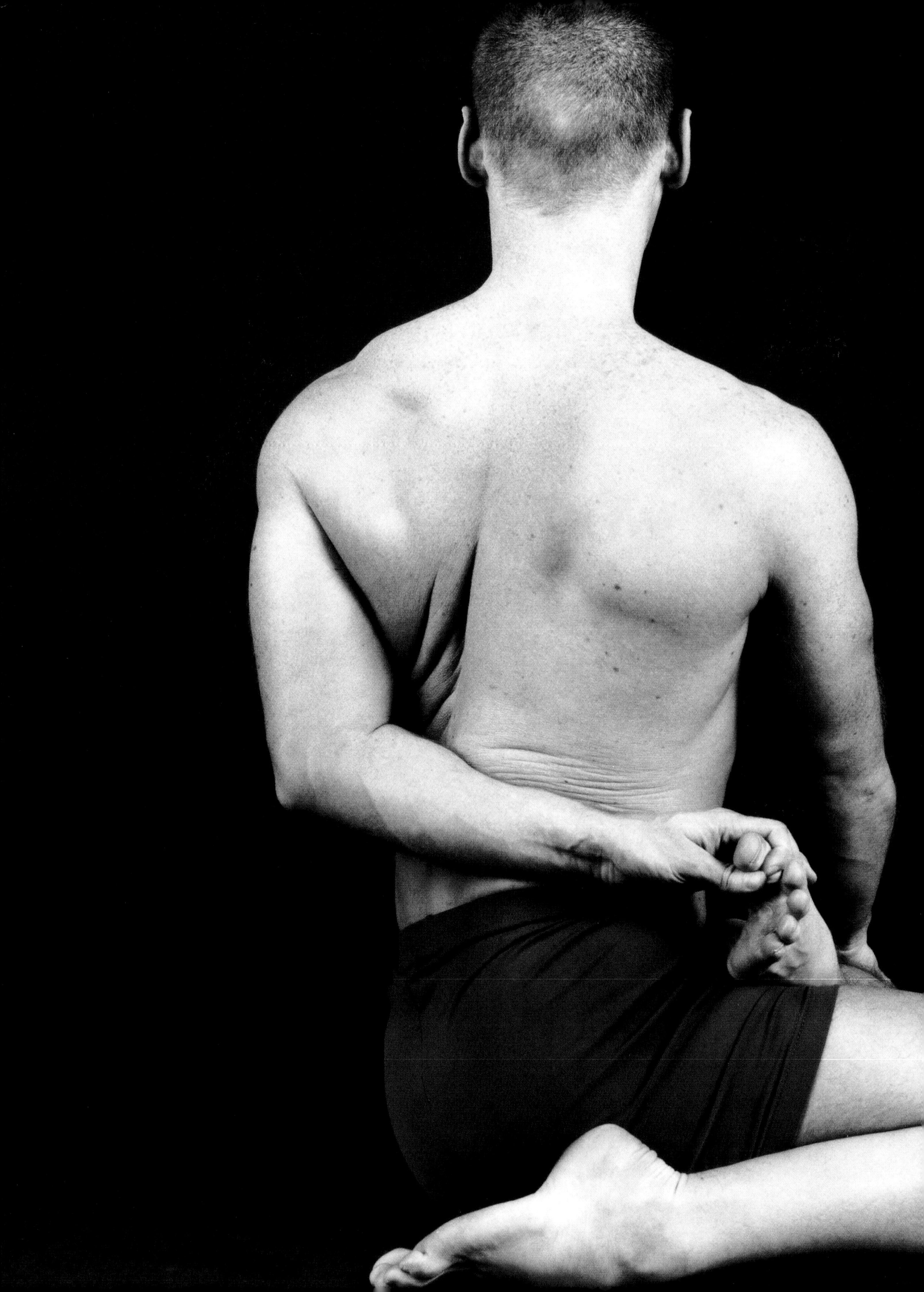

Twists

All lateral extension postures (twists) create flexibility in the spine and shoulders. They activate and nourish the pelvic and abdominal organs, and bring relief to back, hip and groin problems. As the spine becomes more supple, blood flow to the spinal nerves improves, and energy levels are raised. When practising twists, lift the spine first, and then turn the abdomen, chest and finally the head. Moving the shoulder blades into the back will improve the turn.

Standing Maricyasana | STANDING TWIST

This posture reduces stiffness in the neck and shoulders. It improves the alignment of the spine and strengthens the spinal muscles. It also relieves lower back pain and sciatica.

★

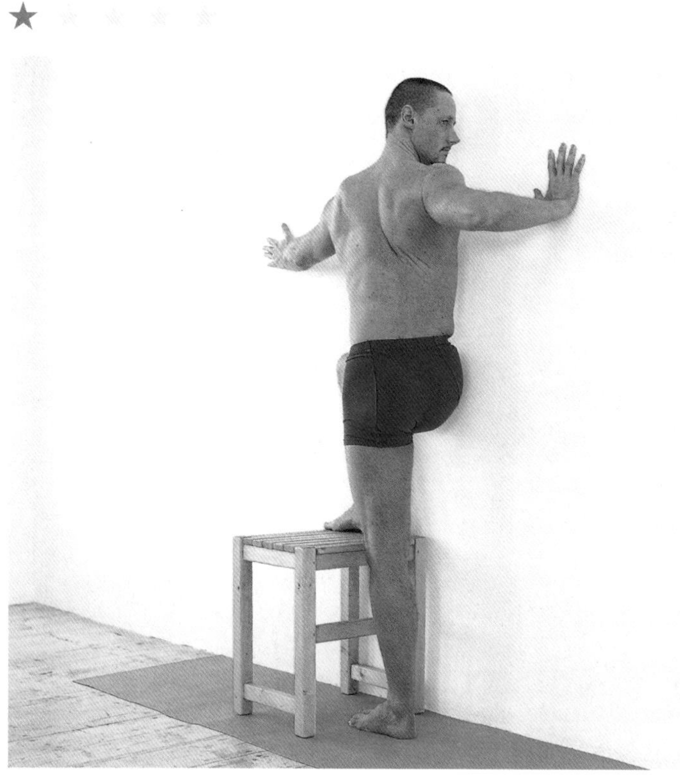

1 Put a stool near the wall. Stand in Tadasana with the wall on your right. Bend the right knee and place the foot on the stool, keeping the right thigh against the wall.

Inhale, stretch the left leg strongly up and keep the toes of this foot facing forwards. Extend the trunk towards the ceiling. Exhale, turn the front body to face the wall, and place the hands on the wall at shoulder level.

Inhale, extend trunk further, exhale, press the hands into the wall to enable the trunk to turn more to the right. Turn as far as you can, look over the right shoulder. Hold for 20–40 seconds, release, and repeat on the other side.

Focus

- Don't allow the front body to lean towards the wall.
- Move the shoulder blades into the body and downwards towards the waist to open the chest.

Sukhasana (twist) | EASY POSE TWIST

In this easy, cross-legged twist, use the breath to lift and turn. Relax the shoulders, moving them away from the ears and into the body.

★

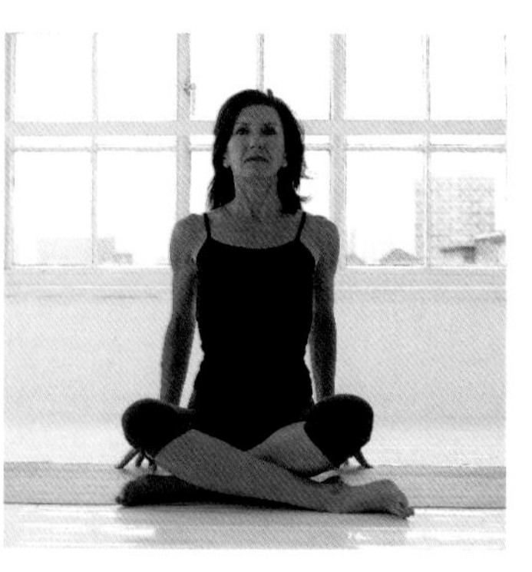

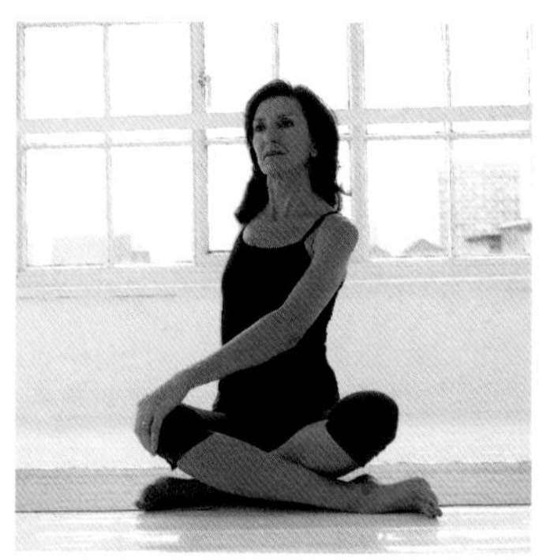

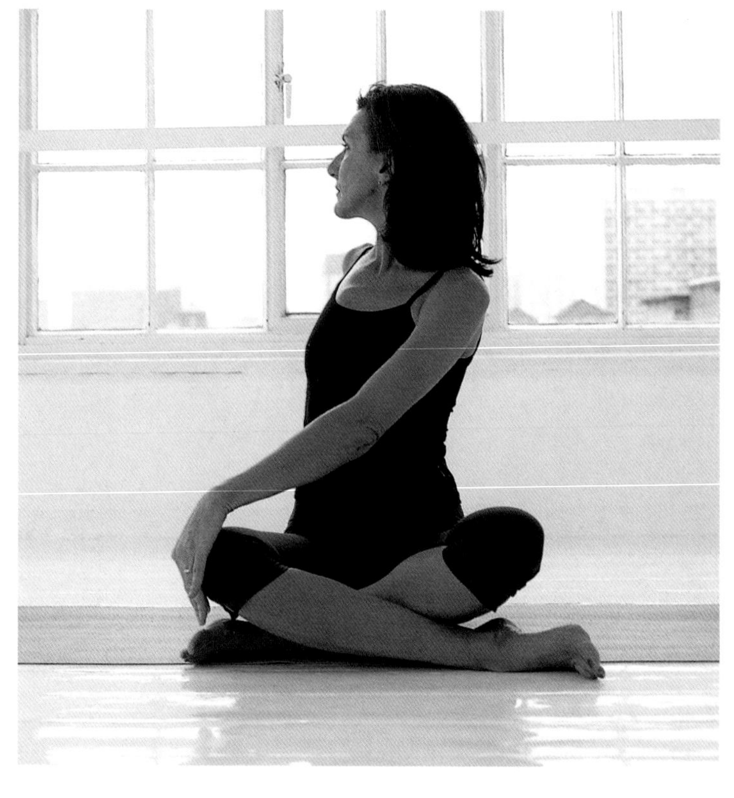

1 Sit in step 1 of Sukhasana, with the fingertips on the floor.

2 Place the palm of the left hand on the outer right thigh. Inhale, press the right fingertips into the floor and extend the spine upwards. Exhale, press the left palm into the thigh and turn towards the right.

3 Look over the right shoulder. Hold for 30–40 seconds, release and repeat to the other side, changing the cross of the legs.

Virasana (twist) | HERO POSE TWIST

This pose strengthens the abdominal muscles and relieves indigestion. Lower backache is eased, the hips become more flexible and the hamstring muscles more supple.

★

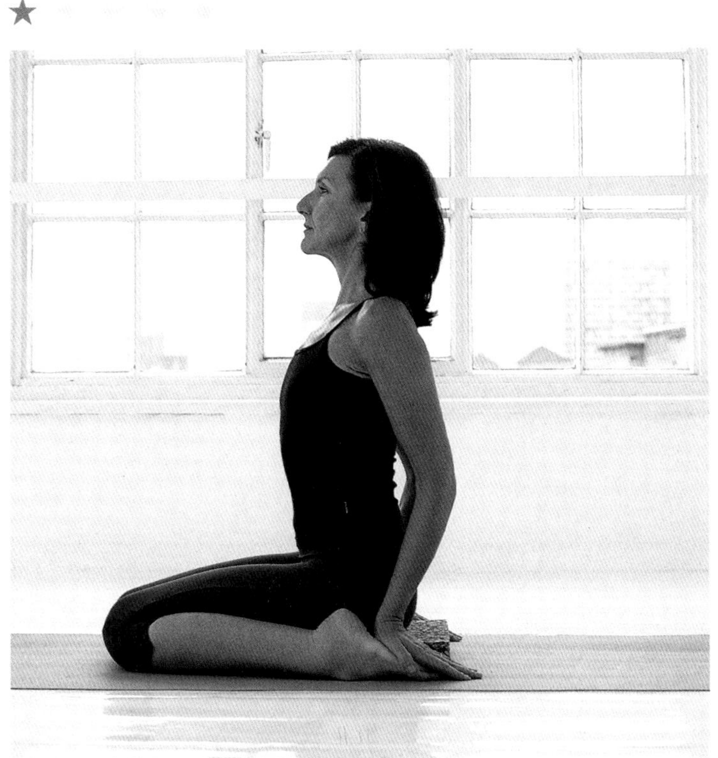

1 Sit in Virasana with the soles of the feet facing the ceiling, and the palms on the feet.

Sit on a foam block or folded blanket if this helps.

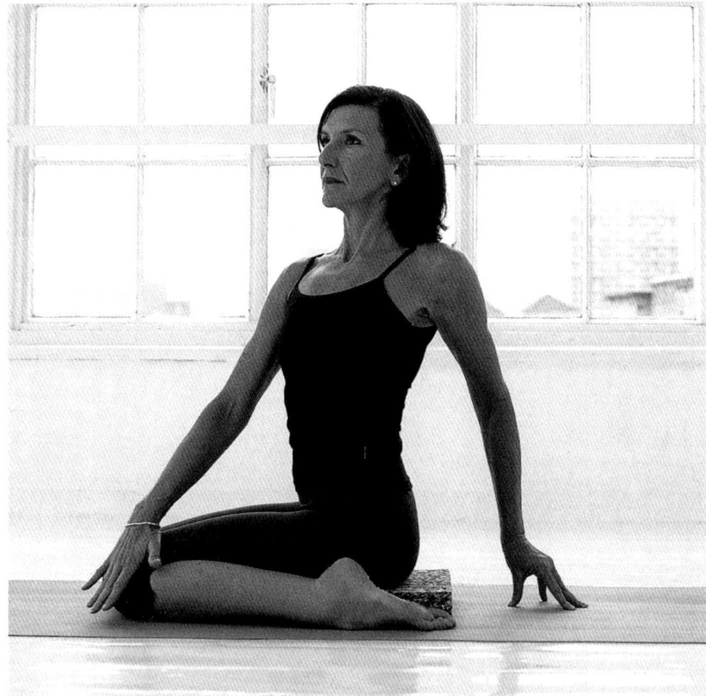

2 Put the left fingertips on the floor/block beside the left hip, and put the right palm on the left thigh.

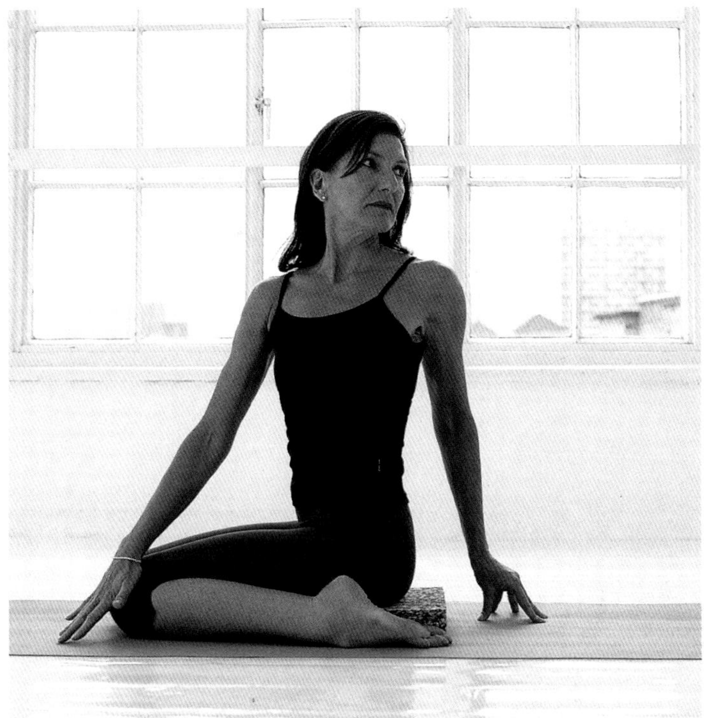

3 Inhale, press the left fingers into the floor and lift the trunk. Exhale, press the right palm into the left thigh and turn to the left. With each exhalation, turn the abdomen, waist, chest and shoulders further to the left and look over the left shoulder.

Hold for 30–60 seconds, release and repeat on the other side.

Focus

- Keep the shoulders relaxed, moving them down, away from the ears and into the body.
- Try to turn a little more with each exhalation.
- Use the breath to lift and turn.

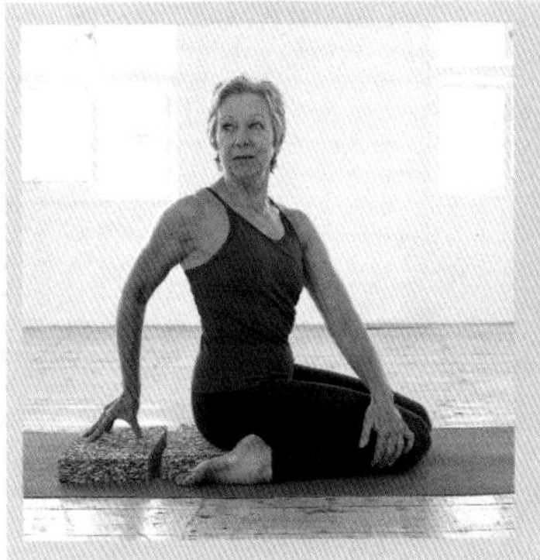

Modification

- Sit on a wooden or foam block and use another block to place the fingertips on, behind the body.
- As with all directional poses, start with the right side and repeat on the left.

Bharadvajasana (chair) | SIMPLE TWIST USING A CHAIR

This twist is an easier version of Bharadvajasana I. The chair is used to allow a safe and effective rotation of the trunk. It makes the muscles of the spine supple, relieves stiff neck and shoulders, improves digestion and exercises the abdominal muscles.

★

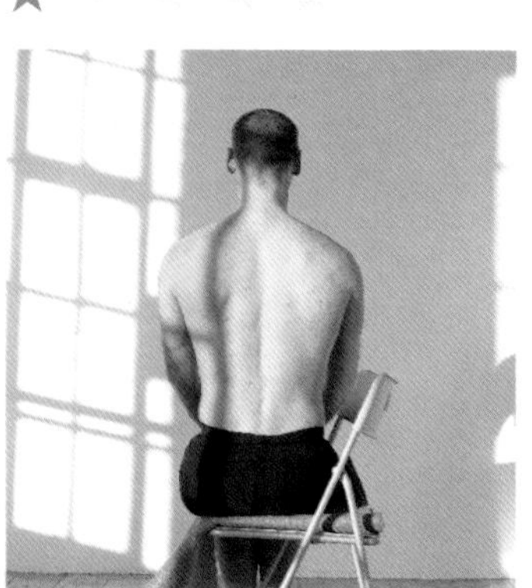

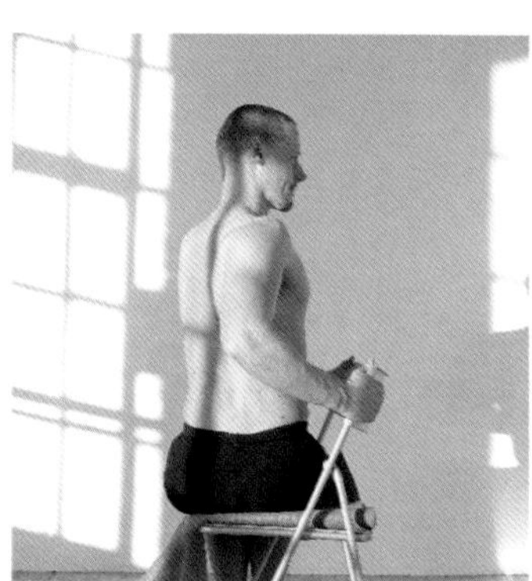

1 Sit on a chair with the right side of the body facing the chair-back. Keep the knees and feet together. Sit up straight and look straight ahead.

2 Inhale, extend the spine up and put the hands on the back of the chair.

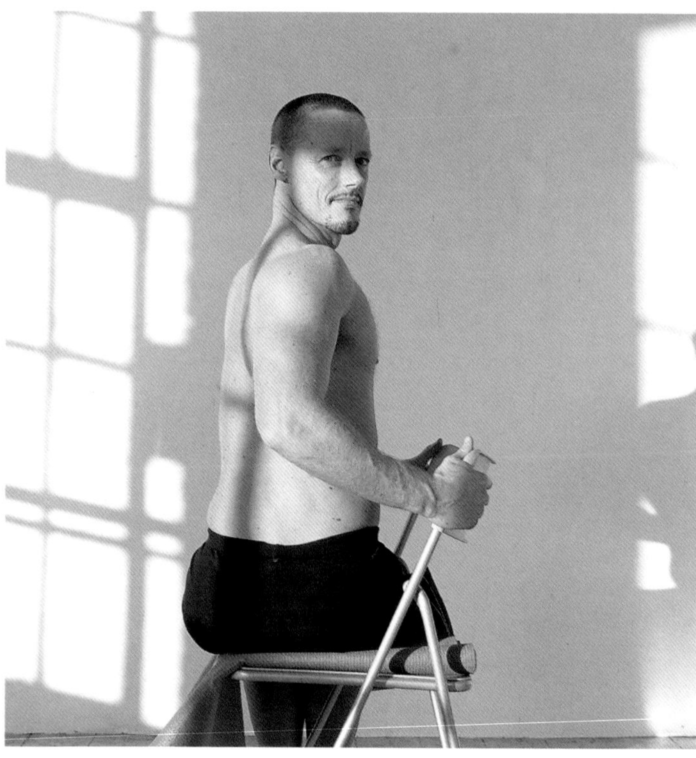

3 Exhale, and turn the trunk to the right, using the hands to help you turn.

Inhale, lift the spine further, take the shoulder blades into the body and open the chest. Rotate the spine further so that the chest is parallel to the back of the chair. Keep the neck free from tension or strain.

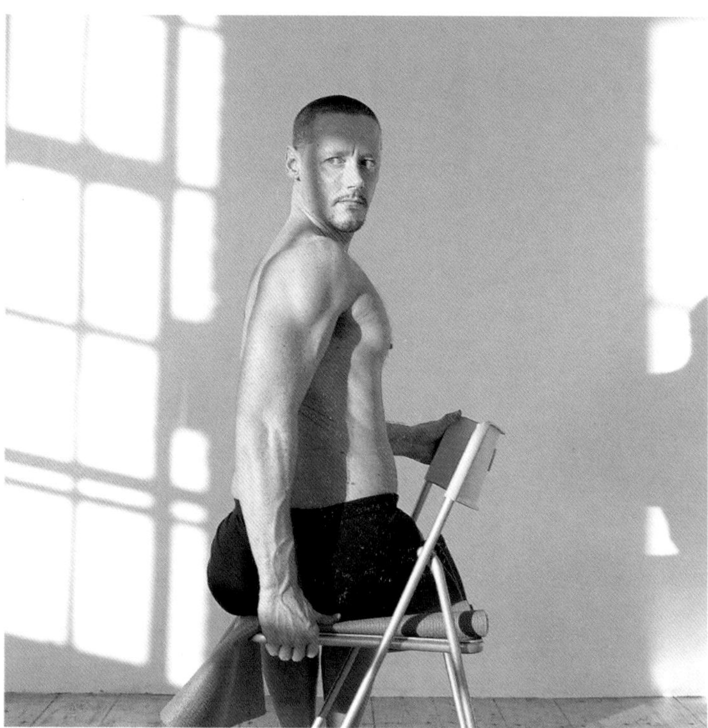

4 Exhale, turn the trunk more and look over the right shoulder. Grip the back of the chair for leverage. Hold for 20–30 seconds, exhale, release the hands, face forwards and repeat on the other side.

Focus

- Press the feet firmly into the floor to lift the trunk.
- Press the left buttock down towards the seat of the chair – it wants to lift. Use the inhalation to extend the spine; use the exhalation to turn it.

Modification

- This twist can be made easier by raising the feet, or by placing a block between the knees.

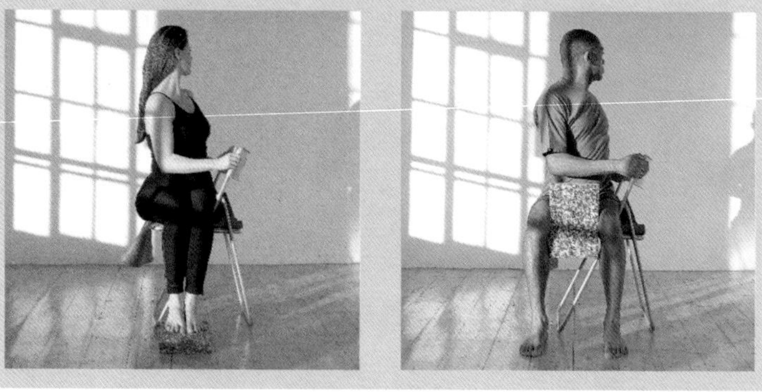

Bharadvajasana I | SIMPLE TWIST

This twisting posture creates flexibility in the neck and shoulders and relieves lower back pain. It reduces pain in the knees and tones and massages the abdominal organs, particularly the kidneys, liver, spleen and gall bladder.

★ ★

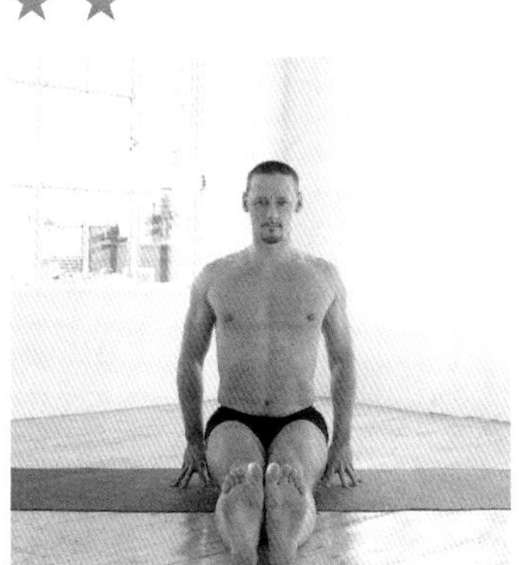

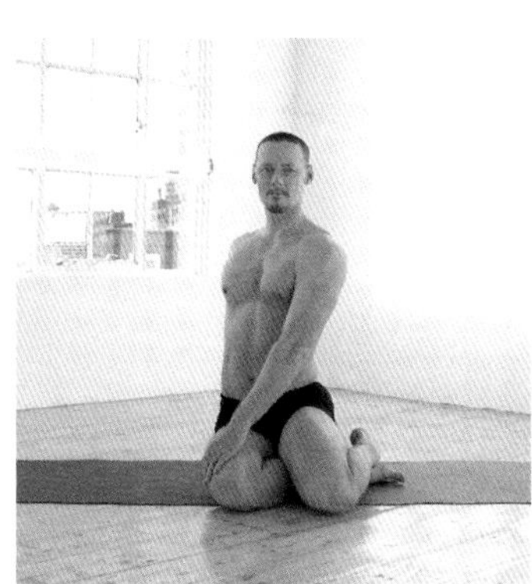

1 Sit in Dandasana on a support.

2 Bend both legs to the left, placing the feet beside the left hip. Put the left foot on top of the arch of the right foot.

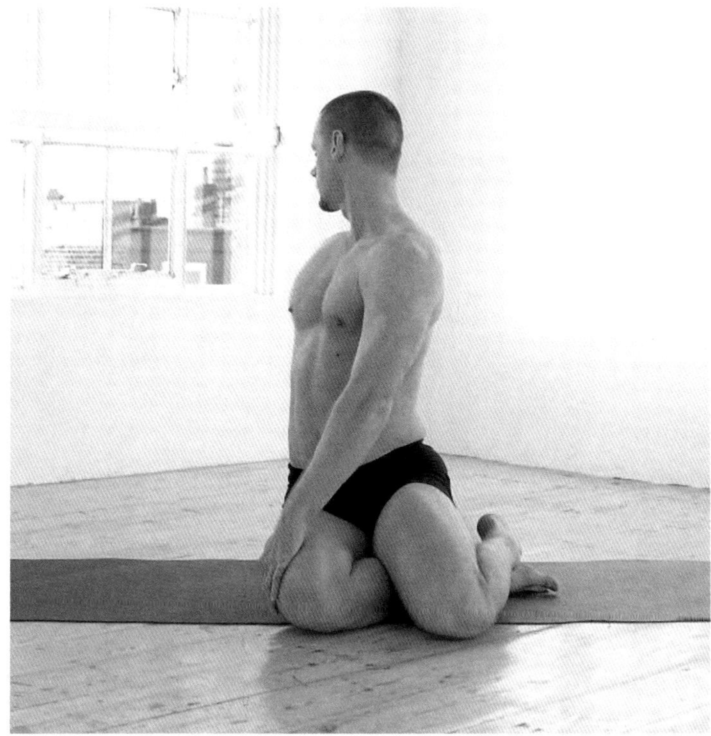

3 Keep the soles of both feet facing the ceiling.

Extend the trunk and spine up. Put the right fingertips beside the right hip and the palm of the left hand on the right knee.

Inhale, press the right fingers into the floor to lift the spine.

Exhale, press the left palm against the right knee to turn the trunk to the right.

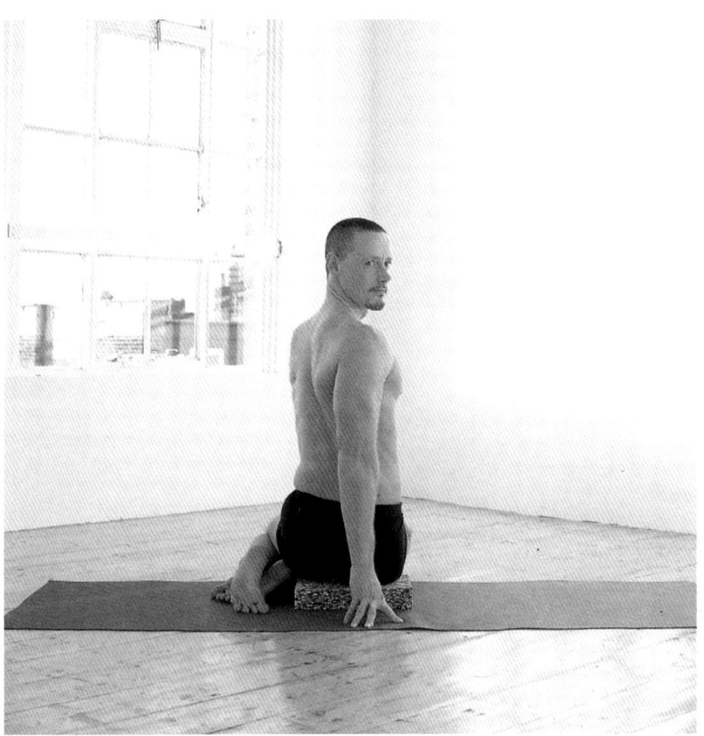

4 Repeat, turning the abdomen, waist, chest and shoulders further with each exhalation.

Look over the right shoulder, hold for 30–40 seconds, exhale, release and repeat on the other side.

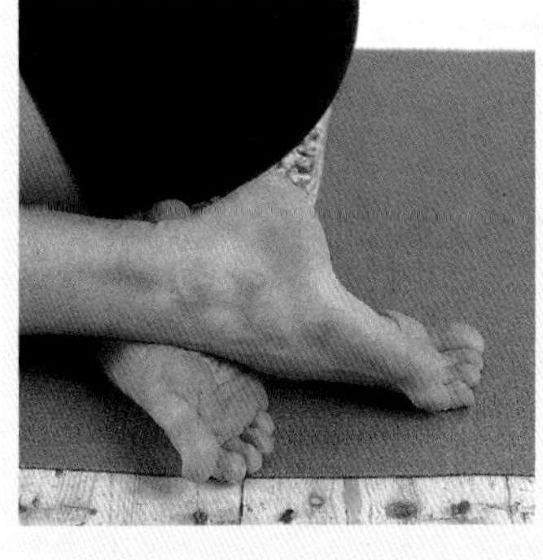

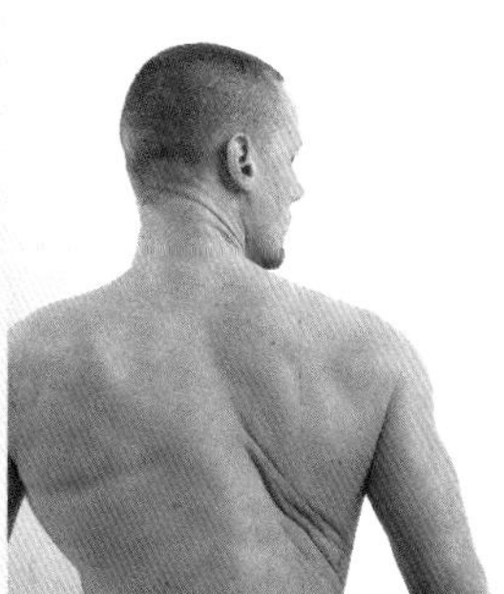

Focus

- Rest the left foot over the instep of the right foot.
- Press the left buttock down towards the floor to get the whole spine turning.
- Use the breath to lift and turn.
- Draw the shoulder blades down and into the body to lift the spine and open the chest.

Maricyasana I (twist only) | CATCHING ARMS BEHIND

This spinal twist removes stiffness in the shoulders and spine and reduces lower backache. As there is an increased blood flow to the abdominal organs, digestion improves and the organs become toned.

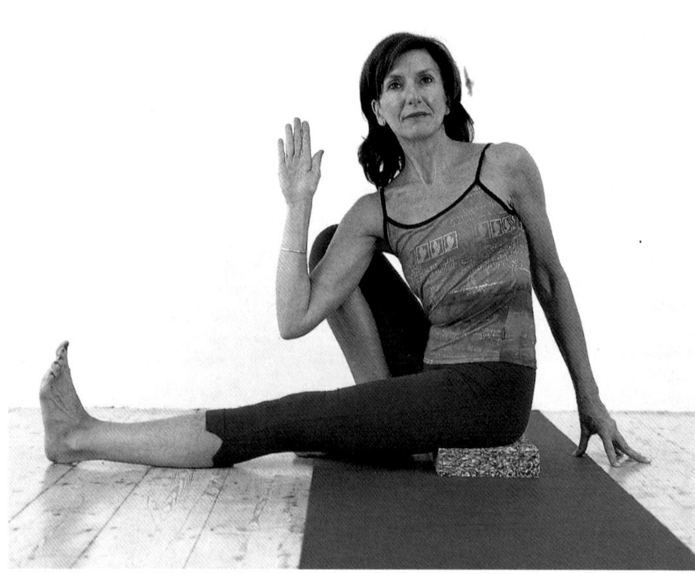

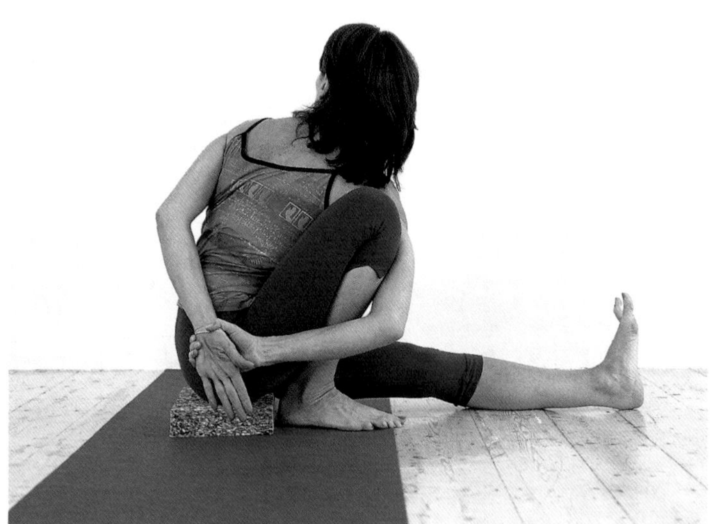

1 Sit in Dandasana on a support. Keep the fingertips pressing into the floor beside the hips. Bend the right leg so that the knee faces the ceiling and the right heel is in line with the right buttock bone, toes pointing forwards.

Extend the left leg along the floor. Turn the trunk to the left and take the right elbow in front of the right knee (fingers pointing to the ceiling). Rotate the trunk more to the left.

Modification

- To ease your body into this posture, use a block under the floor hand and a lift to sit on.
- If you cannot reach your hands behind your back, use a strap. Fold the strap in two and grasp it firmly behind you, pulling the arms around.

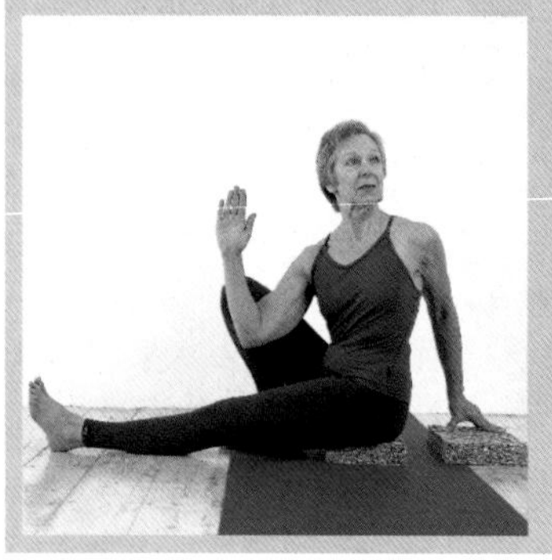

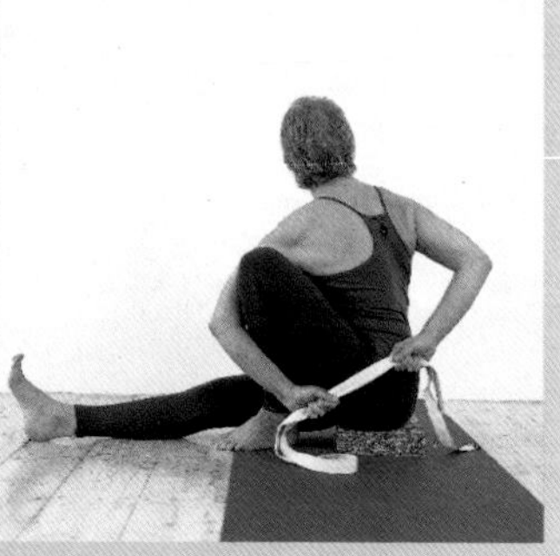

2 Press the left fingertips into the floor to lengthen the spine. Wrap the right arm around the right leg and take it behind the body.

Turn the left shoulder slightly back and swing the left arm behind the back, catching hold of it with the right hand. If the hands don't reach, use a strap.

Turn the trunk as far as possible to the left, turn the head and look over the left shoulder. Move the back ribs and shoulder blades into the body to open the chest, and turn more. Extend the front of the body from the pubis to the chin. Hold for 20–30 seconds, then release and repeat on the other side.

Focus

- Keep the knee of the bent leg facing the ceiling throughout, and the heel close to the body.
- Press the sole of the right foot into the floor to lift the spine as much as possible.
- Move the shoulder blades into the body and down towards the floor to extend and rotate the spine more.
- The full posture, and Maricyasana II, combine a twist with a forward bend suitable for advanced yogis only.

Maricyasana III | SITTING TWIST

This stronger twist increases energy levels. As there is a vigorous rotation, the abdominal organs, such as liver, spleen, pancreas, kidneys and intestines are toned and massaged, improving their performance and function.

★ ★ ★

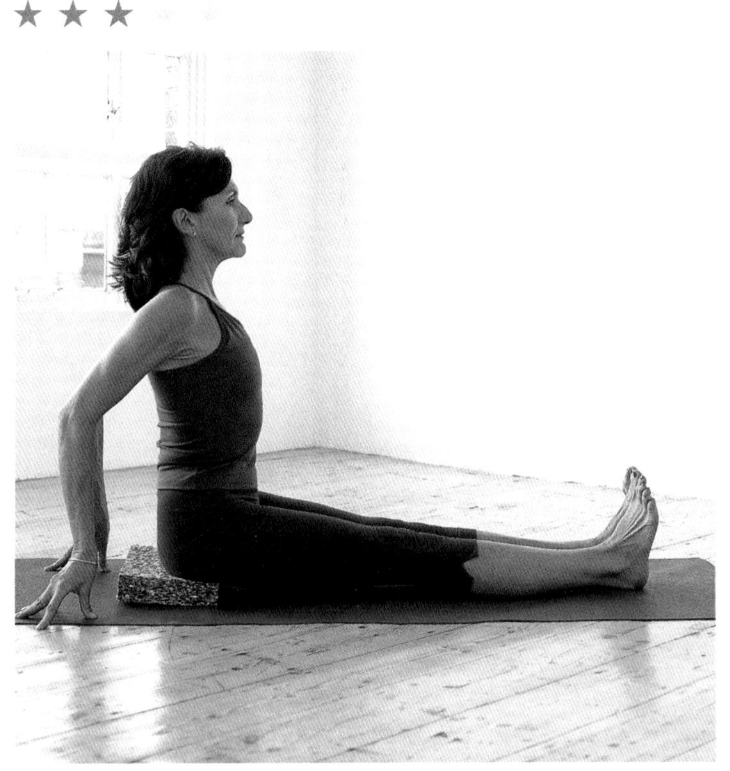

1 Sit in Dandasana on a support. Lift the spine upwards.

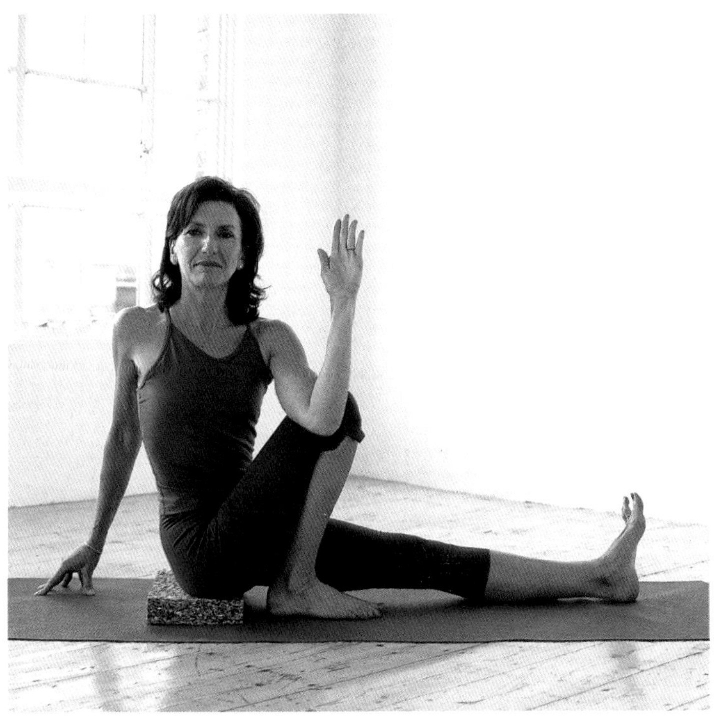

2 Bend the right knee up towards the ceiling, and put the sole of the foot on the floor in line with the right buttock bone. Turn to the right. Put the fingertips of the right hand on the floor/block behind the right hip. Bend the left arm and place the elbow on the outside of the right knee.

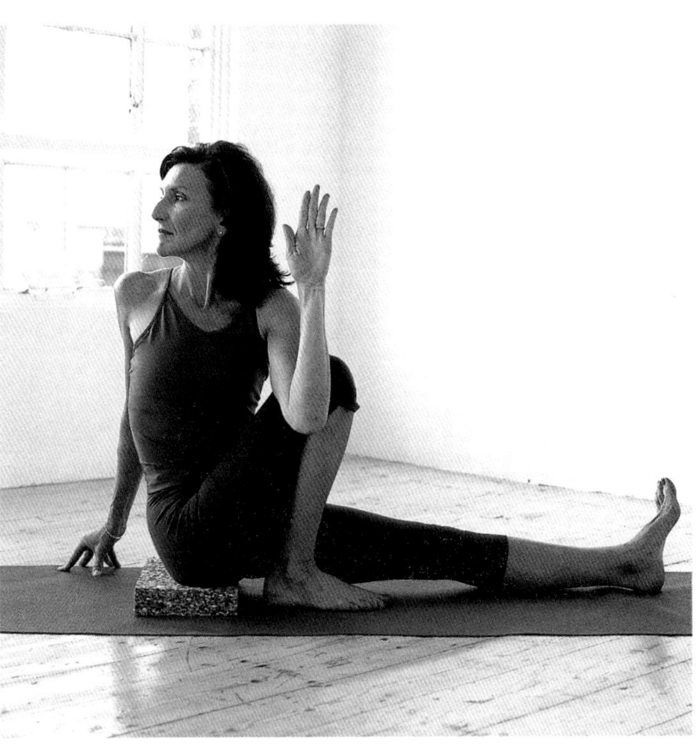

3 Try to get the left armpit closer to the knee. Inhale, press the right fingers into the floor and lift the spine.

Exhale, press the left arm against the knee and the knee against the arm, and turn further to the right.

Repeat the lift and turn. Move the spine into the body, take the shoulder blades into the back and turn further. Look over the right shoulder. Rotate the left side of the ribcage, the left armpit and the left hip towards the right to increase the turn of the spine. Keep the chest lifted and open by moving the shoulders down and the shoulder blades forwards.

Hold for 30–60 seconds, release and repeat on the other side.

Focus

- Press the right foot firmly into the floor, especially the big toes and inner heel, and press the back of the left leg into the floor and stretch it forwards, toes facing up.
- Use the breath to lift and turn.
- Ensure that the bent knee stays facing the ceiling – when placing the bent arm over the knee, don't push it out of alignment.

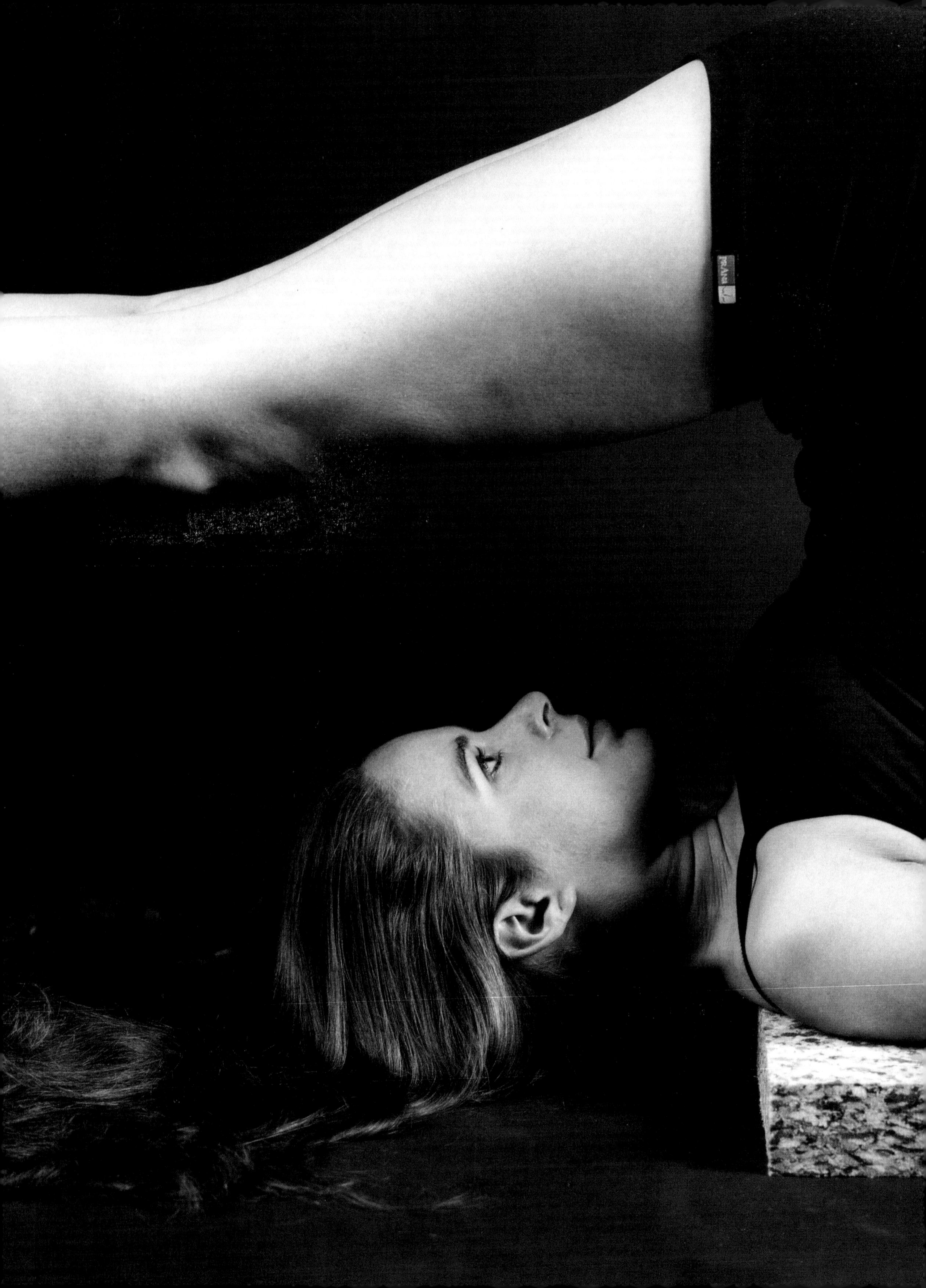

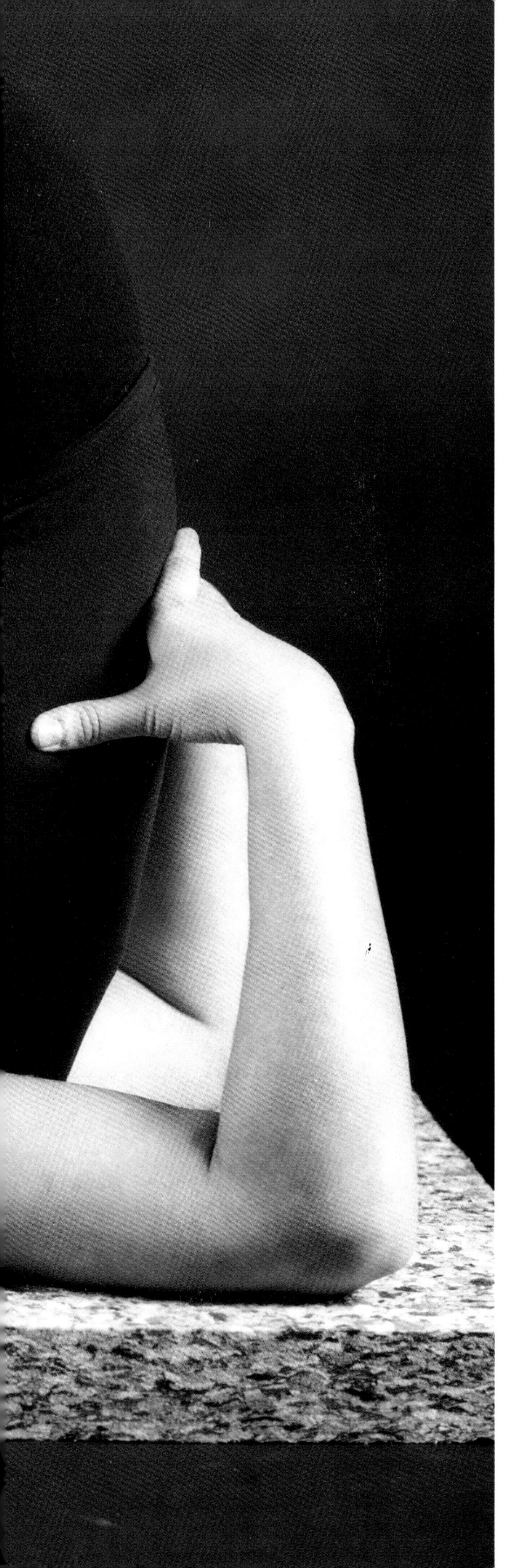

Inverted Asanas

All inverted postures revitalize the entire body system. Because the internal organs are inverted, they become energized, and the brain becomes nourished as the blood flows towards it. Since there is no weight on the legs, inversions bring relief to tired, strained legs. No inversions should be practised during menstruation as this interferes with the natural flow of blood at this time.

Viparita Karani | LEGS UP THE WALL POSE

This restorative pose calms the brain, opens the chest and rests the legs. It helps reduce respiratory problems, eases headaches and relieves indigestion and nausea. It is also beneficial for preventing varicose veins.

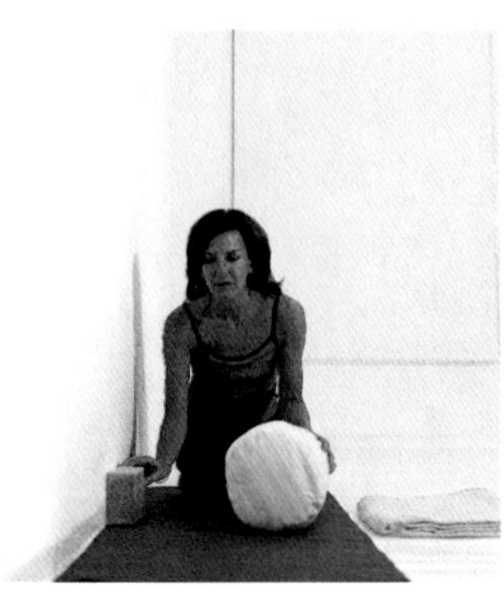

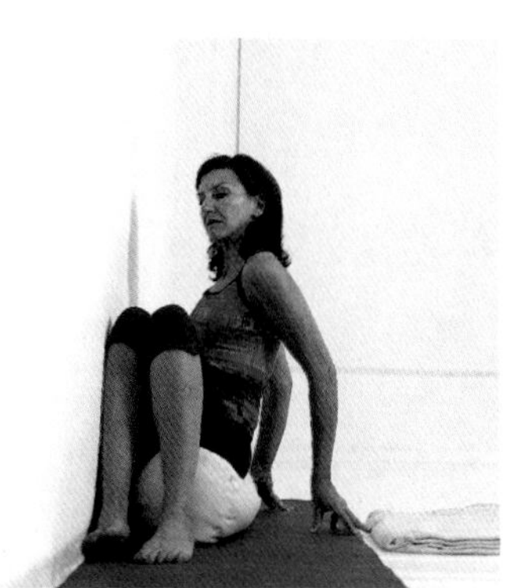

1 Put a wooden block against the wall with a bolster in front and a folded blanket in front of the bolster.

2 Sit on the bolster, sideways to the wall with the hip touching the wall.

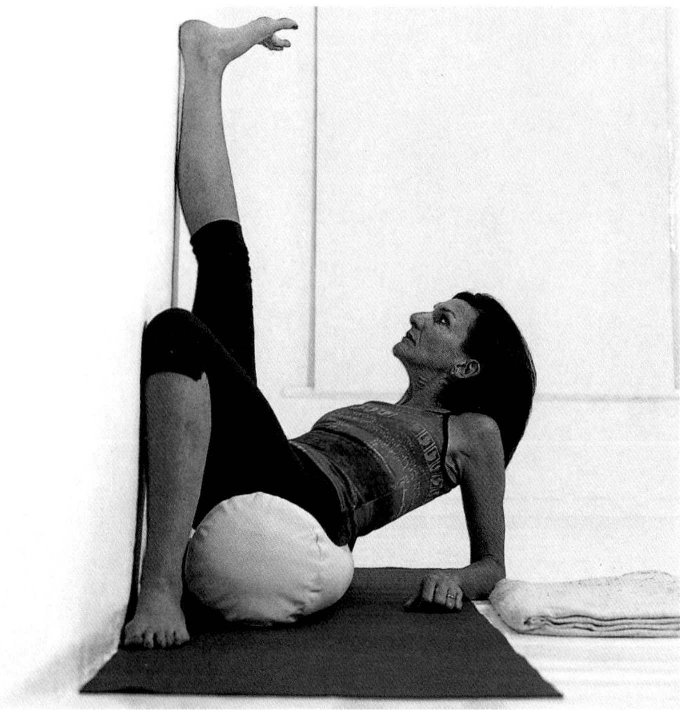

3 Swivel the trunk around, using the hands to balance. Take one leg up the wall, keep the buttocks against the wall and straighten the second leg.

Focus

• Keep the inner edges of the feet together so that the soles of the feet are parallel to the ceiling.

•Keep the abdomen soft and press the shoulders into the floor.

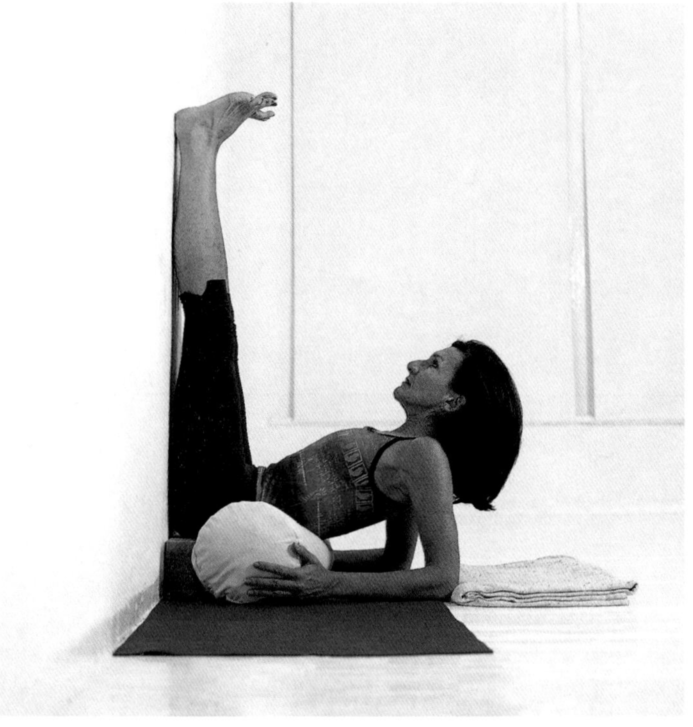

4 Once both legs are up the wall, carefully take the trunk down and lower the shoulders and head on to the floor. Keep the backs of the legs and buttocks against the wall and open the chest.

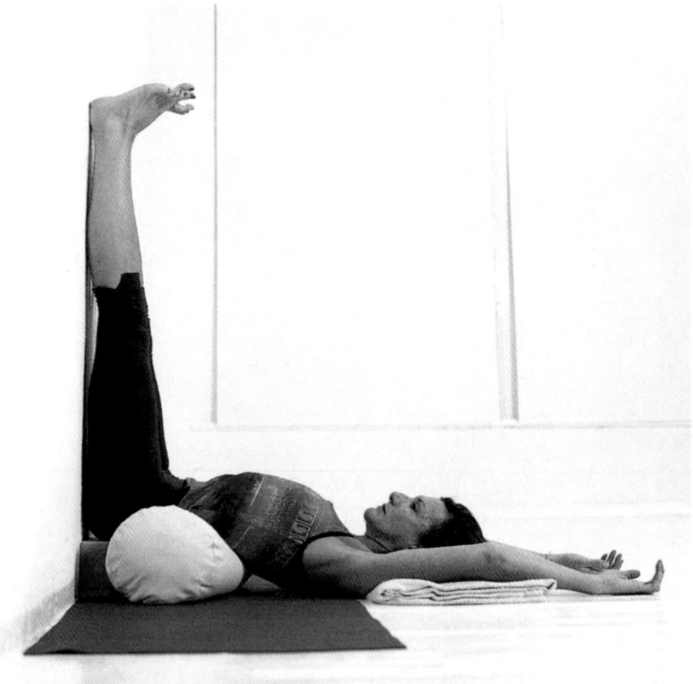

5 Take the arms over the head, breathe evenly and relax. Hold for 5–6 minutes and then come down.

Salamba Sarvangasana | SUPPORTED SHOULDER STAND

This is known as the queen, or mother, of the postures. It soothes and nourishes the internal organs, helps the thyroid gland to function properly and frees the body of toxins. It is beneficial for relieving respiratory problems such as asthma, congestion and sinusitis.

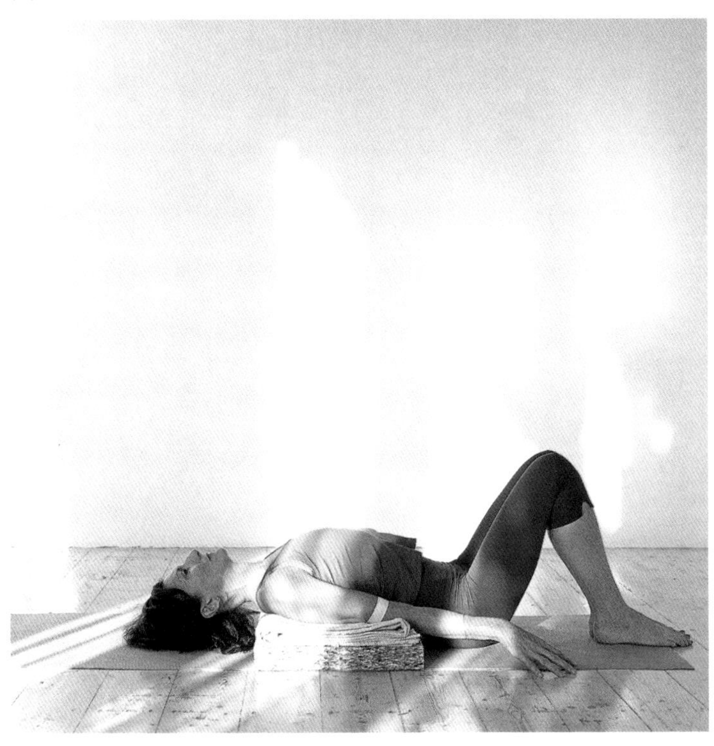

1 Place four small, or one large, foam block and a folded blanket on the mat for comfort. Lie with the shoulders and arms on the support and the head on the floor.

Stretch the arms towards the feet and move the shoulders away from the head.

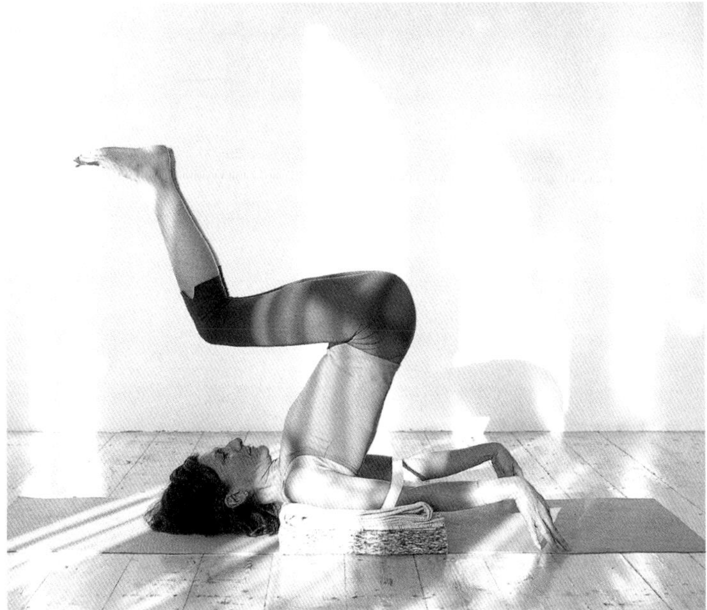

2 Bend the knees towards the chest. Press the fingertips into the floor, and take the knees towards the head.

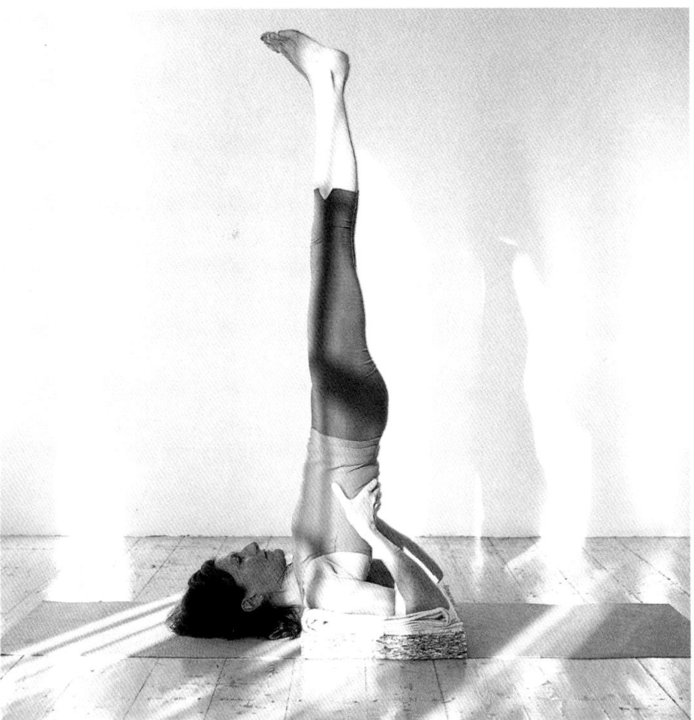

3 Lift the hips and trunk and immediately support the back with the palms of both hands. Straighten the legs and move the hands up the back towards the shoulder blades to increase the lift of the chest. Bring the chest towards the chin and stretch the whole body straight up. Look towards the chest. Hold for 2–5 minutes.

Focus

- Press the hands into the back to move the back ribs towards the front of the chest and to lift the trunk. Press the upper arms into the support.
- If the elbows slip apart, tie a belt around the upper arms (just above the elbows) to keep them shoulder-width.
- Stretch the legs up and keep the soles of the feet parallel to the ceiling – rest the toes on a wall for balance.

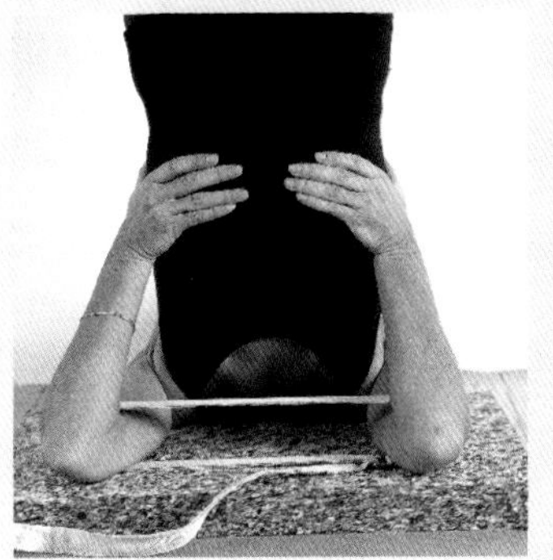

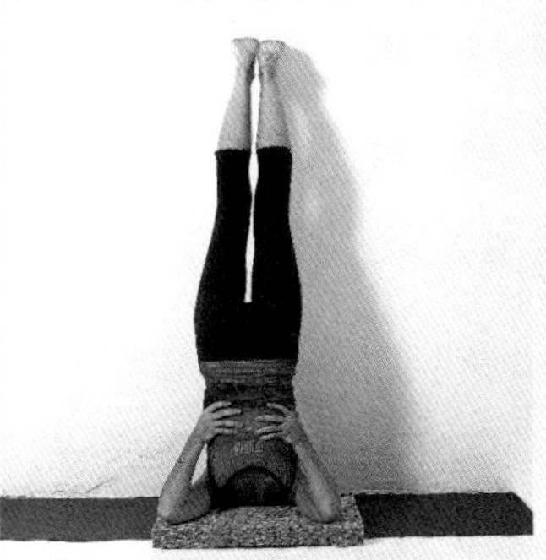

Salamba Sarvangasana (against wall) | SUPPORTED SHOULDER STAND

This is an easier version of the shoulder stand. If pressure is experienced in the head while in Salamba Sarvangasana, come down immediately and try the pose against the wall or using a chair.

★★

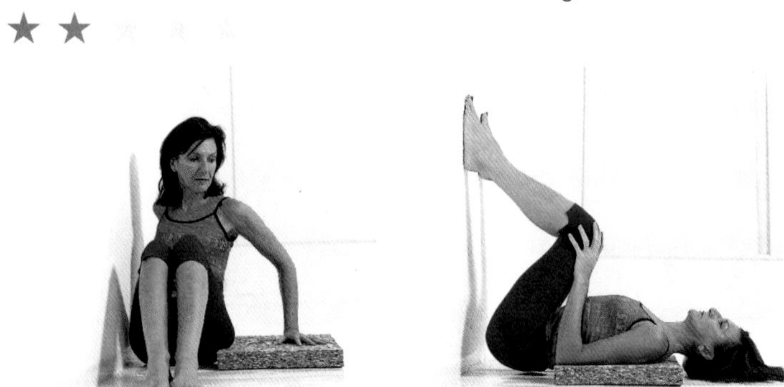

1 Sit as close as possible to the wall and place a foam block just under your left buttock.

2 Lean back, swivel the trunk around and take one leg, and then the second, up the wall. Keep the buttocks against the wall, the shoulders near the edge of the support and the head on the floor.

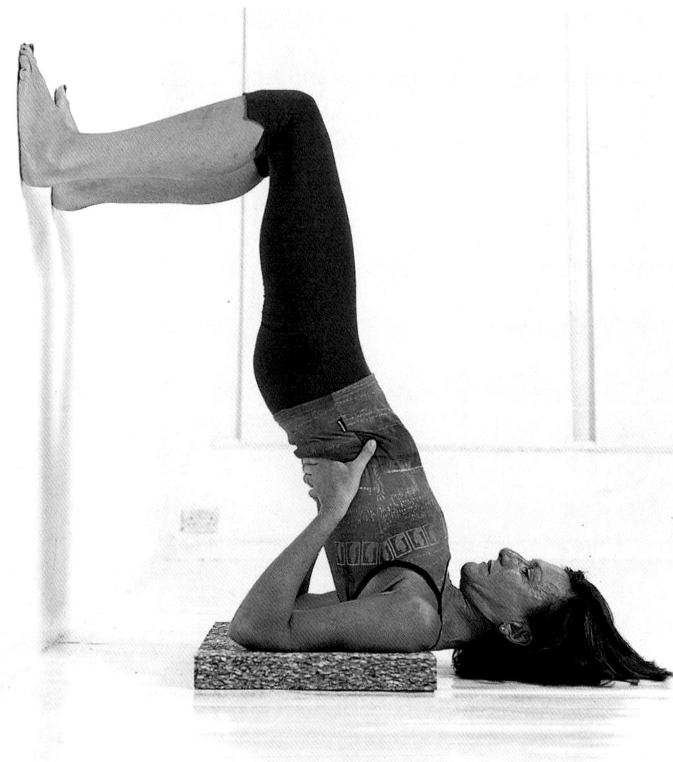

3 Press the feet into the wall and raise the hips and chest. Support the back with the hands and move the elbows towards one another.

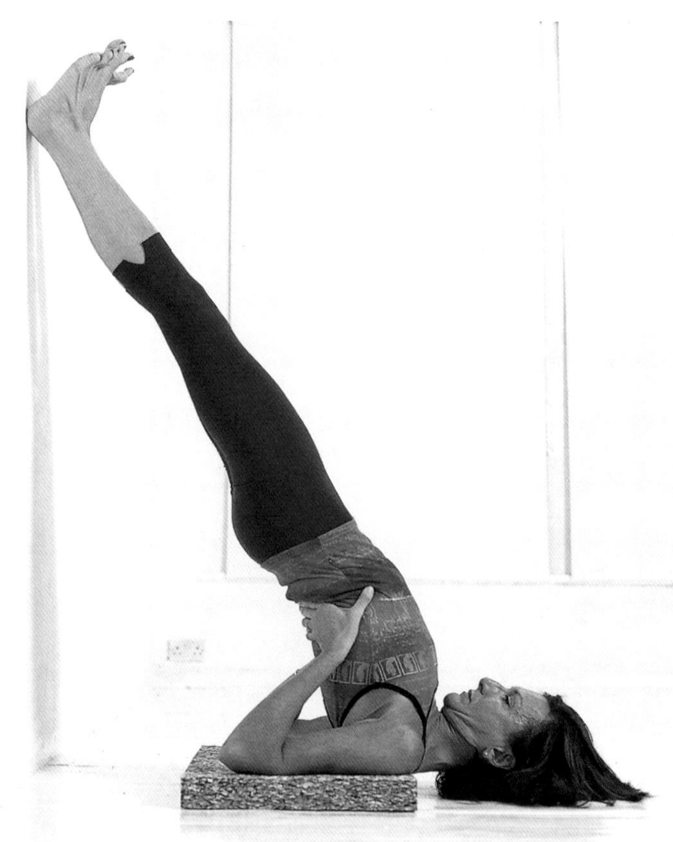

4 Straighten the legs, press the heels firmly into the wall and lift the chest, trunk and hips. Hold for 2–5 minutes, bend the legs and come down.

Modification

- If you cannot manage Salamba Sarvangasana alone or against a wall, get someone to assist you by holding your legs upright. Begin by resting your feet on their thighs, then allow them to correct your alignment.
- Once you have done the posture with help, you may find it easier to achieve on your own.

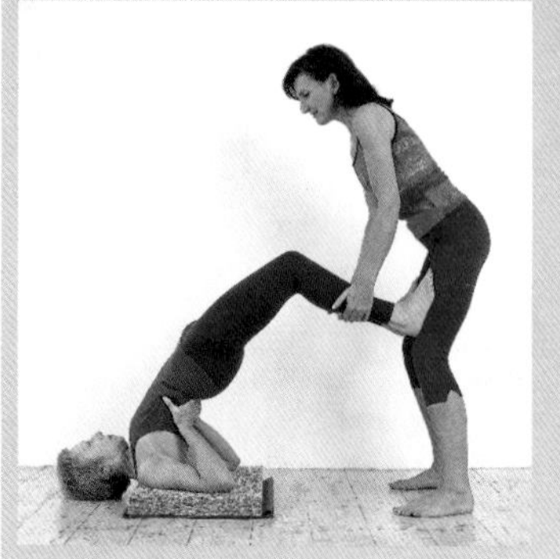

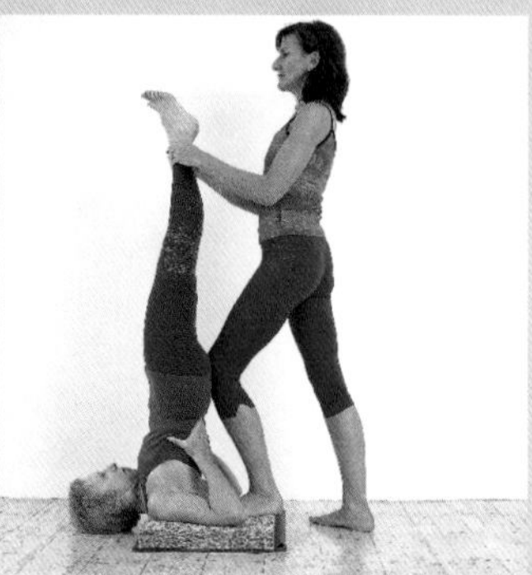

Chair Sarvangasana | SHOULDER BALANCE IN CHAIR

In the classic Salamba Sarvangasana posture, the hands support the back. In this modified version, a chair is used and this allows the pose to be held for longer with minimal strain on the neck and back.

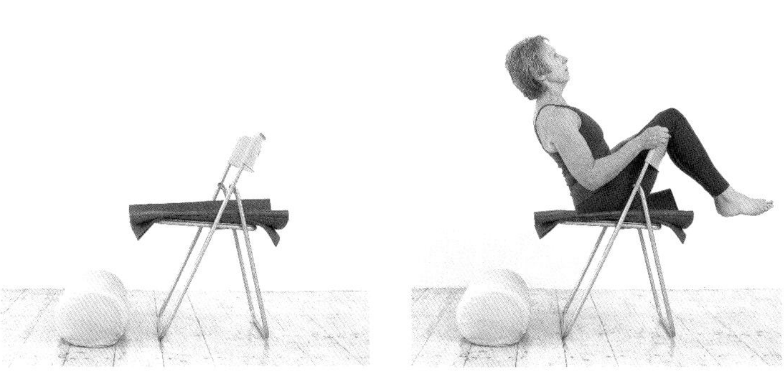

1 Place a bolster on the floor parallel to the front legs of the chair. Fold a mat and put it on the seat of the chair.

2 Sit on the chair and bend the legs over the back of the chair. Hold on to the sides of the chair. Lean the trunk slightly back.

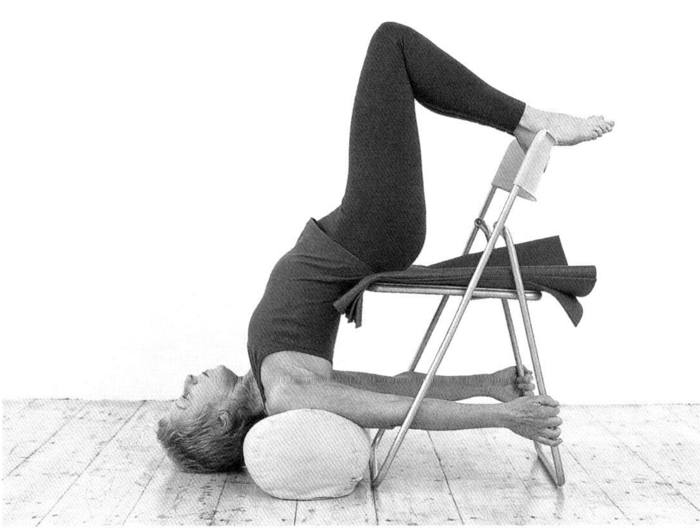

3 Lower the back on to the seat of the chair. Slide the buttocks and back towards the front edge of the chair seat. Carefully rest the shoulders on the bolster and the back of the head on the floor. Hold the back chair legs.

Focus

- As with other inversions, Chair Sarvangasana should not be practised during menstruation.

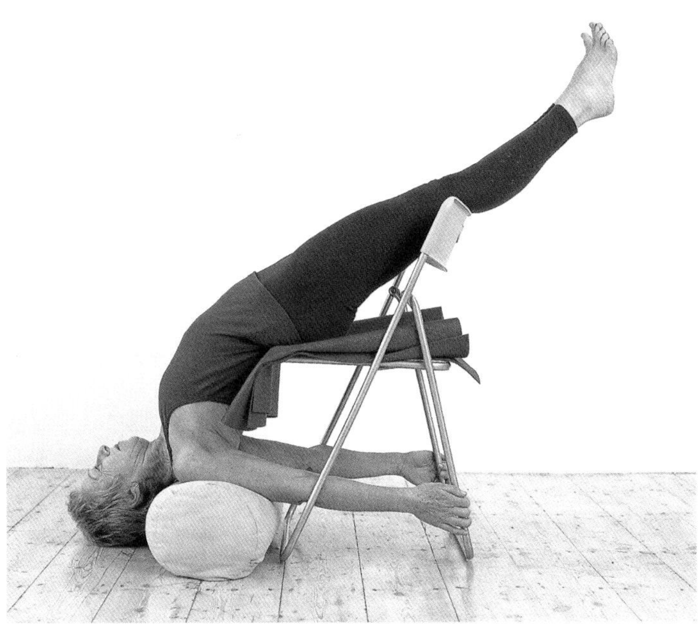

4 Straighten one leg at a time. When both legs are straight, slide the hands further down the back chair legs to increase the stretch of the arms. Move the shoulders away from the ears and the shoulder blades towards the head to open and lift the chest.

Breathe normally and look towards the chest. Hold the pose for up to 5 minutes, keeping the back of the neck soft.

Coming out of the posture

- Return first one leg, then the other, to step 3. Begin to release the grip of the hands on the chair legs and gently push the chair slightly away.
- Slide the back then buttocks on to the bolster, pushing the chair by the seat. Rest for a moment, roll over to the side, slide off the bolster and come up.

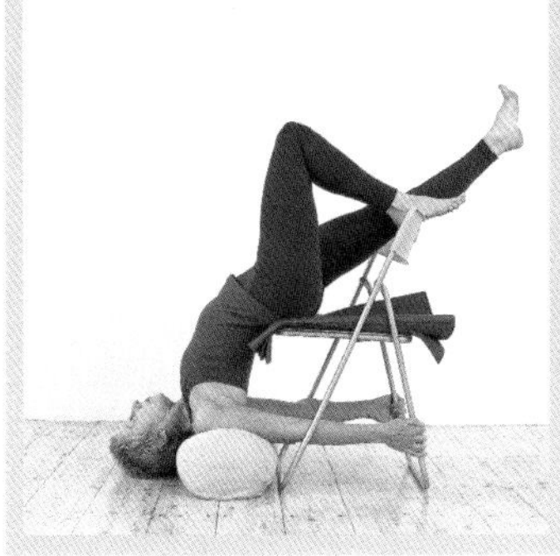

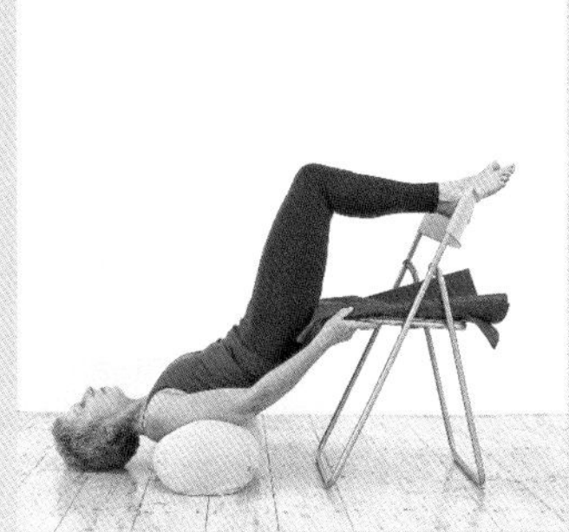

Ardha Halasana | HALF-PLOUGH POSE

This supported version of Halasana is a restorative pose. It reduces the effects of fatigue, anxiety and insomnia, and relieves stress-related headaches. If one has lower back pain, practising Ardha Halasana will not aggravate the condition.

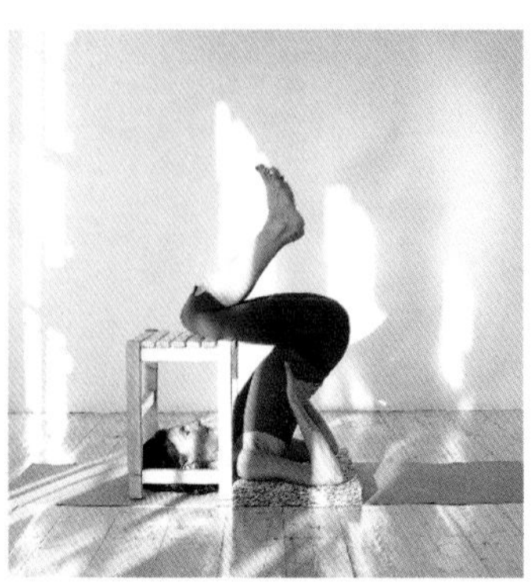

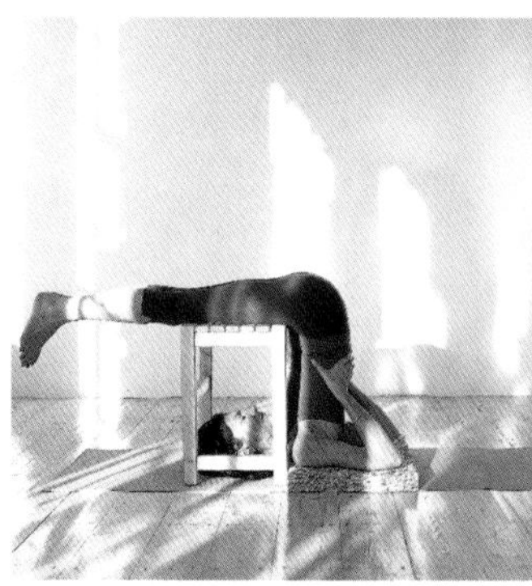

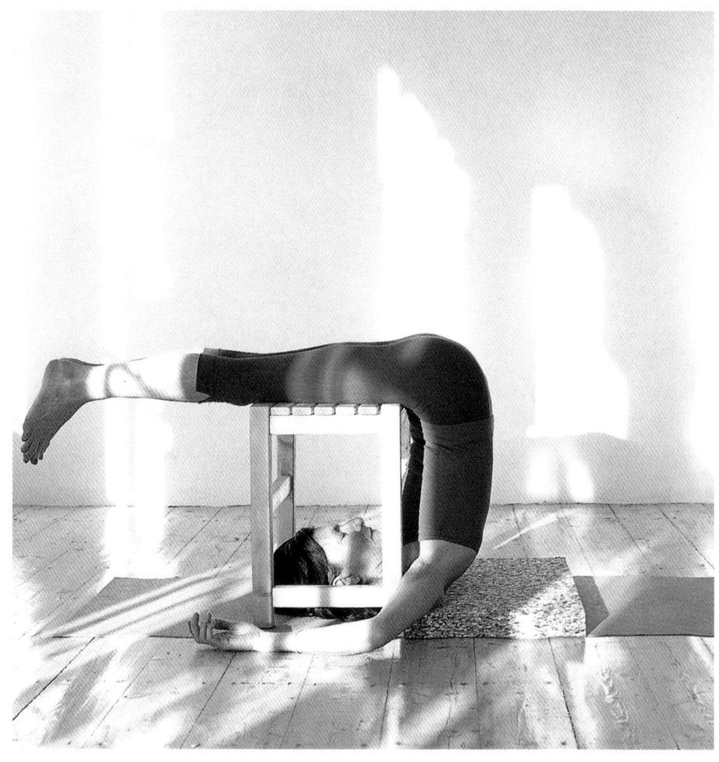

1 Place a chair/stool over the head before going into Salamba Sarvangasana. From this pose, take the legs down on to the stool to support the thighs.

2 Straighten the legs and support the spine with the hands.

3 Take the arms over the head and relax. Hold for 2–5 minutes, bend the knees, slide the thighs off the stool and come down.

Halasana | PLOUGH POSE

This inversion relaxes the brain. It is beneficial to practise it when one has a cold, and improves the functioning of the thyroid and parathyroid glands.

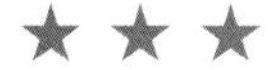

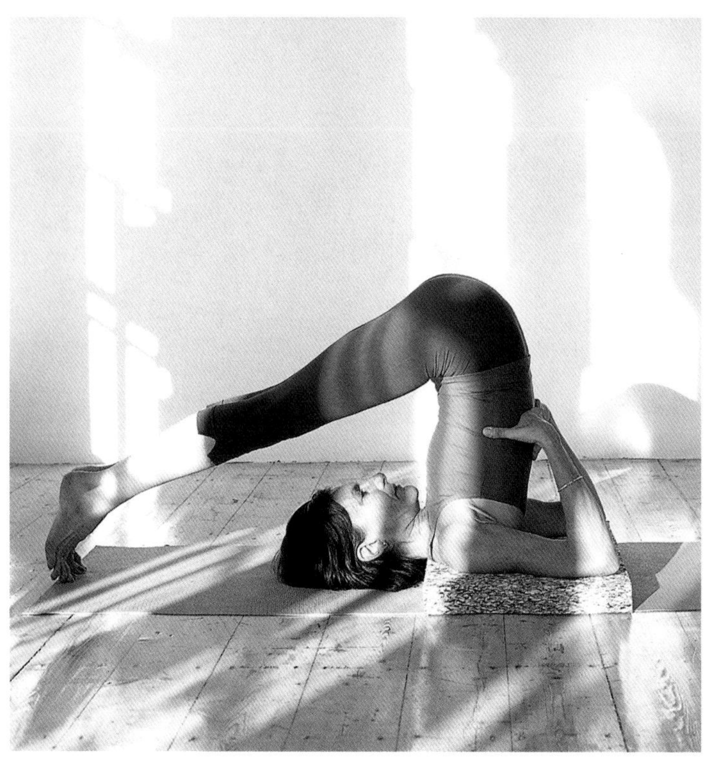

1 Go into Salamba Sarvangasana with the shoulders on a folded blanket or foam support. Take the legs down over the head to the floor and put the feet on the floor.

Keep supporting the back with the hands, lift the back and keep the chest open and lifted. Straighten the legs and extend them away from the hips.

Relax the eyes, hold for 2–5 minutes and come down.

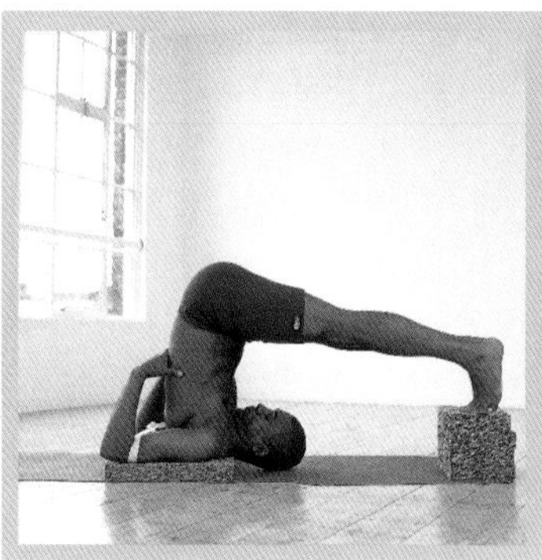

Modification

- If the back hurts, put a support under the toes.
- The tips of the toes press into the floor or bricks.
- Lift thigh bones towards the ceiling and stretch the heels away from the head.

Setu Bandha Sarvangasana (supported) | SHOULDER STAND BRIDGE POSE

This pose opens the chest and gives a mild extension to the spine. It calms the brain, reduces depression and relieves headaches. The abdominal muscles are stretched, digestion is improved and the internal organs are strengthened.

★ ★

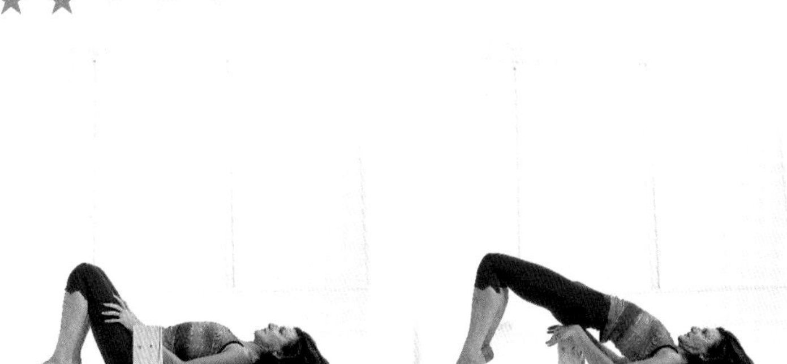

1 Lie on the floor with the knees bent and the toes pointing towards the wall.

2 Keeping the head, neck and shoulders on the floor, press the feet down and lift the hips from the floor. Put a wooden block vertically under the sacrum near the tailbone.

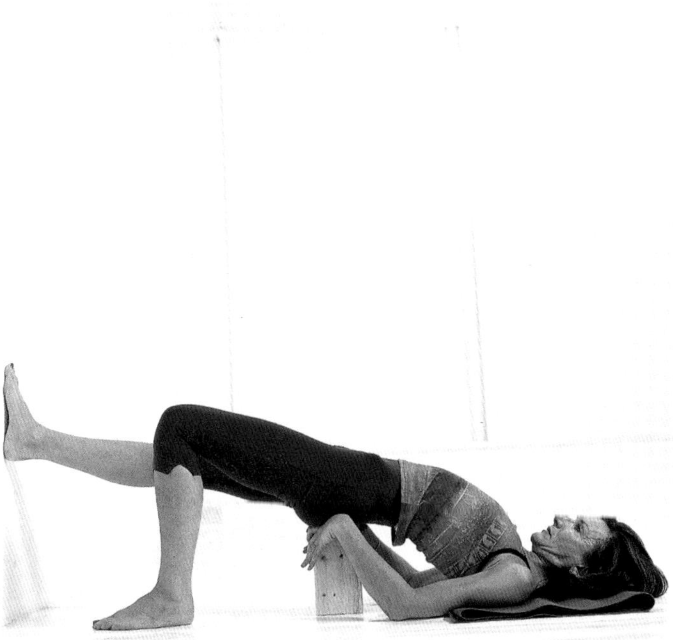

3 Straighten one leg at a time and place the feet on the wall at whatever height is comfortable for the lower back.

Focus

- Maintain a strong stretch on the back of the legs from the buttock bones to the heels.
- There should be no tension in the neck.
- Lift the breastbone towards the chin.

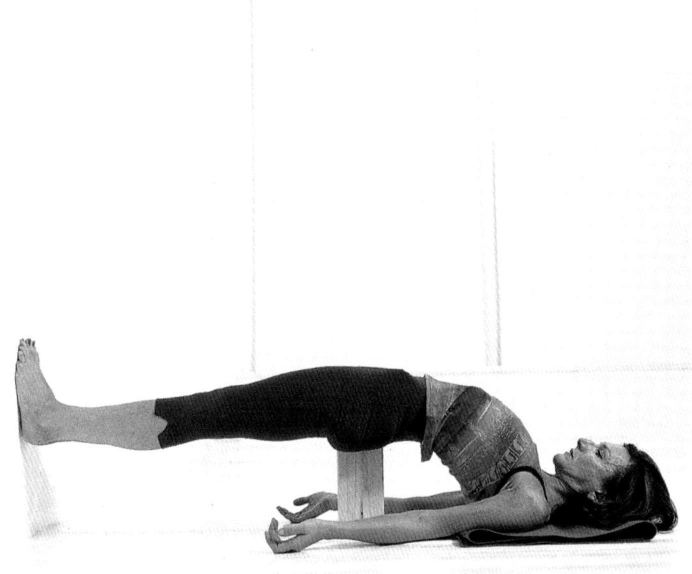

4 Open the chest, and extend the arms towards the feet, which are pressing firmly into the wall. Roll the tops of the shoulders towards the floor and move the shoulder blades towards the front of the body to open the chest.

Hold for 1–2 minutes, bend the legs, remove the block and come down.

Modification

- If the wooden block is uncomfortable on the sacrum (lower back), use four stacked foam blocks.
- If the lower back hurts, support the feet on wooden blocks or a bolster.

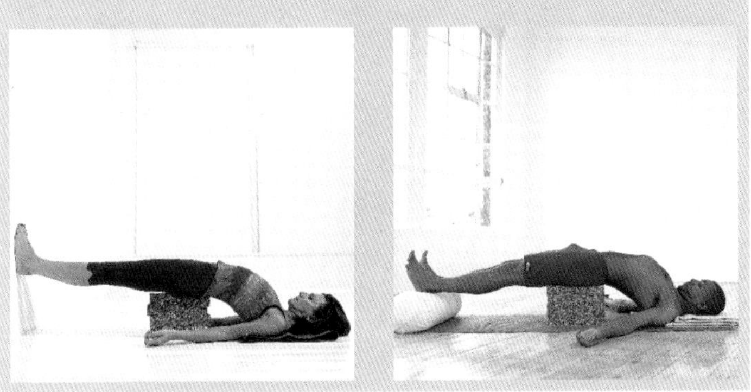

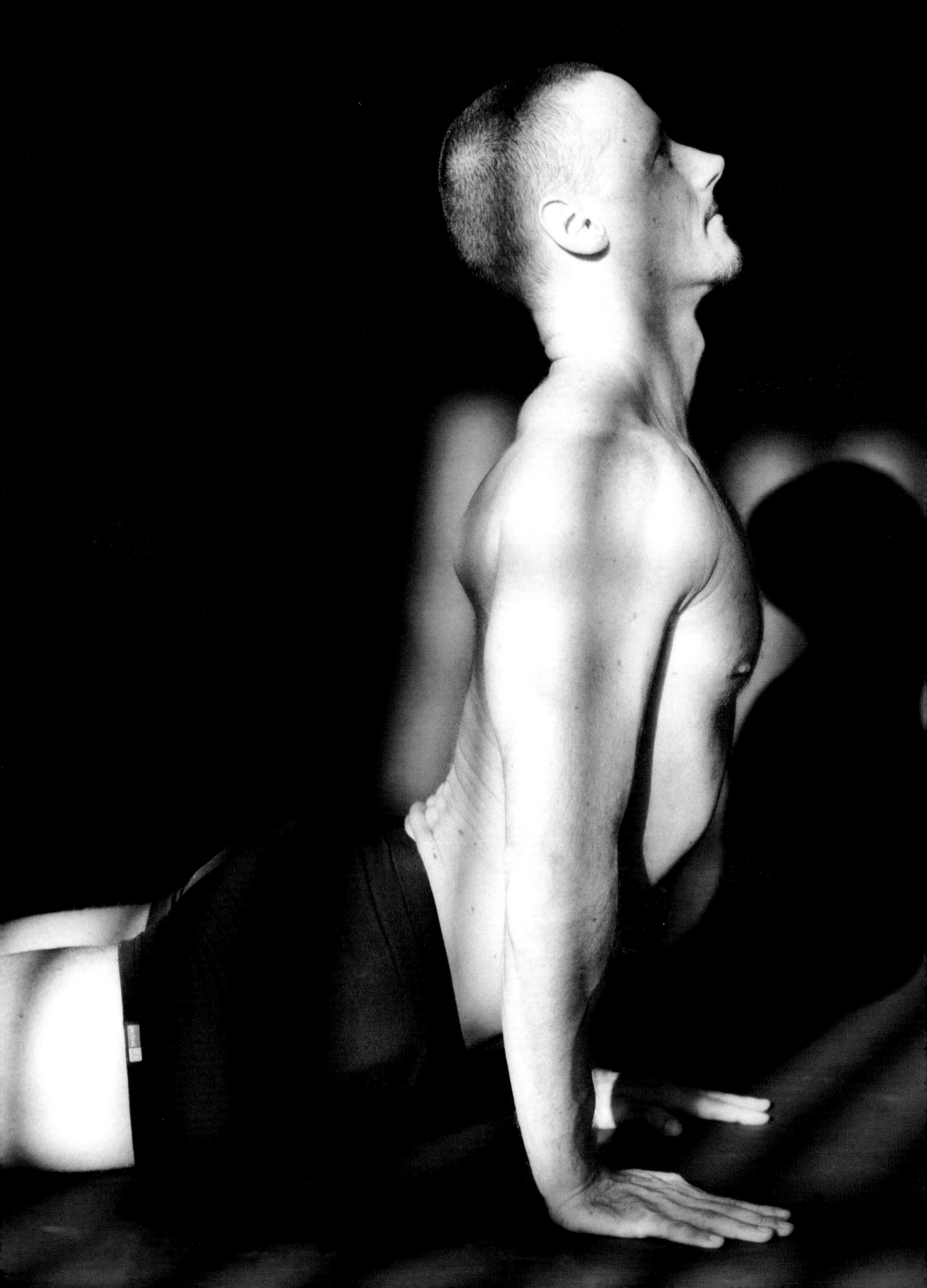

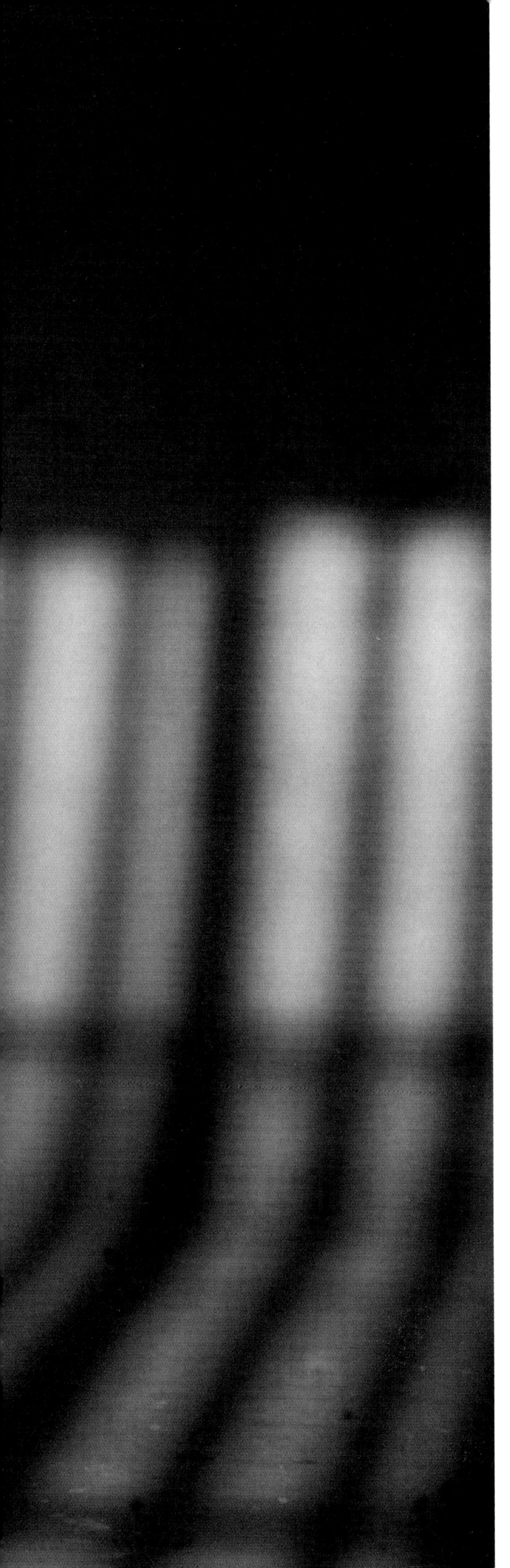

Supine and Prone Asanas

There are two types of supine/prone postures: some are restful and used for recuperation, while others strengthen the back, arms and legs. In all of them, the abdomen is stretched and the spine and hips gain flexibility.

Matsyasana (simple) | FISH POSE

Here the muscles of the spine and abdomen are fully stretched. Flexibility in the hips, knees and ankles develops and the chest lifts and opens, so the depth of the breath improves.

★

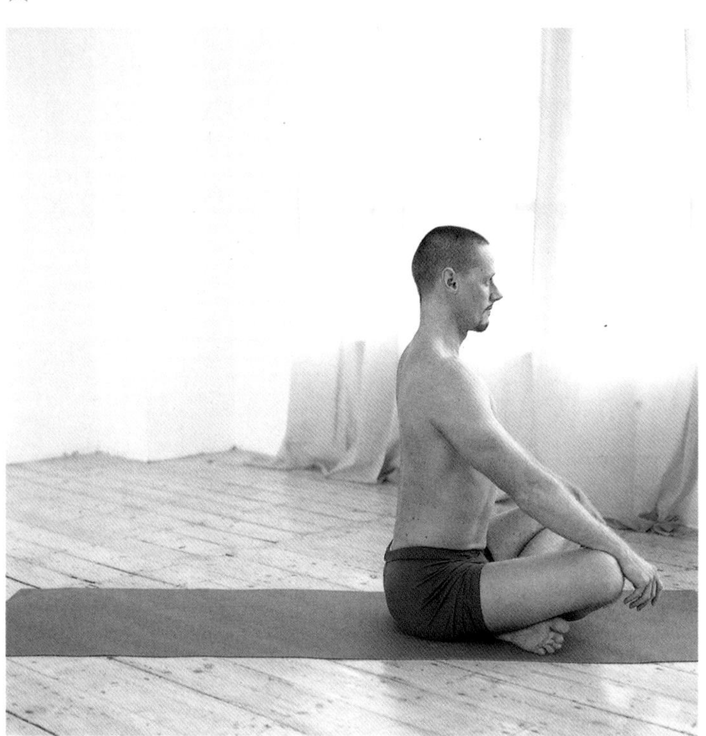

1 Sit in Sukhasana (simple cross legs), crossing the right shin-bone over the left.

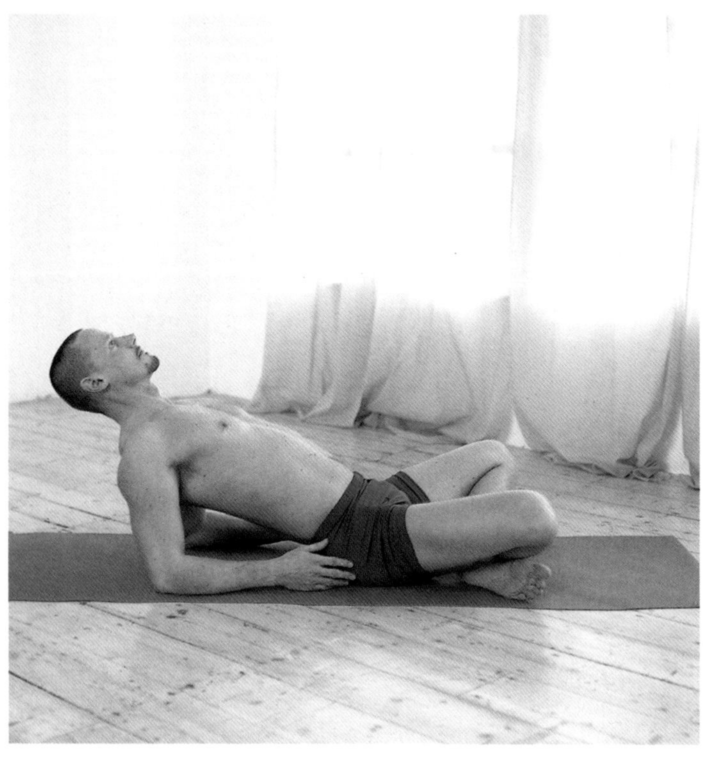

2 Lean back by resting on the elbows and then lie down. Soften the groin to allow the knees to release towards the floor.

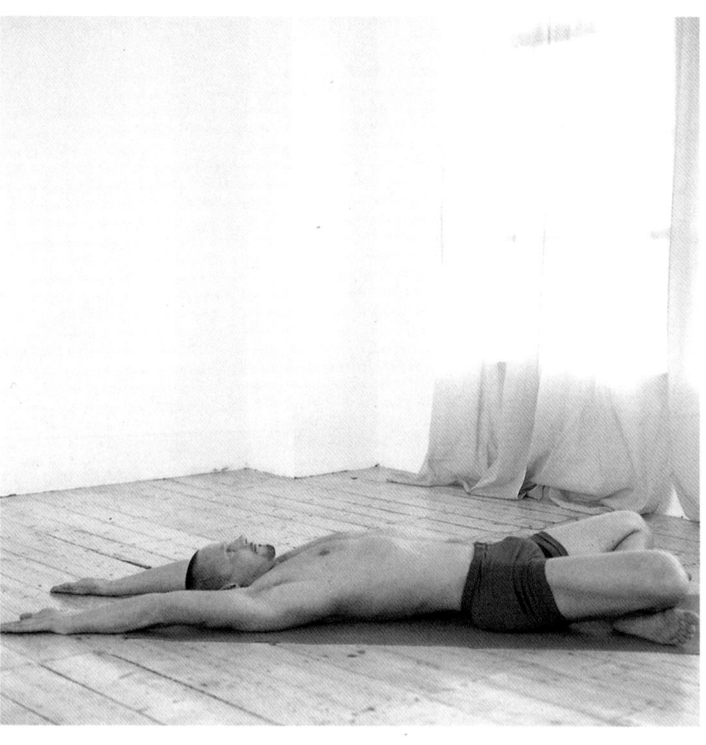

3 Take the arms over the head, straighten the elbows and extend the arms strongly back.

Extend the trunk towards the head and the knees away from the head. Keep the lower back long (don't arch it) and move the shoulders away from the floor and towards the ceiling to lift and open the chest.

Hold for 1–2 minutes, come up, change the cross-over of the legs and repeat.

Modification

- If the groin is painful, support each knee with a foam block or bolster.

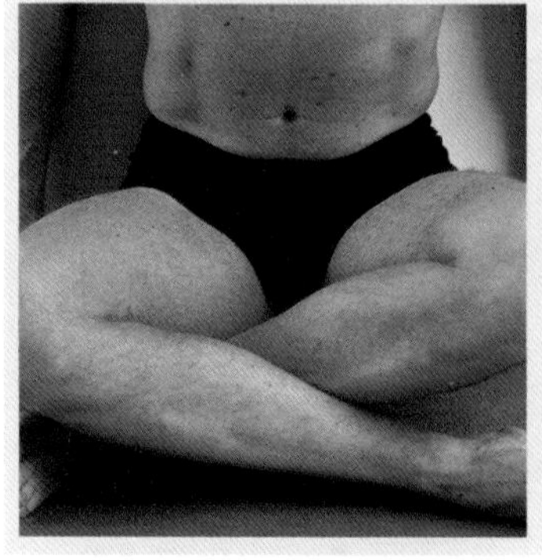

Focus

- Cross the legs evenly at the shins, not at the ankles, and change the cross.
- Don't overarch in the lower back – lengthen it by extending the sacrum towards the feet.

Cross Bolsters

This pose gently stretches the back and soothes the brain. As the back ribs are supported by the vertical bolster, the chest opens and breathing deepens, the abdomen extends and the whole body relaxes.

★

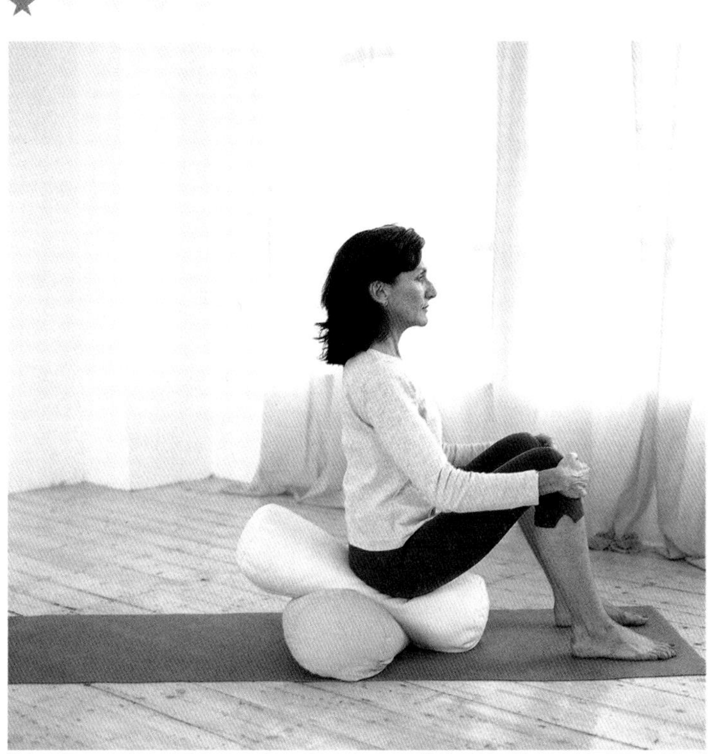

1 Place two bolsters on the floor, the first one horizontal and the second lengthways on top. Sit on the top bolster where it crosses over the bottom one, and bend the knees.

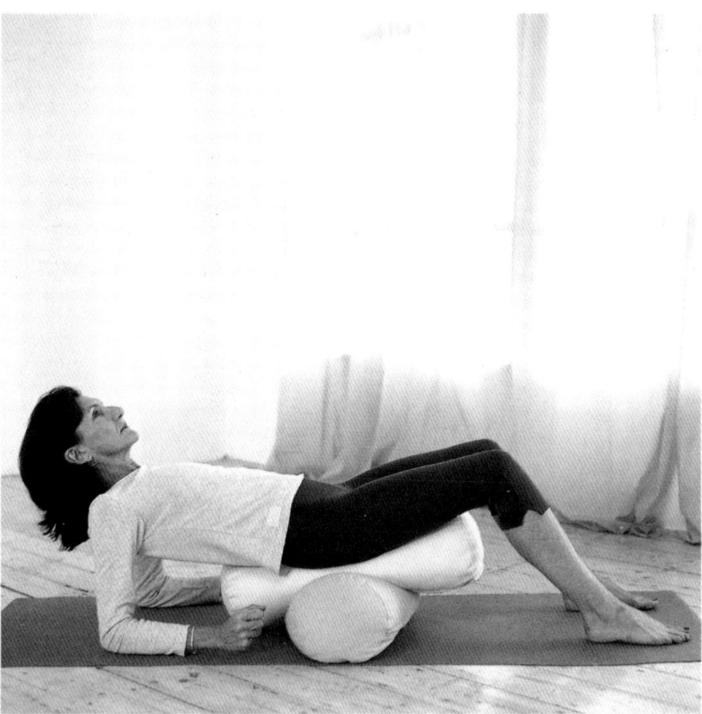

2 Lie back, placing the lower back on the highest part of the top bolster and lowering the shoulders down on to the floor.

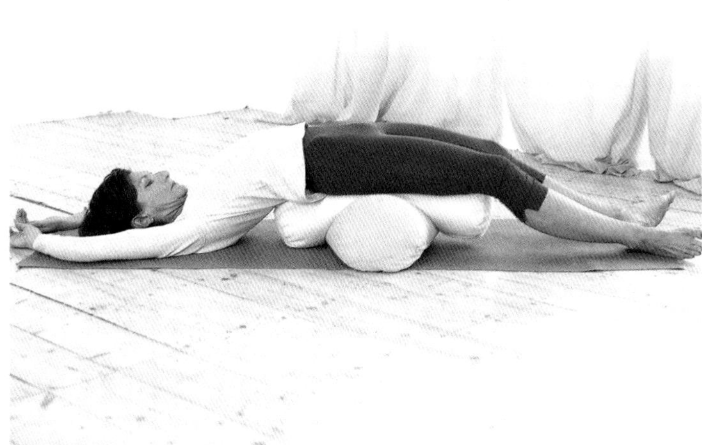

3 Extend the legs forwards, take the arms over the head and relax them.

Hold for 2–5 minutes, bend the knees, slide back towards the head, roll over to the side and get up.

Modification

- The shoulders must rest on the floor. If this is difficult, put a folded blanket underneath them.
- If the lower back aches, lift the feet and place them on two or three foam blocks. It may be easier to lie on top of the bolsters placed separately lengthways.
- To make the posture more relaxing, tie two straps around the legs, one at the ankles and one across the middle of the thighs.

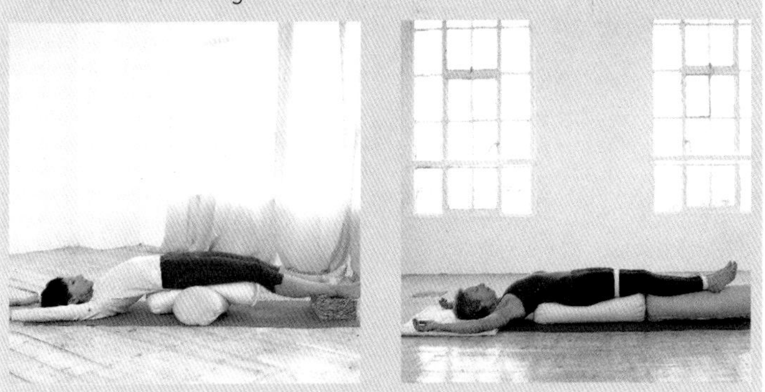

Supta Baddhakonasana | SUPINE COBBLER POSE

This recuperative pose is particularly useful for women, especially during menstruation. The strap around the lower back lengthens the spine, and the bolster lifts the chest. This pose also helps sciatica.

★ ★

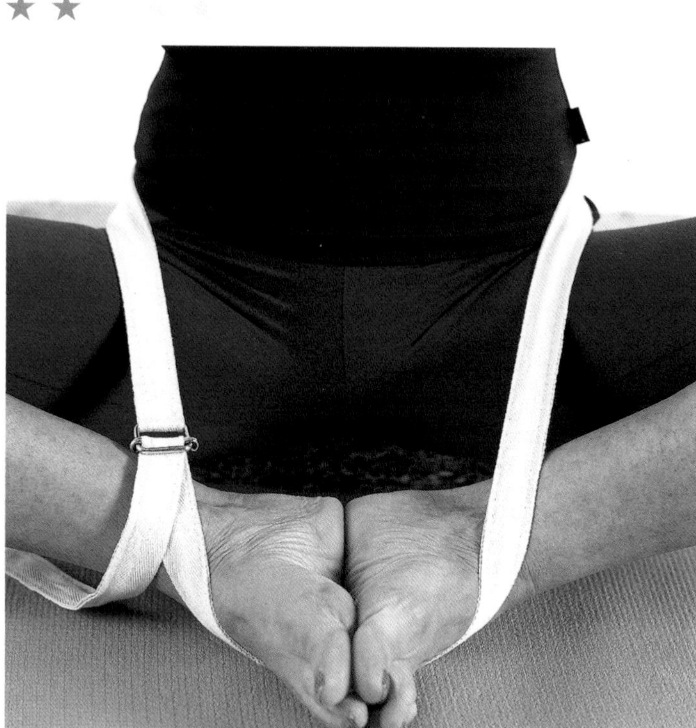

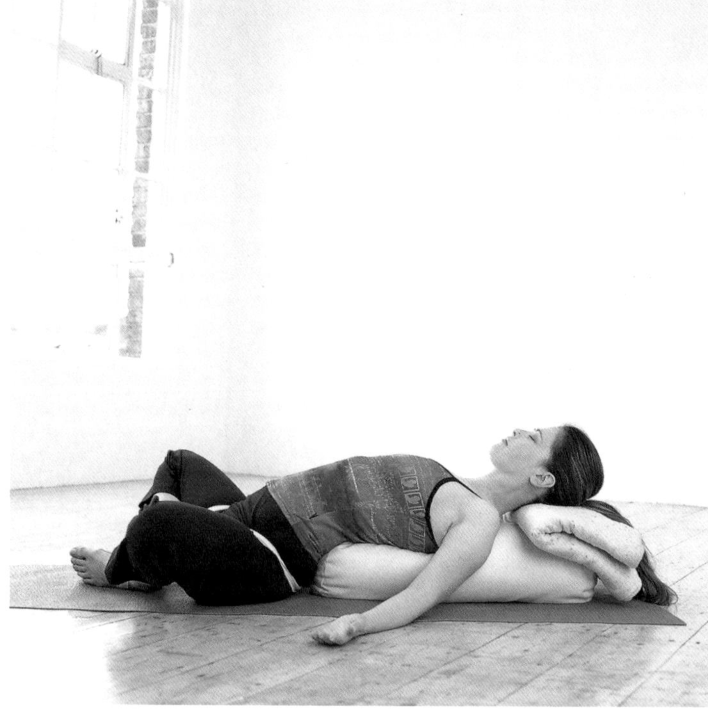

1 Place a bolster lengthways on the floor with a folded blanket at the top end. Sit in front of the bolster with the edge in contact with the lower back. Bend the knees out to the sides, take the soles of the feet together and draw the heels as close to the pubis as possible. Loop the strap across the lower back, over the hips and bind the soles of the feet together at the ankles.

Modification

- If the back is aching, put more support on the bolster and under the head.
- If the groin is uncomfortable, support each knee with a foam block or bolster.
- If the back aches in this posture despite the extra support, come out of it and lie over the bolster with the legs crossed as in Sukhasana.

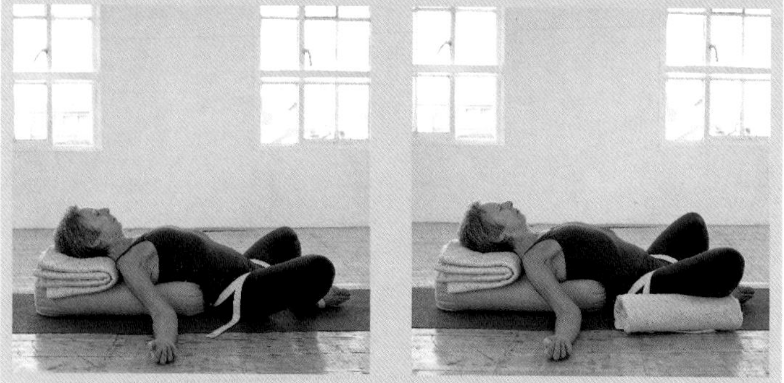

2 Lie back over the bolster, keeping the edge touching the lower back, and support the head and neck with the folded blanket.

Feel the bolster gently moving the spine into the body and the resultant broadening, lifting and opening of the chest. Allow the shoulders to roll down towards the bolster. Keep the face, mouth and throat relaxed.

Take the arms out to the side, keeping the palms facing upwards. Relax them and close the eyes.

Hold for 2–5 minutes, focusing on the breathing, then open the eyes and come up.

Focus

- Make a circle with a strap and place it over the head. Bring it down to the hips, and hook it over the feet.
- As you lie back, the strap will keep the feet as close to the body as possible.

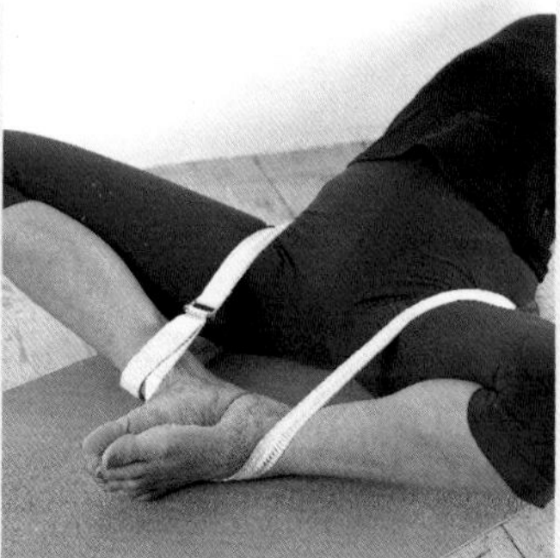

Supta Virasana | RECLINING HERO POSE

This restful posture stretches the abdominal organs and the pelvic region. It also relieves aching legs and is good for digestion. If the back aches in this posture despite the extra support, come out of it and lie over the bolster with legs crossed.

★ ★ ★

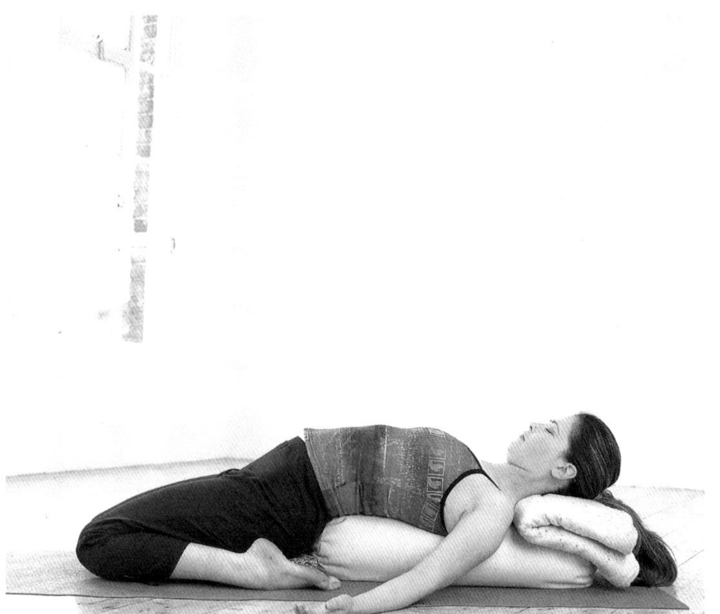

1 Place a bolster lengthways on a mat with a folded blanket at the top end to support the head. Sit in Virasana on a foam block placed against the bolster.

Hold the bolster against the lower back and lie over the bolster, supporting the head and neck on the folded blanket. Take the arms out to the side, palms facing upwards. Hold for 3–5 minutes and come up.

Modification

- If the knees or lower back are painful, put another bolster under the first one.
- Keep the shoulders back the chest open and raised.
- If necessary, place more blankets under the head.

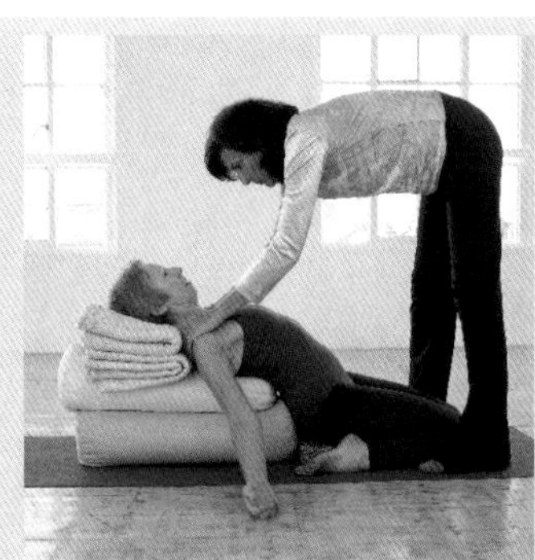

Urdhva Prasarita Padasana | LEGS STRETCHED TO 90 DEGREES

This pose strengthens the lower back and gives relief to tired legs. The brain stays calm while focusing on the breath.

★ ★

1 Sit sideways to the wall and move the right hip and buttock as close to the wall as possible. Lean back, swivel the trunk around and take both legs up the wall. The head should be in line with the tailbone.

Lie down and allow the wall to support the legs. Extend both arms over the head, keep the hips down, and stretch the legs up the wall. Hold for 40–60 seconds and come up.

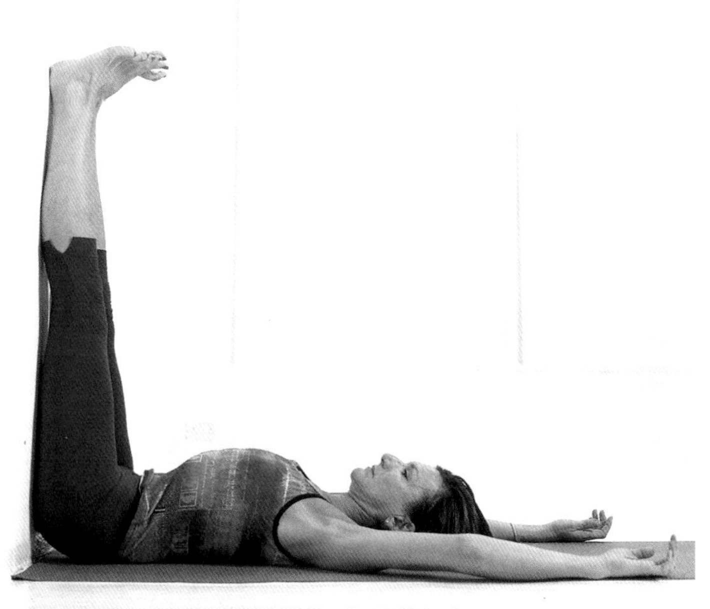

Focus

- Extend the backs of the legs towards the ceiling and press them into the wall.
- Keep the lower back and hips moving towards the floor.
- Take the shoulder blades into the body to open the chest.
- This is considered a supine, relaxing pose, while Viparita Karani raises the hips and back off the floor, and is therefore considered an inverted posture.

Supta Padangusthasana I & II | PRONE LEG STRETCH

Supta Padangusthasana I & II are good for stretching the hamstring muscles. Both postures strengthen the knees and hip joints, and help to relieve sciatica. The pelvic area is aligned, which removes stiffness from the lower back and eases backache.

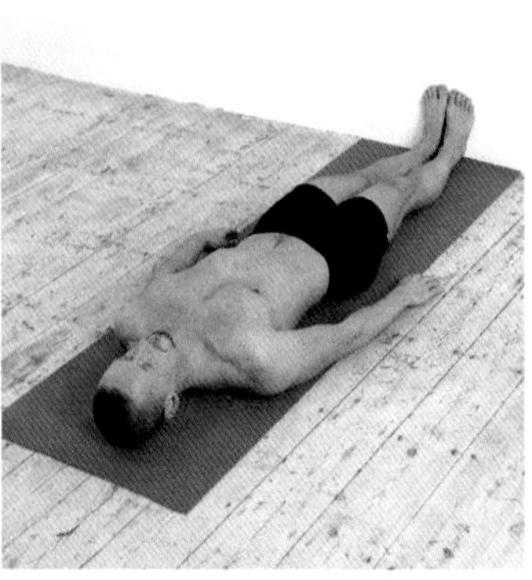

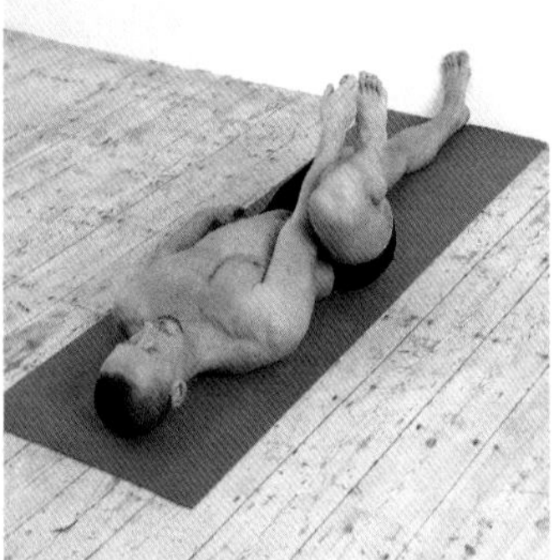

1 Lie down on a mat or blanket, with the soles of both feet touching the wall.

2 Bend the right knee towards the chest, and grab the big toe with the thumb and forefinger.

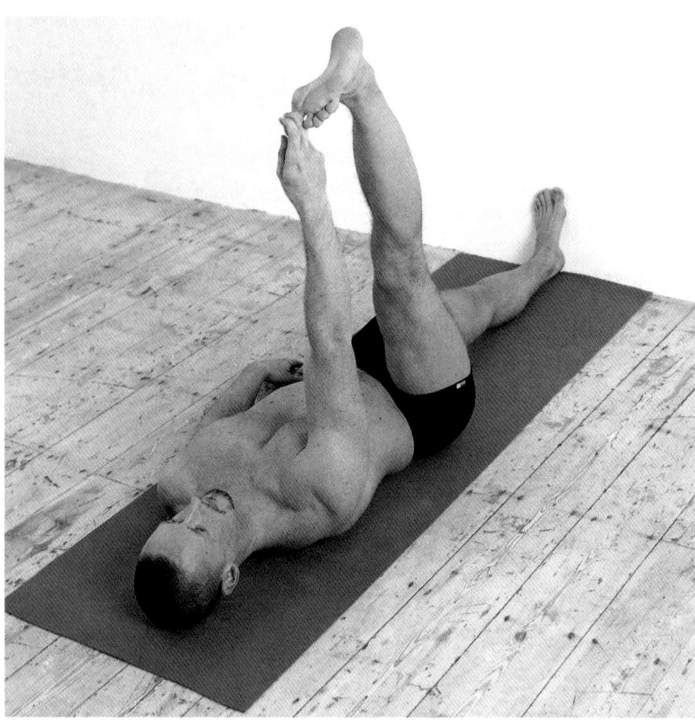

3 Supta Panangusthasana I – Stretch the right leg straight up towards the ceiling while pressing the sole of the left foot more firmly into the wall. Keep the right leg at a 90-degree angle. (If the back is painful, take the leg to a 60-/70-degree angle.)

Lengthen the back of the right leg from the buttock bone to the heel. Press the back of the left leg into, and along, the floor. Pull on the foot to open the chest. Hold for 30–40 seconds, come down and repeat with the left leg.

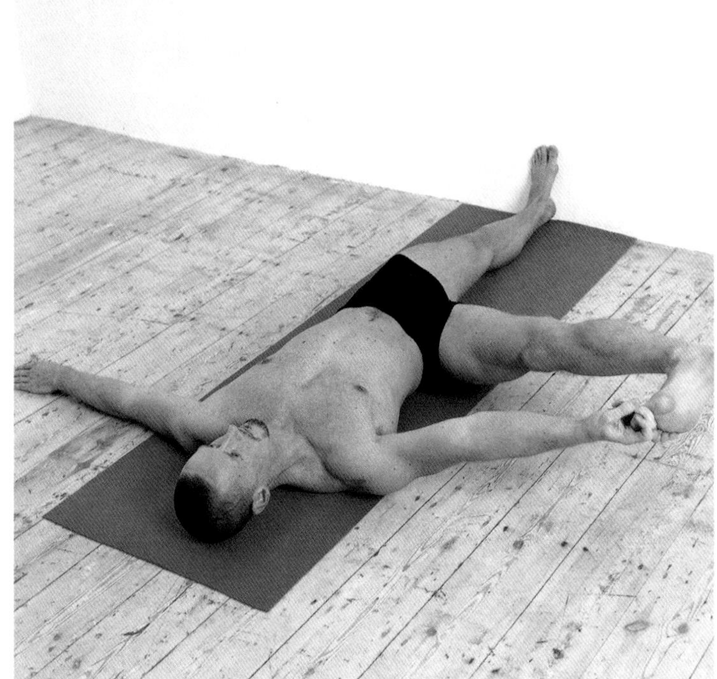

4 Supta Padangusthasana II – follow the instructions as before, extend the leg up to 90 degrees and then stretch the right leg and arm sideways to the right. Take the right leg towards the floor without disturbing the head, trunk or left leg.

Press the sole of the left foot into the wall and the back of the leg into the floor. If the whole body rolls over towards the right, put a support under the right foot to control the descent of the leg (if using a strap, pull on it with the right hand) and extend the left arm out to the side.

Open the chest. Hold for 30–40 seconds and repeat on the other side.

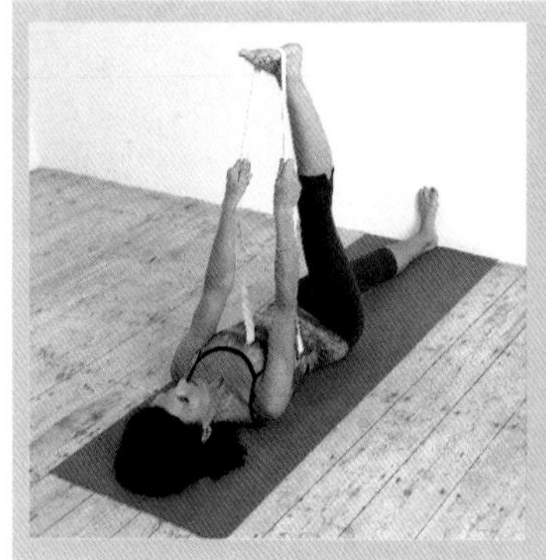

Modification

- Students with tight hamstrings can use a strap around the foot, rather than catching the big toe.
- If difficulty is experienced with the leg to the side, rest the thigh on a bolster.

Adho Mukha Svanasana | DOG POSE

Dog pose is a good all-over stretch. It extends the legs and strengthens the ankles. It also eases stiffness in the neck, shoulders and wrists. Staying longer in this pose removes fatigue and restores energy.

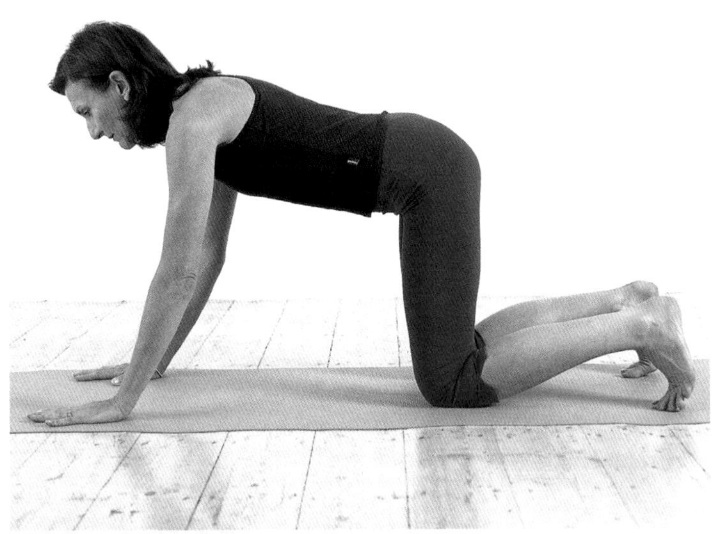

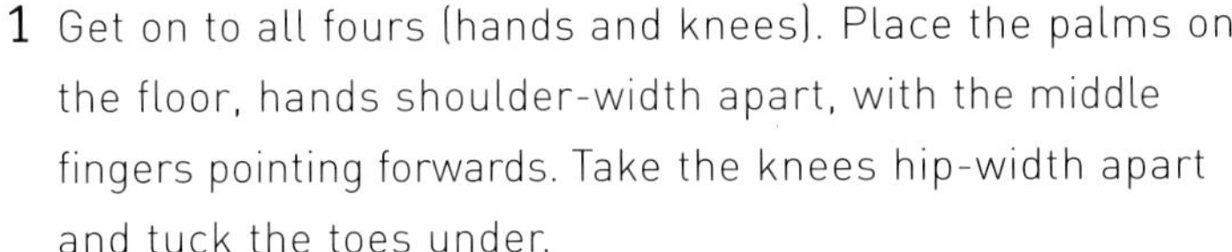

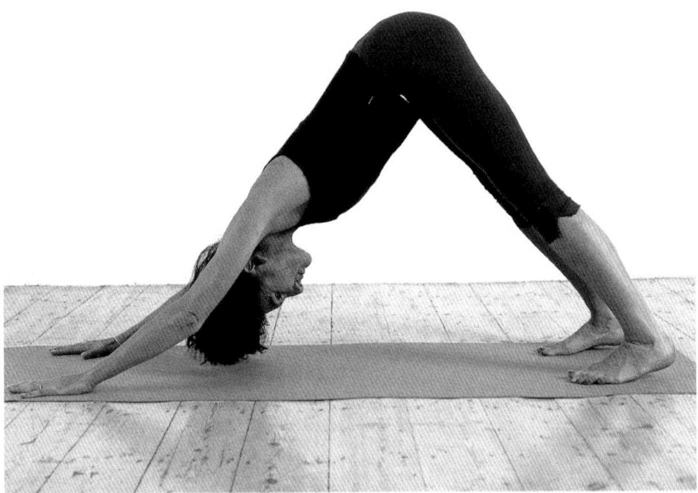

1 Get on to all fours (hands and knees). Place the palms on the floor, hands shoulder-width apart, with the middle fingers pointing forwards. Take the knees hip-width apart and tuck the toes under.

Press the hands firmly into the floor, particularly the thumbs and index fingers. Fully straighten the arms, extending them from the floor towards the shoulders. Move the shoulders away from the ears and the shoulder blades into the body to open the chest.

2 Raise the hips, straighten the legs and extend the heels towards the floor. Press the thighs back. Straighten both elbows, lift the shoulders towards the waist and stretch the trunk up.

Relax the head towards the floor. Keep the arms and legs firm. Push the heels towards the ground.

Hold for 20–30 seconds, bend the knees and come down.

Modification

- For an easier version of this posture, work with the hands or feet supported by a wall.
- Turn the hands out and place the palms on the floor with the index fingers and thumbs against the wall.
- Alternatively, start with the back to the wall, rest the heels up the wall and come into the pose.
- If there is strain in the head or neck, rest the forehead on a bolster for a more restful version of this posture.

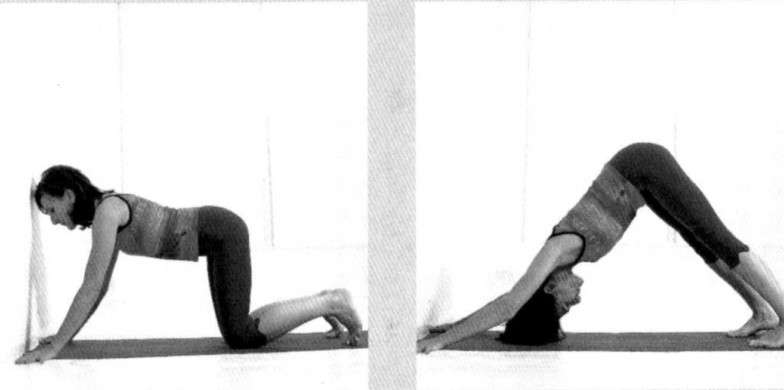

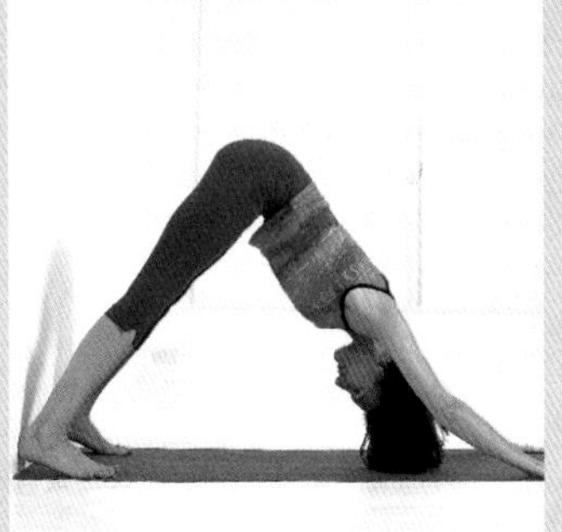

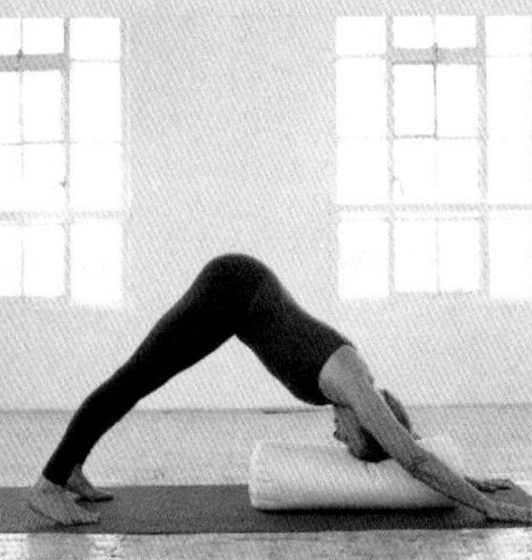

Urdhva Mukha Svanasana | DOG POSE (HEAD UP)

This pose strengthens the spine and relieves backache and sciatica. Increased blood flow to the pelvic area nourishes and tones the internal organs. It also helps to expand the chest and increase flexibility in the neck and shoulders.

★ ★ ★

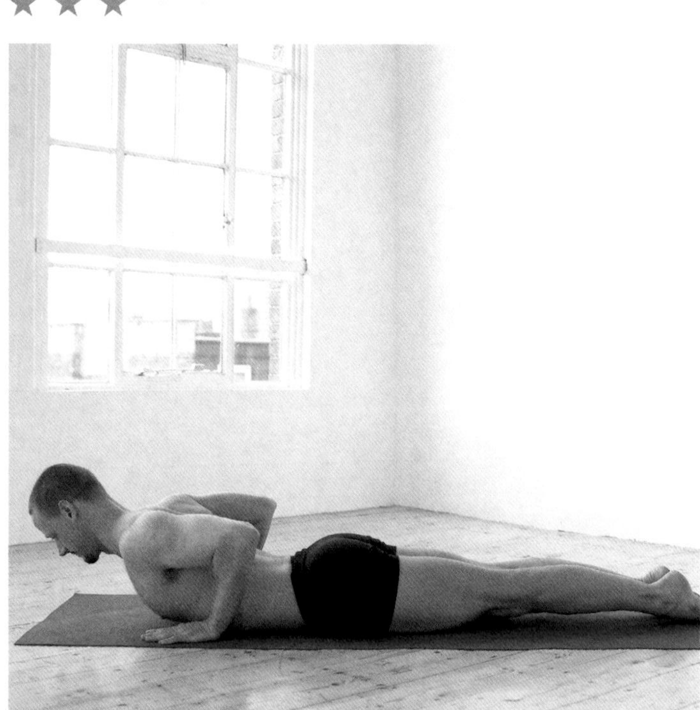

1 Lie face down on the floor and stretch both legs back, pressing the tops of the feet into the floor. (If the lower back hurts, tuck the toes under.) Place the palms on the floor beside the chest and spread the fingers.

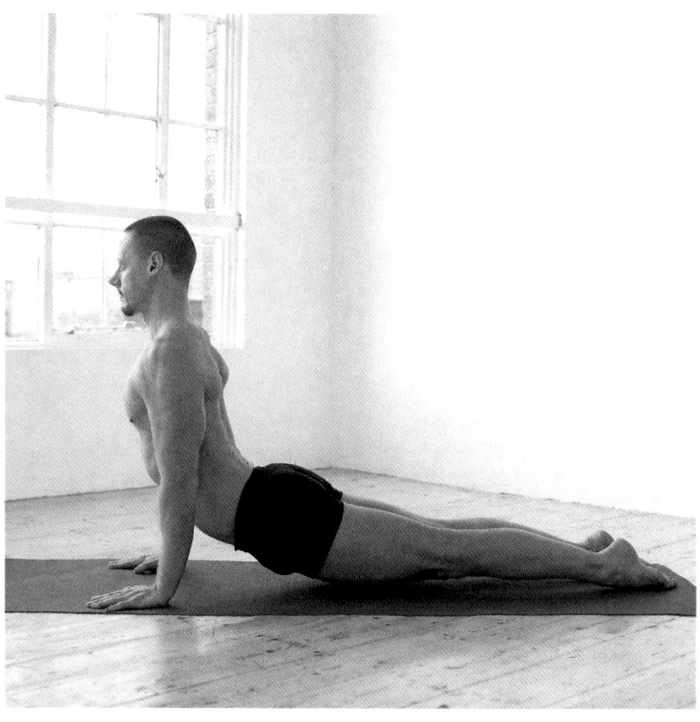

2 Inhale, raise the head and chest, straighten the arms and lock the elbows.

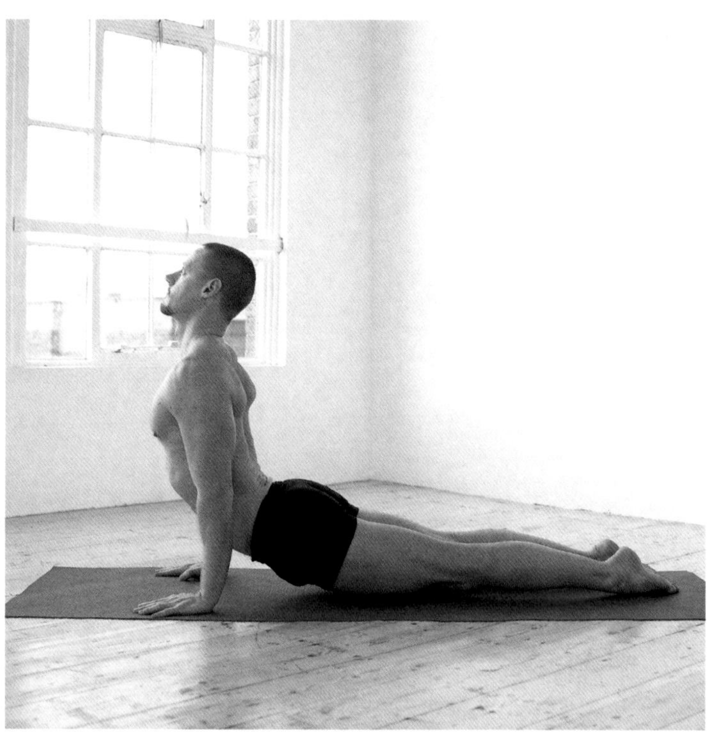

3 Lift the hips, thighs and knees a few centimetres/inches off the floor, bringing the tailbone and sacrum forwards.

Keeping the elbows straight, roll the shoulders back, lift the chest further and curve the trunk back between the arms. Lengthen the back of the neck, take the head back slightly and look up. Stay for 30–40 seconds, breathing evenly.

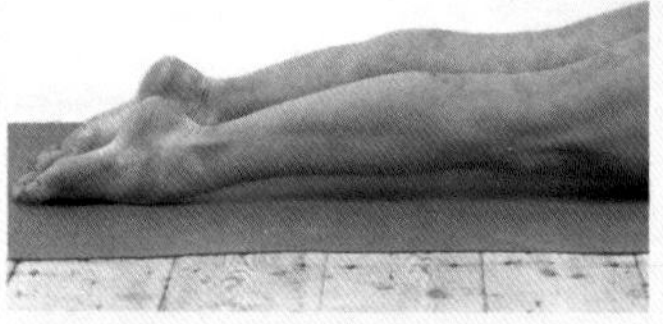

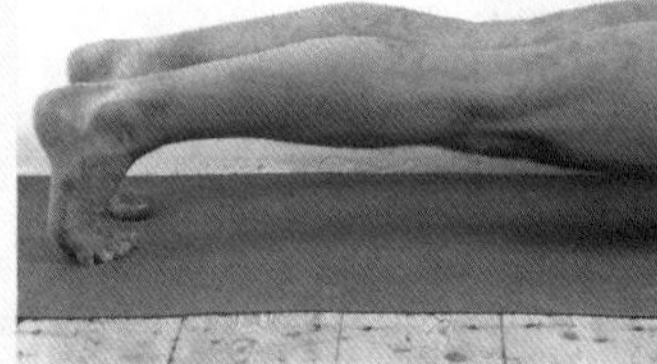

Focus

- Keep the toes pointing backwards, and lift the legs off the floor. If difficulty is experienced lifting the legs off the floor, tuck the toes under and then lift up.
- To lift the trunk and chest more, put each hand on a wooden block.

Salabhasana I | LOCUST POSE

Salabhasana strengthens the back and improves flexibility in the spinal muscles. The abdominal muscles become stronger, it improves digestion and relieves gastric conditions. Stiffness is reduced in the neck and shoulders.

★ ★ ★

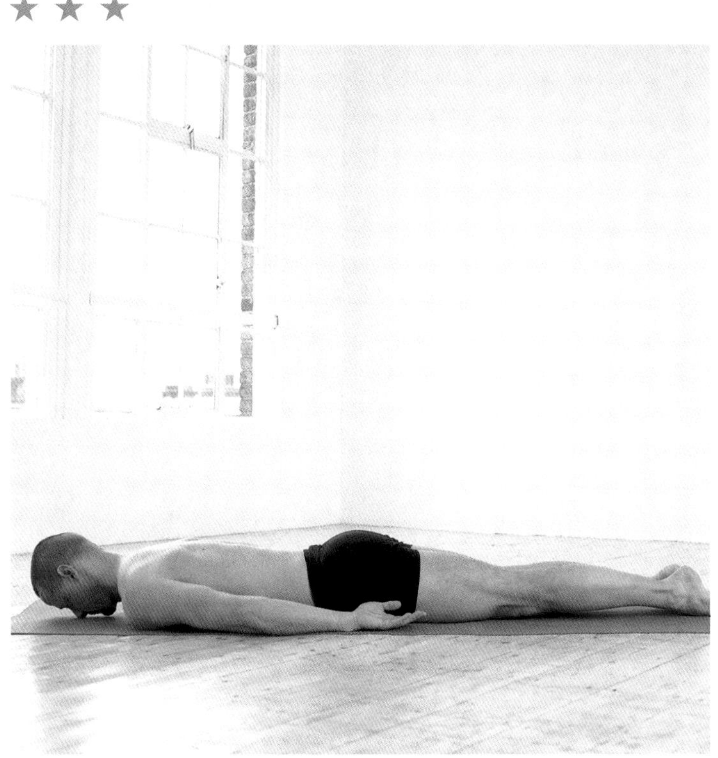

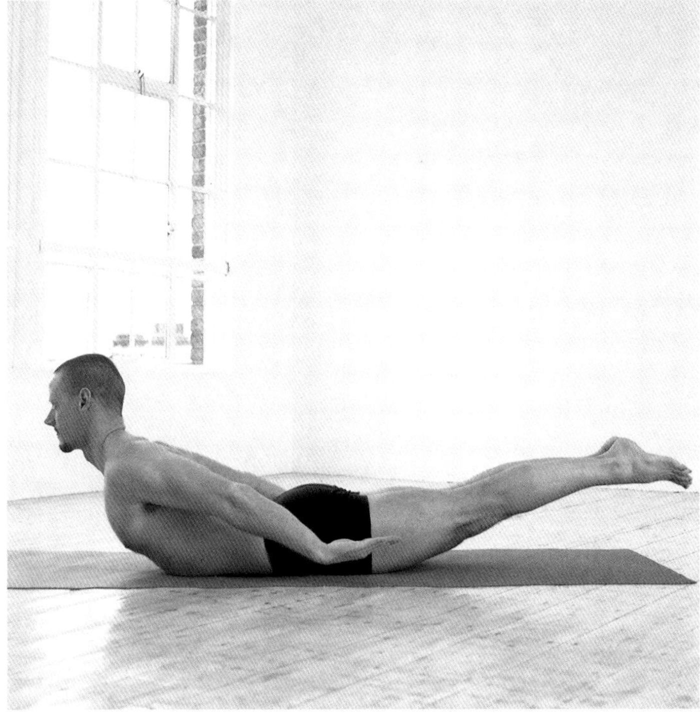

1 Lie face down on the floor with the arms beside the trunk, feet together, knees straight and the toes stretching back. Turn the palms up. Stretch the arms and raise them so the hands are parallel to the floor. Press the sacrum down and raise the head, chest and legs as high as they will go without causing any back pain.

2 Extend the trunk forwards, the legs and arms back and lift the chest.

Balance on the lower abdomen, look straight ahead and breathe normally. Hold the pose for 20–30 seconds and then release.

Focus

• In everyday life we are continually bending forwards, but have little reason to bend backwards. Back bends help to extend the heart muscles, stretch the front side of the lungs and maintain flexibility in the respiratory muscles, thereby increasing lung capacity. They are also useful for nourishing and toning the abdominal organs and stimulating the adrenal glands.

• Back bends have not been featured here, as they are advanced postures that should be carried out only under the supervision of an experienced and qualified teacher. For a preliminary back bend try Ustrasana, over the page, in the moderated version at first.

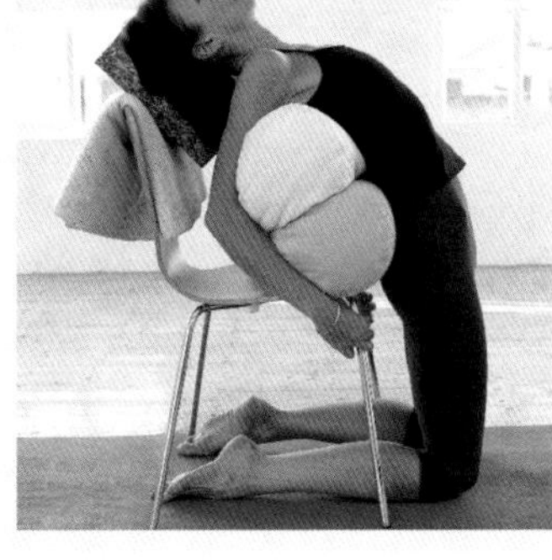

Modification

• Don't raise the arms and legs too high, as this will cause pain in the lower back.

• Stretch the shoulders back, keeping the arms parallel.

• Keep the legs together and the knees straight.

• If it is difficult to do the pose with the feet together, place a foam block between the feet, press the inner edges of the feet into the block and lift the legs.

• In order to open the chest more, and increase the extension in the arms, put a wooden block on the palm of each hand. Imagine the blocks are heavy weights, and without actually lifting the hands any higher, push the palms into the blocks as if trying to lift them.

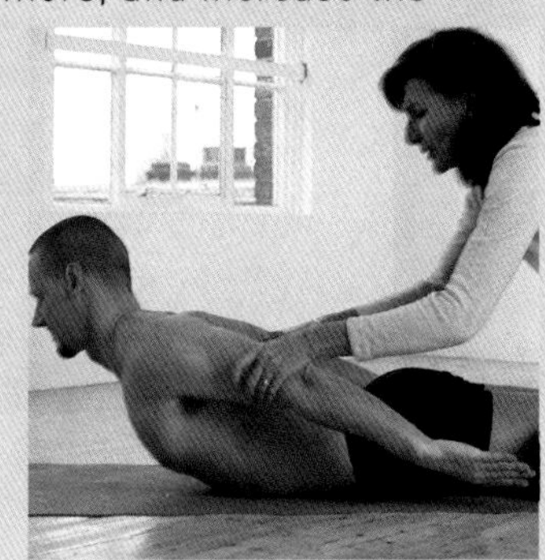

Ustrasana | CAMEL POSE

Although neither supine nor prone, this posture is preparation for more advanced back bends. It makes the shoulders more flexible, strengthens the muscles of the spine and opens the chest, and enables one to understand the curvature of the spine.

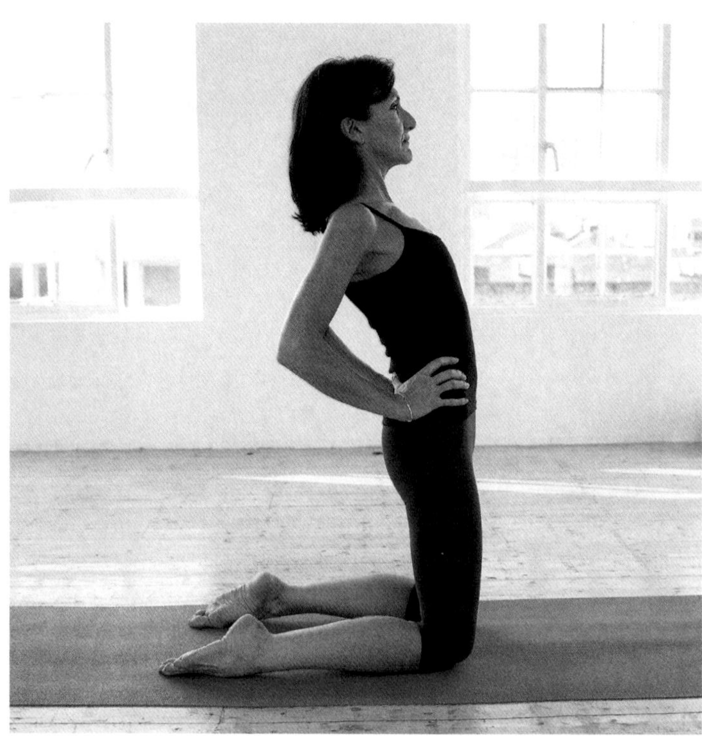

1 Kneel with the knees and feet hip-width apart. Press the shin-bones and tops of the feet firmly into the floor. Place the hands on the waist, and lengthen the trunk up.

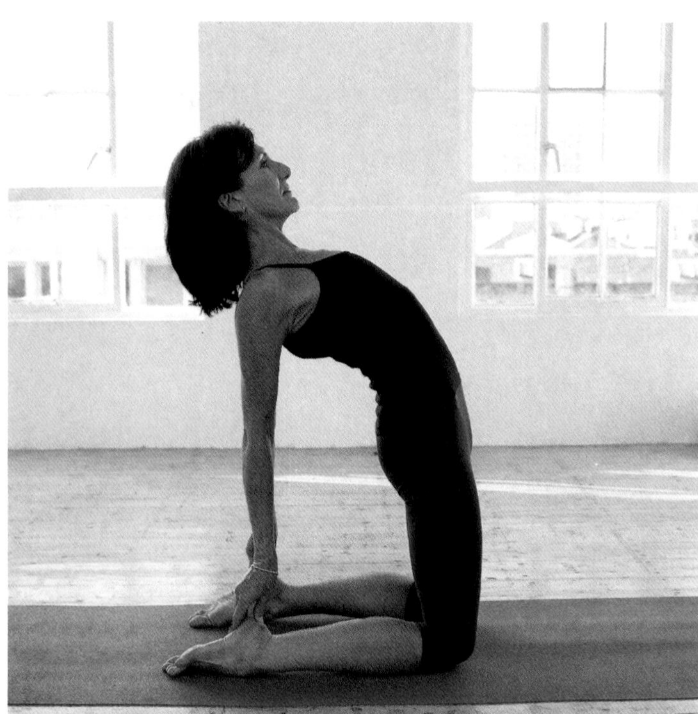

2 Exhale, keep the chest lifting and curve the spine back, moving the spine deeply into the body. Extend the arms towards the heels and hold the heels with the hands.

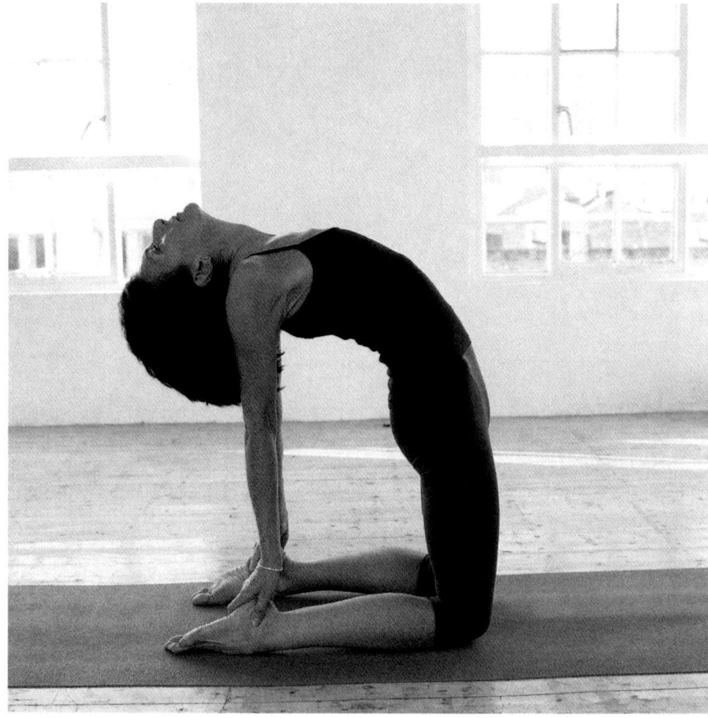

3 Keep the neck long and take the head back. Look behind you. Keep lifting and opening the chest.

Hold for 15–20 seconds, inhale, raise the head, release the hands and lift the trunk.

Focus

- Move the back ribs and shoulder blades more deeply into the back to open the chest more.
- Straighten the arms and hold the heels more firmly to activate the shoulders.
- Finish this pose by leaning forwards to extend the spine in the opposite direction.
- Keep the thighs perpendicular to the floor.

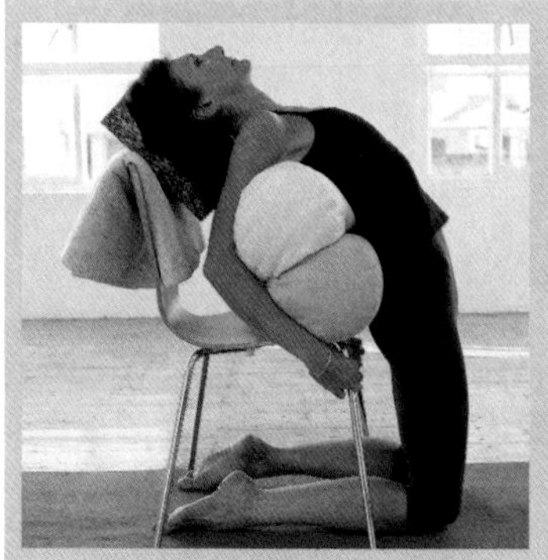

Modification

- Students who cannot reach their heels can arch over bolsters propped on a chair, or place a rolled-up blanket under the tops of their feet so the heels are easier to reach.

Savasana | CORPSE POSE

The Corpse pose is also known as Relaxation. It helps to release tension in the muscles after performing the asanas, settle the breathing and calm the mind. Energy flows into and through the body, recharging it and removing stress.

★

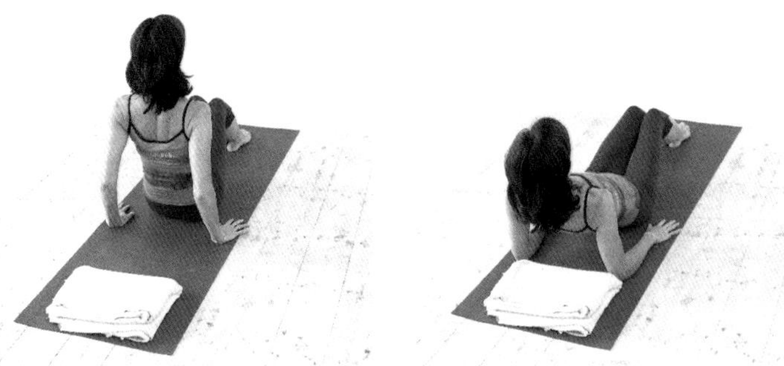

1 Sit in the centre of the mat with the knees bent and the feet on the floor. Put a folded blanket at the head end of the mat.

2 Lower the trunk down, rest on the elbows and check the body alignment, then carefully lower the trunk on to the floor. Place the centre of the back of the head on the support.

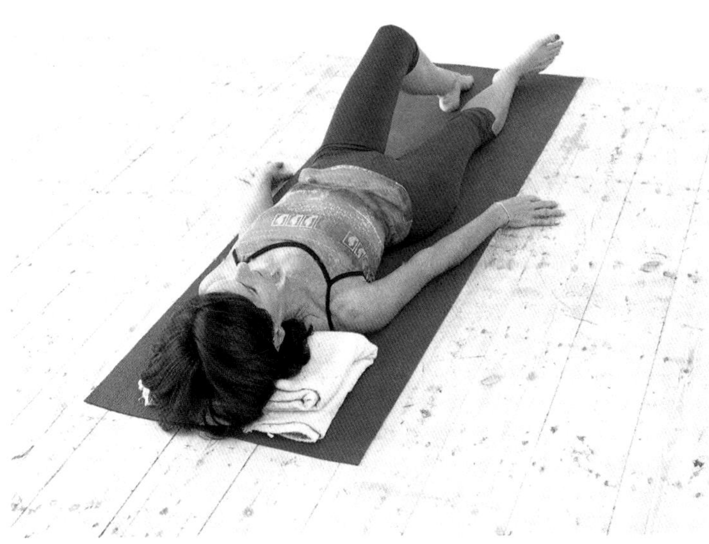

3 Straighten one leg at a time and, when straight, keep the legs and feet together.

Release the tension in the legs and allow the feet to drop out to the side.

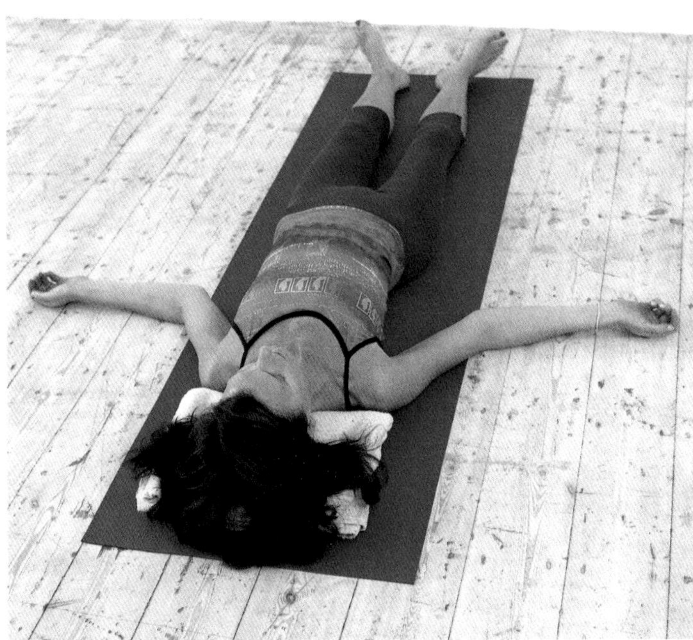

4 Stretch the arms out to the side, slightly away from the sides of the trunk, and turn the palms so that the knuckles of the little fingers are on the floor as much as the knuckles of the index fingers. Shut the eyes by lowering the upper eyelids towards the lower eyelids.

Relax the eyes and facial features and allow the body to sink into the floor. Breathe evenly and focus on the breath in order to keep the brain calm and passive. Don't go to sleep.

Hold for 5–10 minutes, slowly open the eyes, bend the knees, roll over to the side and slowly come up.

Focus

- Let your body go and surrender to the floor.
- Relax the fingers and palms of the hands.
- Keep the head straight, with the bridge of the nose facing the ceiling.
- Relax the thigh muscles and let the legs roll away from one another.
- Draw the organs of perception (eyes, ears and tongue) inwards so that the mind and body become one and inner silence is experienced.

Ujjayi Pranayama | BREATHING

In Pranayama the brain becomes quiet which allows the nervous system to function more effectively. It generates a store of energy in the body, while strengthening and increasing the capacity of the lungs. Beginners should master the postures and gain control over the body before attempting Pranayama.

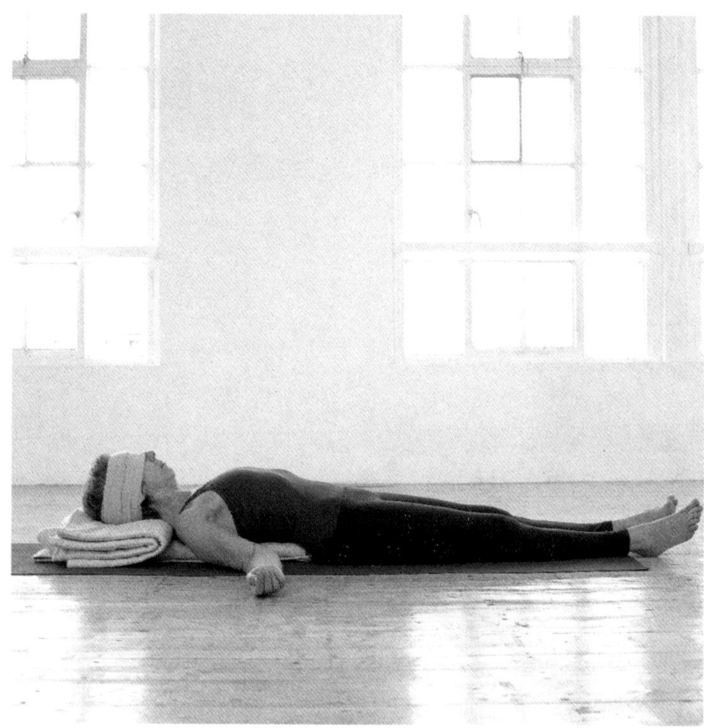

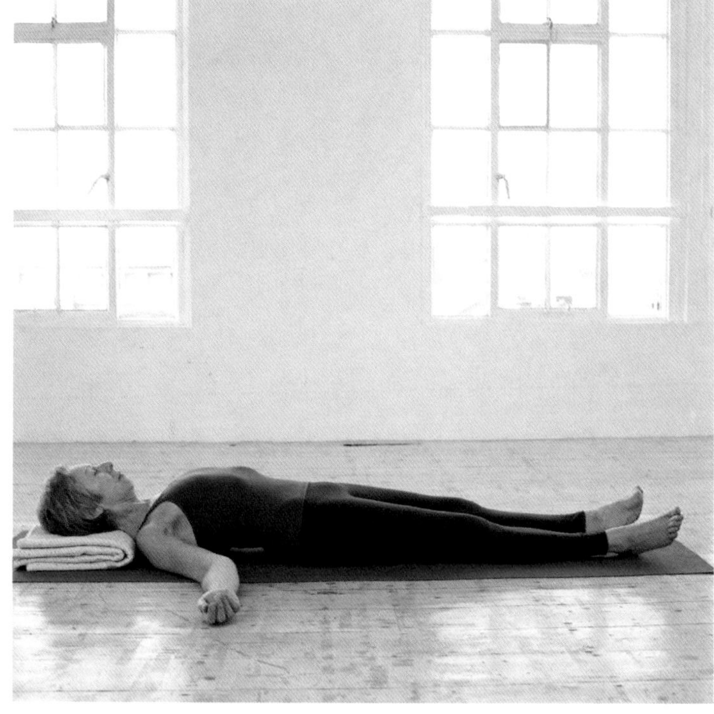

1 Normal Inhalation/Extended Exhalation

Lie in Savasana on a bolster or blanket, with another folded blanket under the head. Cover the eyes with a bandage. Spend a few minutes becoming aware of your normal breathing. Exhale, relax the abdomen. Inhale normally.

Exhale slowly, quietly and smoothly, lengthening the breath without straining. Inhale normally again. Exhale slowly, deeply and smoothly.

If breathlessness or fatigue is experienced in between cycles, take a few normal breaths before proceeding. Continue in this manner for 5 minutes. Return to normal breathing to allow the lungs to recover.

Focus

- Keep the face and eyes relaxed during Pranayama.
- Relax the mouth, tongue and throat.
- Keep the chest and ribcage lifted throughout.
- Keep the shoulders moving away from the ears.
- Keep the abdomen soft in inhalation and exhalation.
- Soften the palms of the hands and relax the fingers.
- If the mind is racing, an eye bandage will aid calmness.

2 Extended Inhalation/Normal Exhalation

Exhale, completely emptying air from the lungs.

Take a slow, soft inhalation, filling the lungs from the bottom to the top.

Don't strain or jerk the chest, breathe smoothly and lengthen the breath calmly.

Exhale normally. Inhale once more, slowly drawing the breath into the lungs.

Exhale normally.

Repeat these two cycles for about 5 minutes, then return to normal breathing. Once you've returned to normal breathing, check that there is no tension in the shoulders, throat, mouth or hands.

Exercise caution when practising Pranayama – incorrect practice may strain the lungs and diaphragm.

These two cycles can be practised separately or together and should be done for a few months before proceeding to breathing with extended inhalation and extended exhalation.

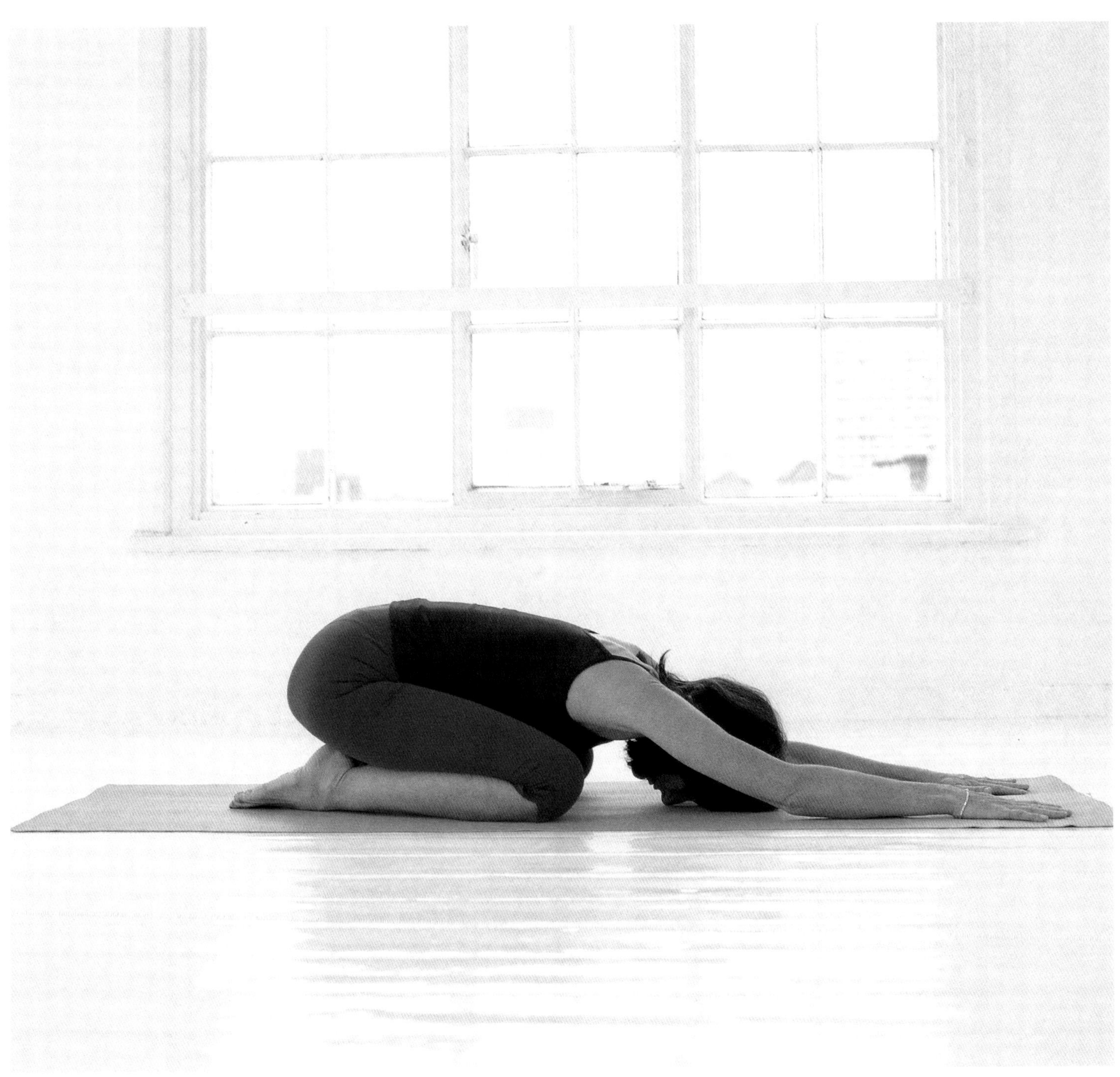

3 **Extended Inhalation/Extended Exhalation**
Exhale, completely emptying the lungs of air. Inhale slowly and smoothly, lengthening the breath.

Maintain the lift of the chest, and exhale slowly and deeply without straining the throat.

Control the flow of breath so that the body doesn't shudder or strain. Take a few normal breaths.

Repeat for about 5 minutes. Return to normal breathing.

To end the above cycles, bend the knees, roll over to the side and remove the bolster. Lie flat, with the head still supported, in Savasana for 5 minutes, keeping the brain quiet and releasing the body to the floor. Slowly open the eyes, turn to one side, stay for a moment, then turn to the other side. Come up and sit in Adho Mukha Virasana before getting up.

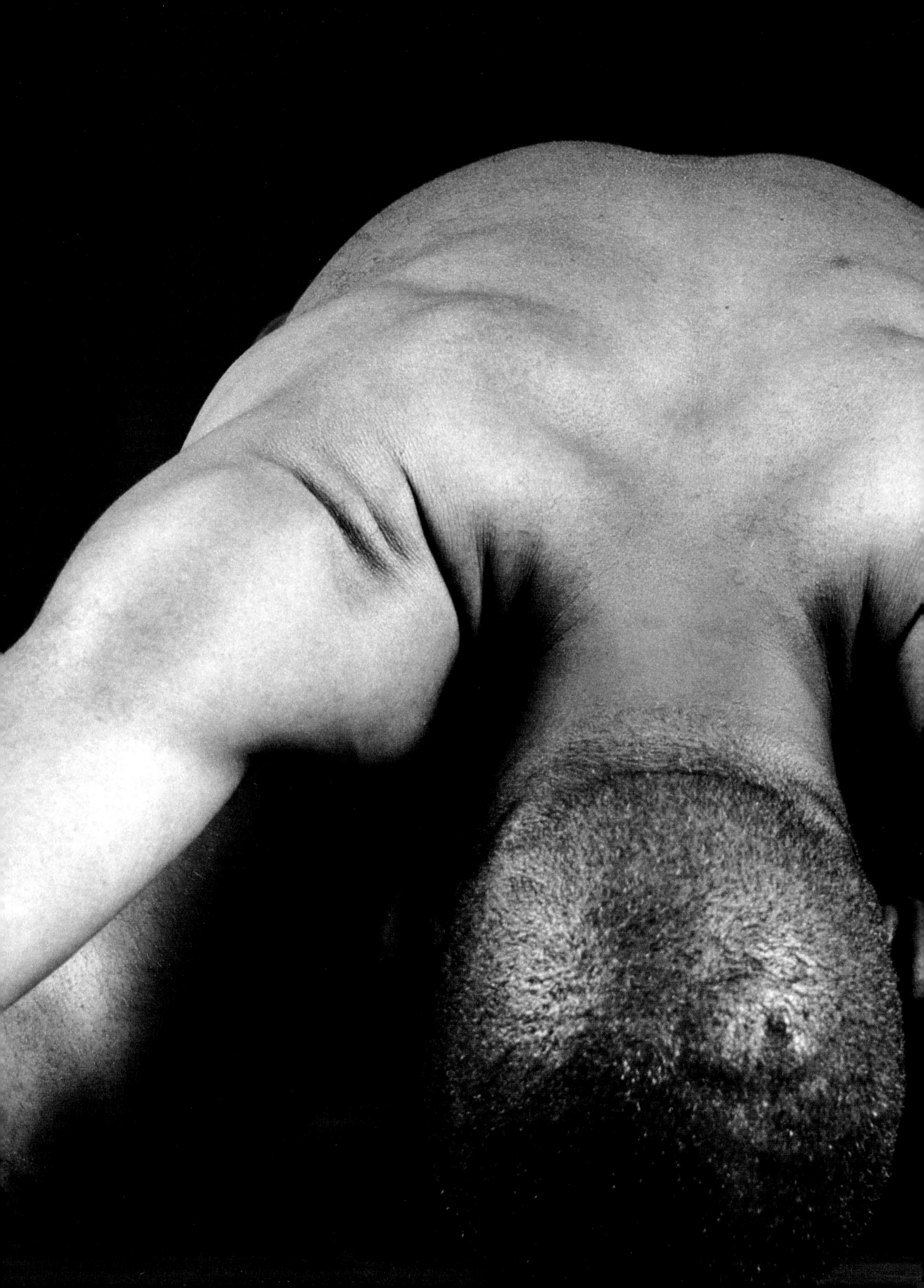

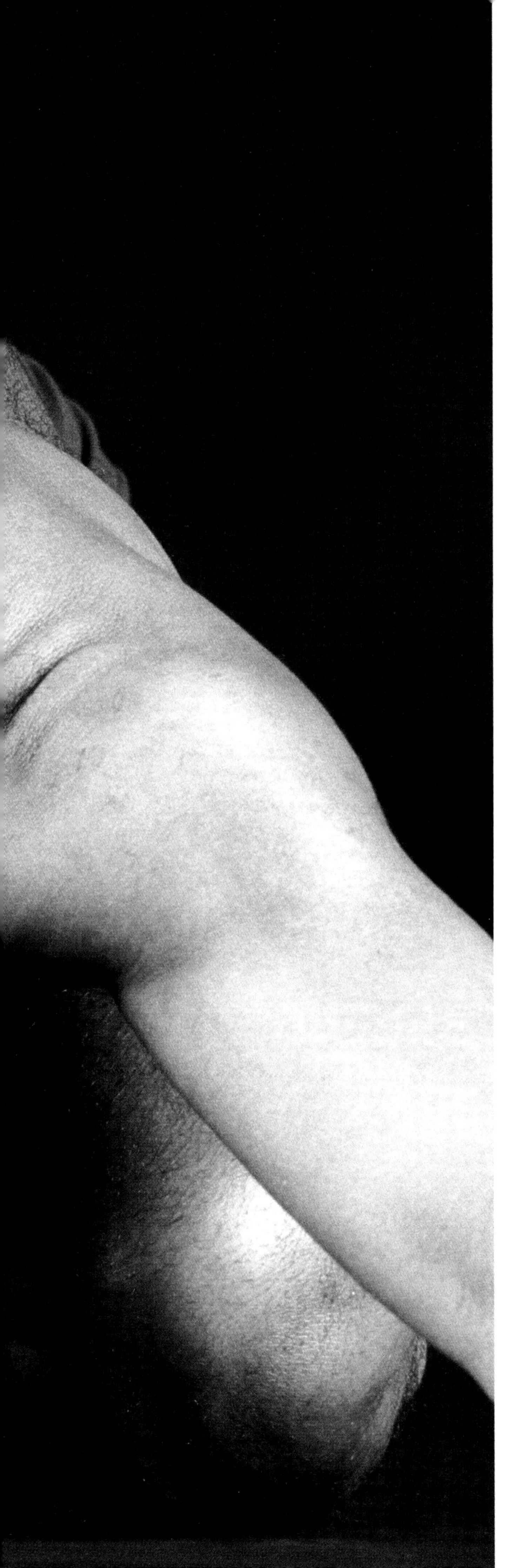

Routine Practice

The sage Patanjali states in *Yoga Sutra* 11.47: "Perfection in an asana is achieved when the effort to perform it becomes effortless, and the infinite being within is reached."

Practising postures in a set order increases their effectiveness as well as the student's understanding of each posture. The subtleties and details of the poses and their effect on the mind and body become more obvious as one's practice becomes more established.

Routines and Sequences

The practice of postures has a beneficial impact on the entire body. The postures tone the muscles, tissues, ligaments, joints and nerves, as well as maintaining and improving the health and functioning of all the body systems. It is important to keep practising until one becomes familiar with, and comfortable in, the postures. When this happens, the full benefits are felt. That is why we practise routines as often as possible.

CLASSIFICATION OF POSTURES

Broadly speaking, standing postures are dynamic and exhilarating. They refresh both body and mind by removing tension, aches and pains. The standing postures form the basis of all other postures, and, through them, practitioners become familiar with various parts of their bodies, their muscles and joints and use their intelligence to bring action and awareness to these parts. Most routines begin with standing postures in order to waken the physical body – the arms, legs and spine – and stimulate the brain by connecting movements to specific areas of the body. They also build stamina and strength as well as determination.

The seated postures are introduced after standing postures to rest and remove strain from the legs. Seated forward bends are calming. They remove fatigue, soothe the nerves and calm the mind. In standing postures the brain is stimulated; in seated postures an agitated, fluctuating mind becomes passive.

Twisting postures extend and rotate the spine. These postures are good for relieving backache and stiffness in the neck and shoulders. The internal organs are stimulated as the trunk turns, and this improves digestion.

Inverted postures energize the entire system. They relieve strain in the legs, activate and nourish the inner organs, stimulate the brain and improve the respiratory, circulatory and nervous systems. Standing, seated and twisting postures prepare the body and mind for inversions. Women should not practise inversions while menstruating.

Supine, prone, or lying-down postures are also known as abdominal postures, and a routine should never begin with these. Standing postures tone the stomach muscles so they can be used correctly, and inverted postures protect the organs so they are not damaged when doing abdominal postures, so these should be done before attempting abdominal postures.

Savasana (relaxation) should be done for 5–10 minutes (depending on time) at the end of each routine.

SUGGESTED PRACTICE PLAN

The following routines are suggested to enable students to practise systematically and progressively. It is more beneficial to practise for a shorter time each day than a longer session once or twice a week. Attend a regular yoga group with a qualified teacher, as they can make sure you are progressing at the correct pace.

Each routine can be practised daily, starting with Sequence 1 on the first day and progressing to Sequence 5 by the end of the week. Repeat the first 5 sequences over a 2–3 week period to consolidate the postures, then continue with the Sequences 6–10. Ultimately one's discrimination should be used with regard to the length of time and which postures

Left Try to get to an organized class, led by a qualified teacher, at least once or twice a week, and supplement this by practising at home every day, and you will feel the difference very quickly.

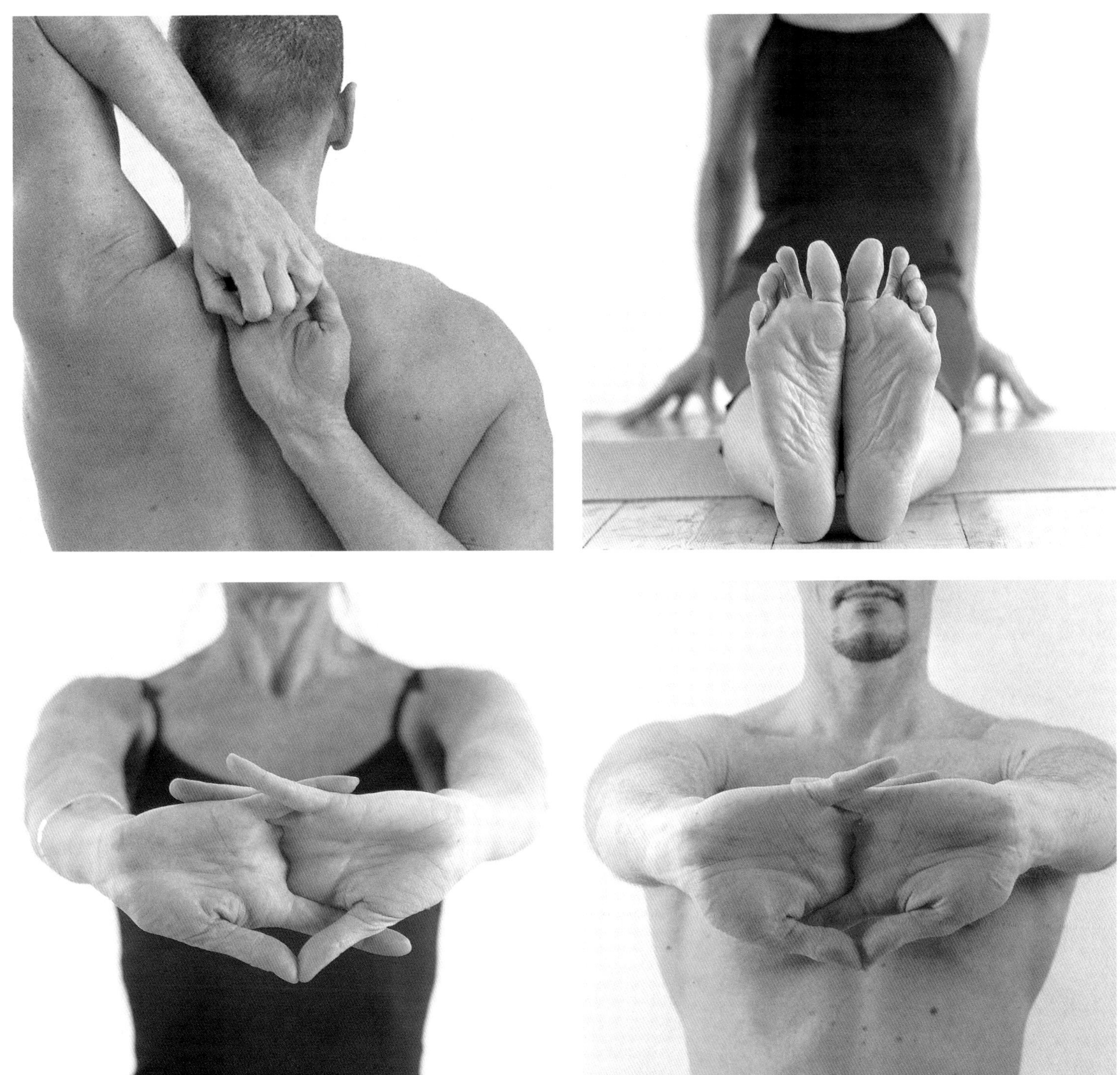

Above Time and patience are required to understand the subtleties and technical requirements of the postures.

to practise, the aim being to have a physical and spiritual rhythm to one's practice. Confidence is gained by working at an even pace, learning about the postures and their effects on the body, and then proceeding with knowledge and understanding on to the next routine. Move on to the next set of routines, only as you feel able and capable to do so.

As one progresses in one's practice, flexibility and stamina improve and the postures can be held for longer periods of time. The effects of the postures are not instant, and timing is dependent on energy, intelligence and awareness. However, if time doesn't permit it, one can tailor one's practice to suit the circumstances.

Sequence 1 – Simple Standing Postures

In this first sequence, the shape of the postures should be studied and worked on. Then, as this becomes more familiar, detailed instructions should be incorporated to make the posture more correct and to feel the effects. Think about keeping the spine long in all the postures. If fatigue or exhaustion is felt, do supported Uttanasa I to recover.

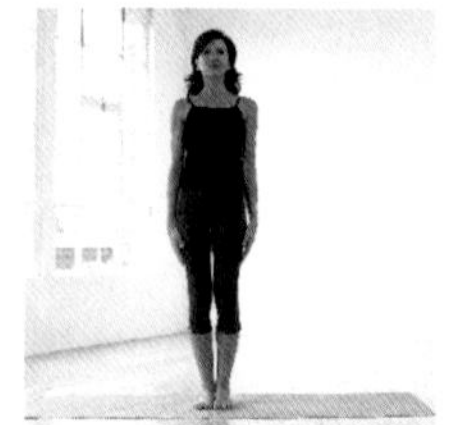
1 **Tadasana**

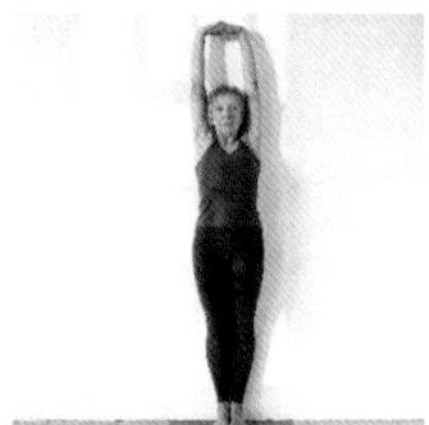
2 **Tadasana** with hands in Parvatasana

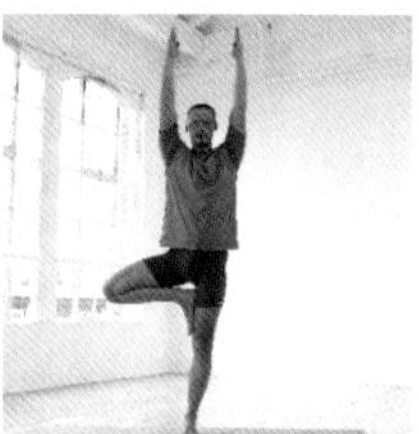
3 **Vrksasana**

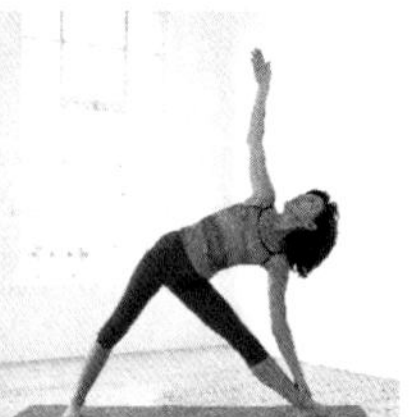
4 **Utthita Trikonasana**

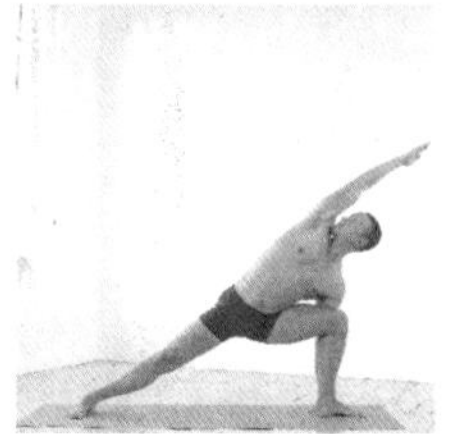
5 **Utthita Parsvakonasana**

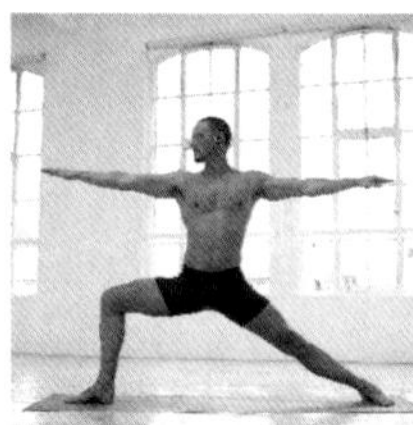
6 **Virabhadrasana II**

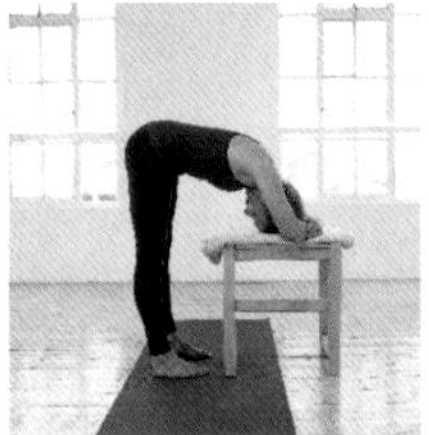
7 **Uttanasana I** (s)

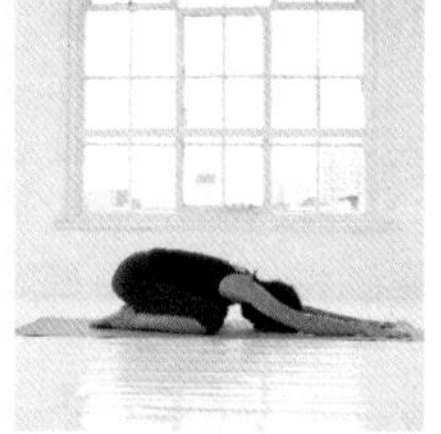
8 **Adho Mukha Virasana**

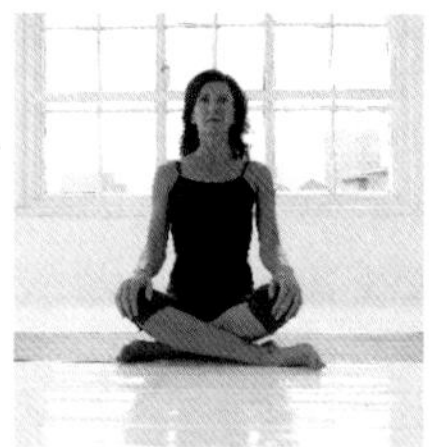
9 **Sukhasana**

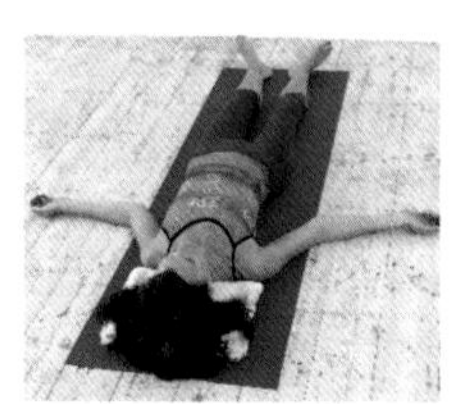
10 **Savasana**

Focus

- Where the moderated posture is used it is marked (s) for supported or (w) if the wall is used.

Sequence 2 – Simple Seated Postures

In this group of seated postures, one supine pose (Adho Mukha Svanasana) and two inverted postures (Setu Bandha Sarvangasana and Viparita Karani) have been introduced. The inversions should not be done if one is menstruating. It is advisable to sit on a support in the seated postures, as this helps to lift and extend the spine. The lower back should not be arched forwards, but lengthened upwards towards the head. In Virasana, ensure that the support under the buttocks is high enough so that there is no pain in the knees. If any discomfort is felt in the lower back in Setu Bandha Sarvangasana, raise the feet higher so as to remove strain from the lumbar region.

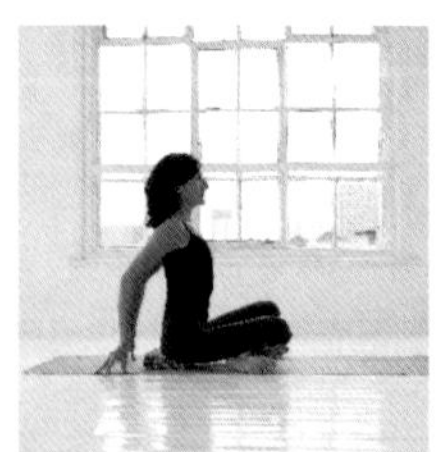
1 **Sukhasana**

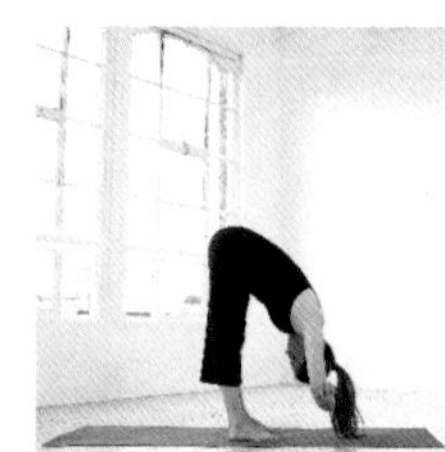
2 **Uttanasana I**

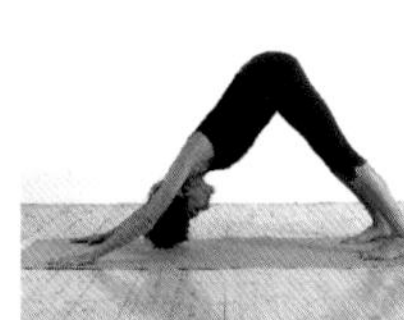
3 **Adho Mukha Svanasana**

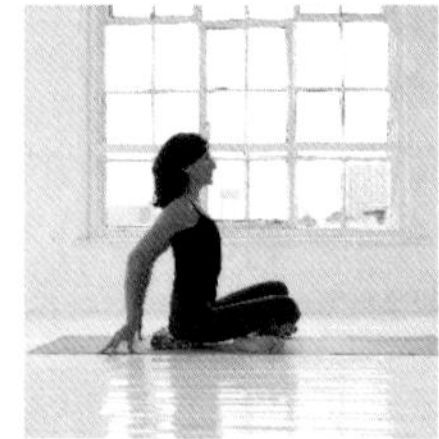
4 **Sukhasana**

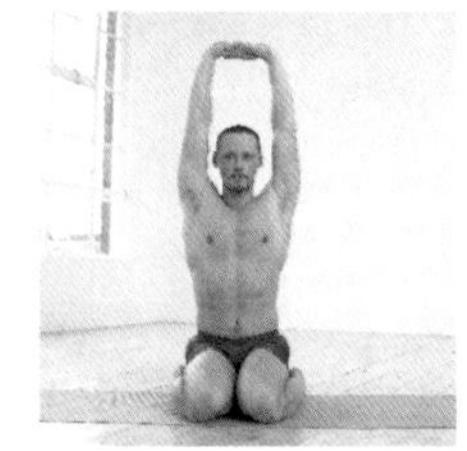
5 **Virasana with Parvatasana**

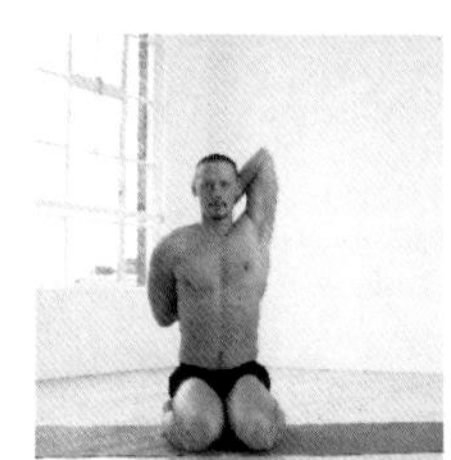
6 **Gomukhasana**

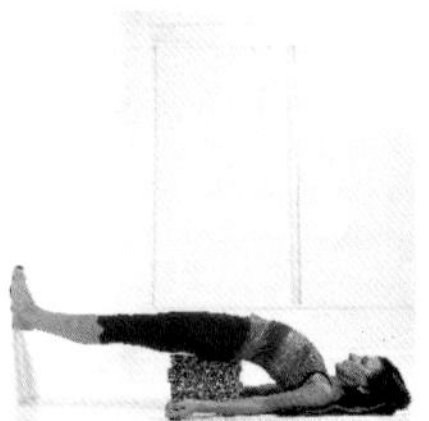
7 **Setu Bandha Sarvangasana**

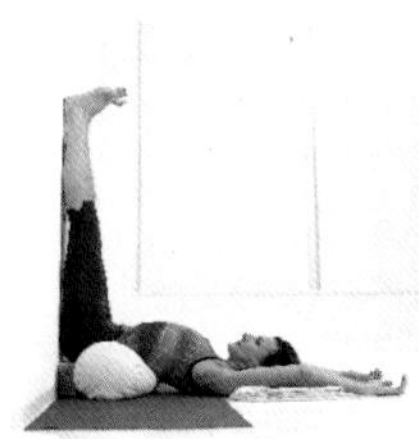
8 **Viparita Karani**

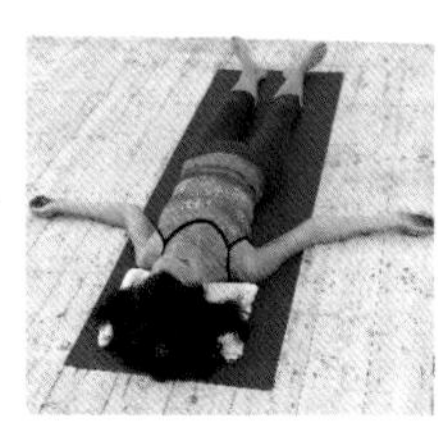
9 **Savasana**

Focus

- Each routine can be practised daily, starting with Sequence 1 on the first day and progressing to Sequence 5 by the end of the week. Then repeat over a 2–3 week period before progressing to sequences 6–10.

Sequence 3 – Consolidation of Simple Standing Postures

Parsvottanasana has been introduced here, and the back foot is turned in much more than with the other standing postures. Ensure that both hips are level and facing in the same direction. Use wooden blocks to support each hand in this posture, and lengthen and extend the spine upwards. Begin to increase the timings in these postures.

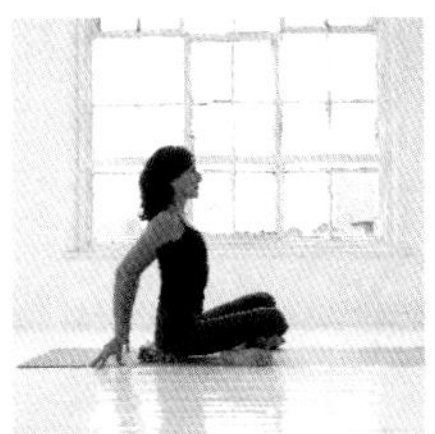
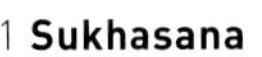

1 **Sukhasana**

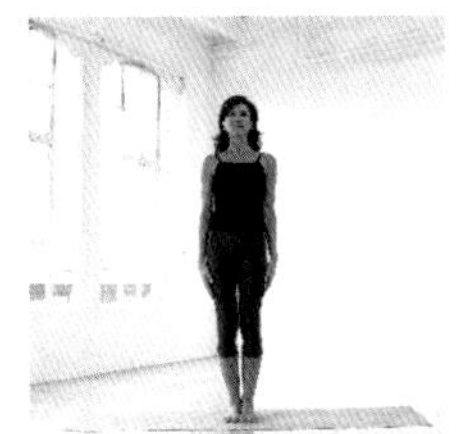

2 **Tadasana**

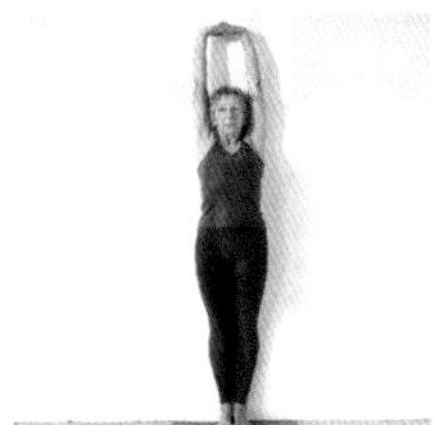

3 **Tadasana** (Parvat.)

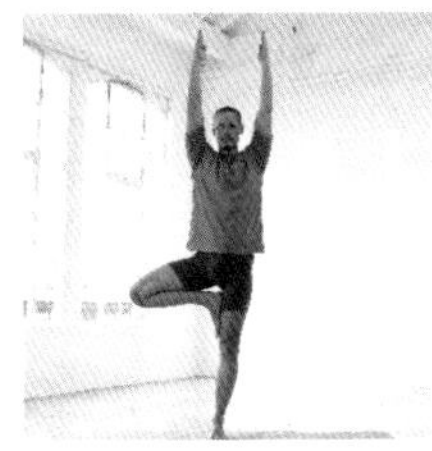

4 **Vrksasana**

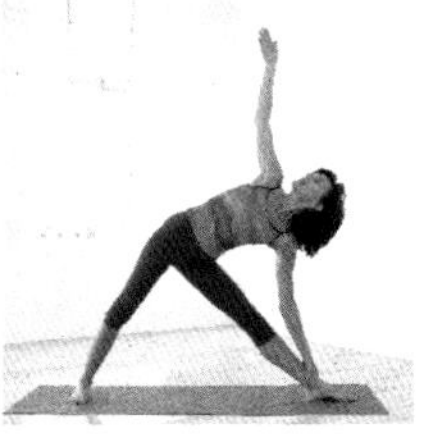

5 **Utthita Trikonasana**

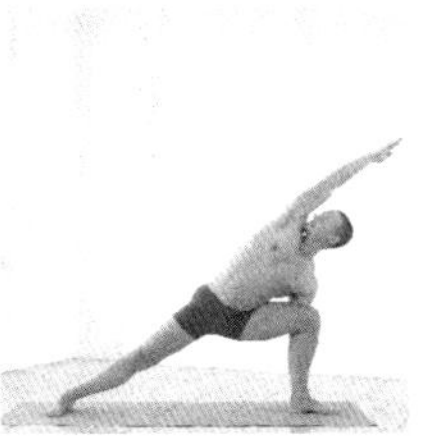

6 **Utthita Parsvakon.**

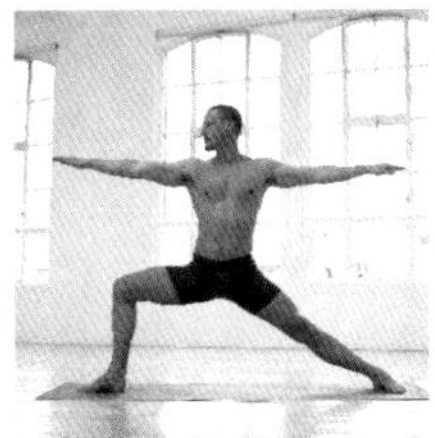

7 **Virabhadrasana II**

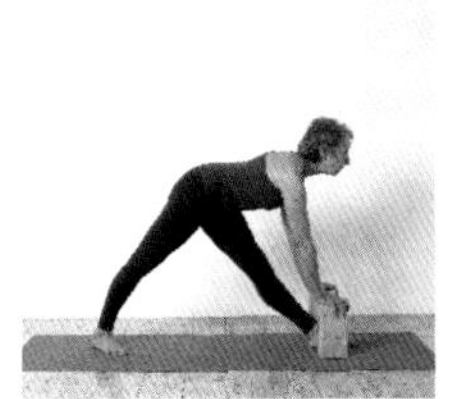

8 **Parsvottanasana** (s)

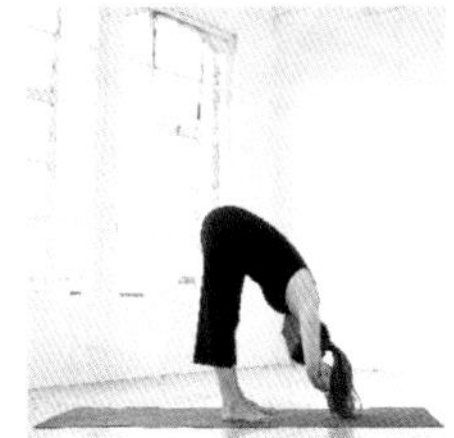

9 **Uttanasana I**

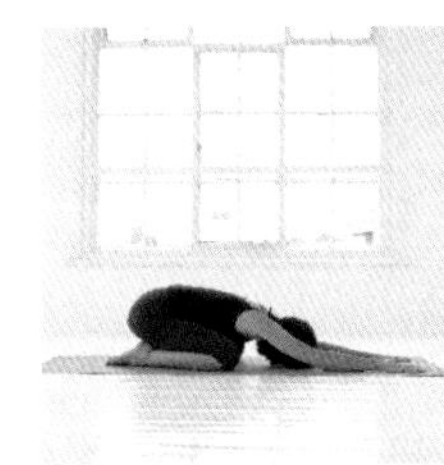

10 **Adho Mukha Vir.**

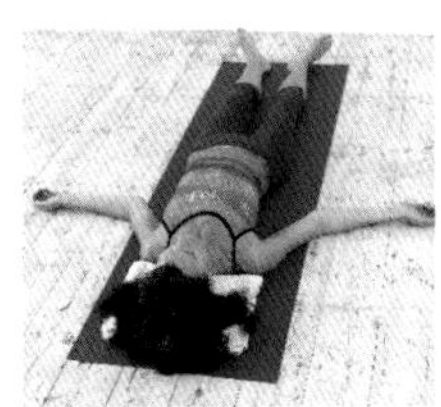

11 **Savasana**

Sequence 4 – Introduction of Salamba Sarvangasana and Ardha Halasana

Virabhadrasana I is brought into this routine as a slightly more challenging standing posture. It is very important to have the back leg well turned in and both hips turned to their maximum in this pose. The back leg in all standing postures is strong and stable – this leg is the "brain" of the posture. If Salamba Sarvangasana is uncomfortable, just lie with the legs up against the wall. Do not do Salamba Sarvangasana or Ardha Halasana if you are menstruating.

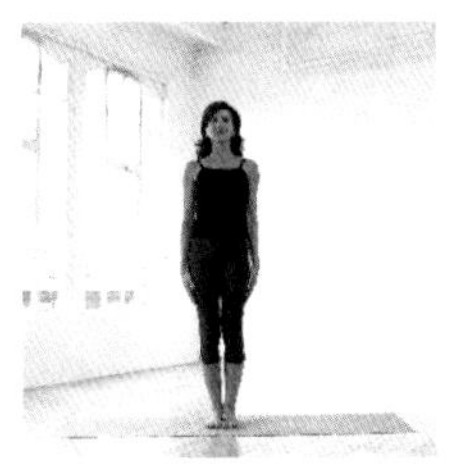

1 **Tadasana**

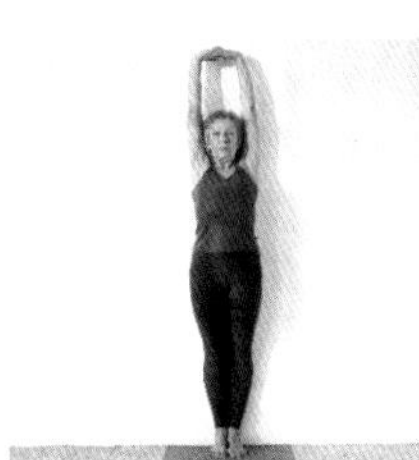

2 **Tadasana** (Parvat.)

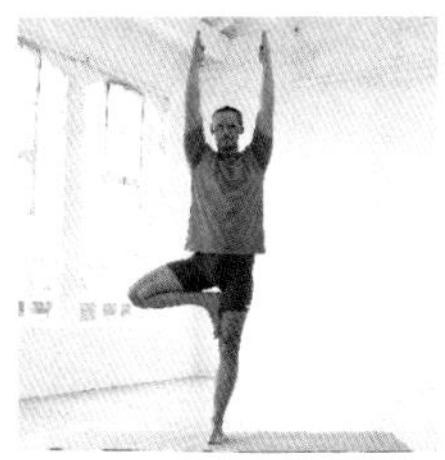

3 **Vrksasana**

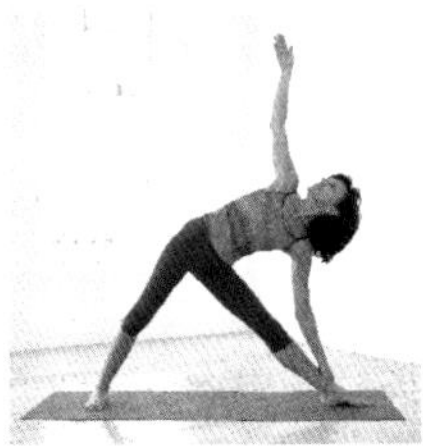

4 **Utthita Trikonasana**

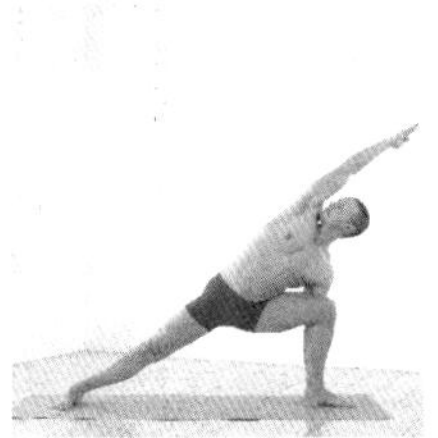

5 **Utthita Parsvakon.**

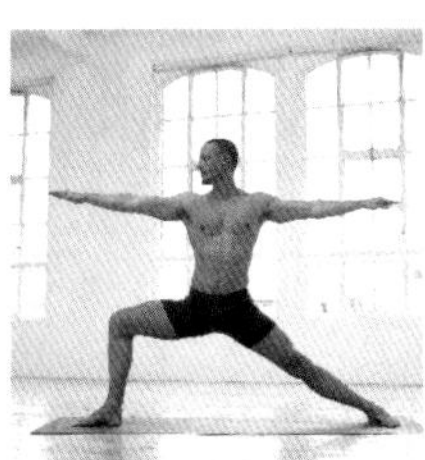

6 **Virabhadrasana II**

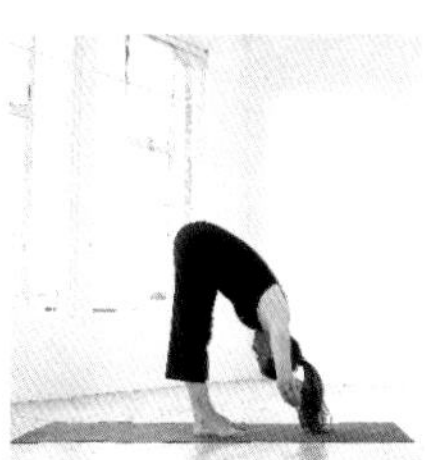

7 **Uttanasana I**

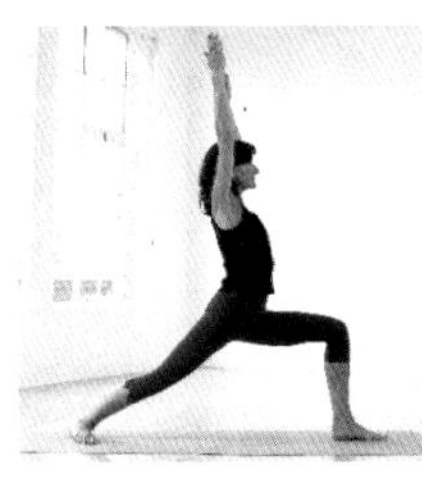

8 **Virabhadrasana I**

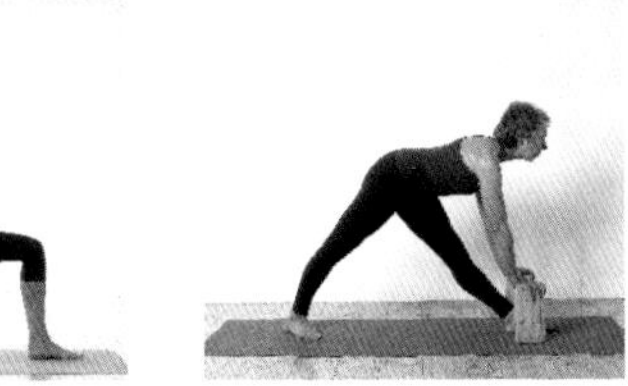

9 **Parsvottanasana** (s)

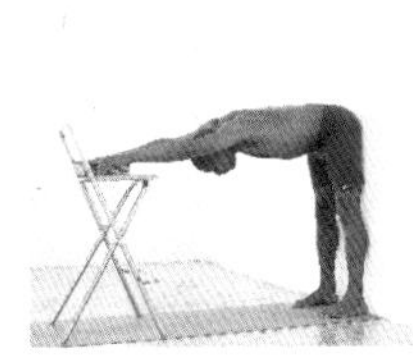

10 **Uttanasana I** (s)

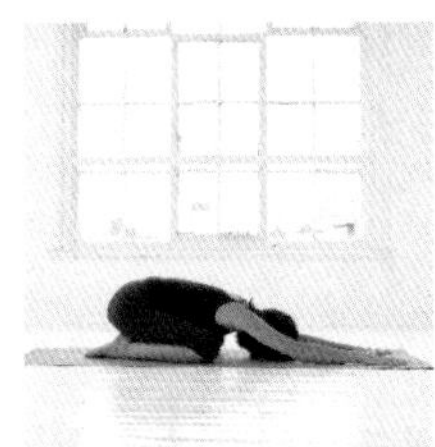

11 **Adho Mukha Vir.**

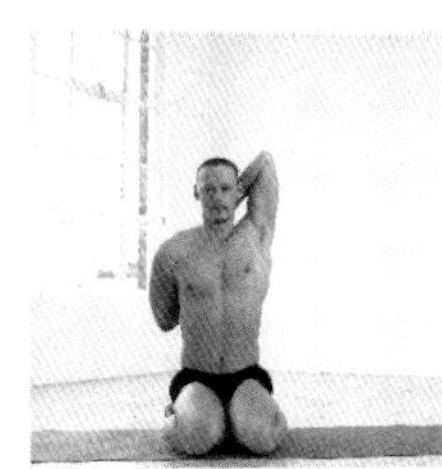

12 **Gomukhasana**

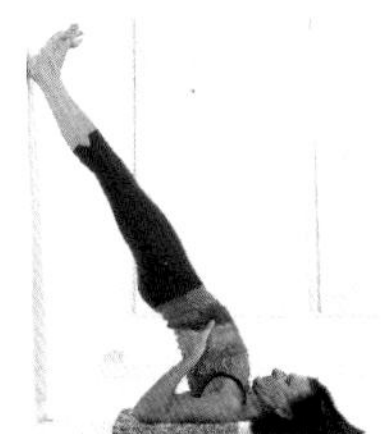

13 **Salamba Sarv.** (w)

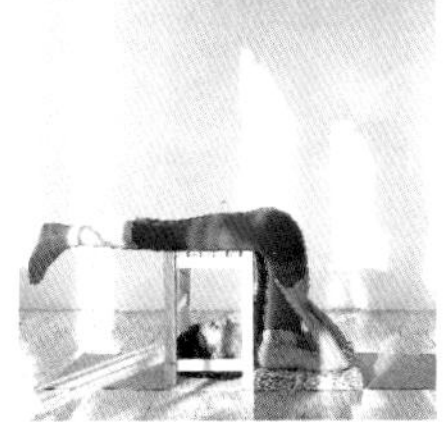

14 **Ardha Halasana**

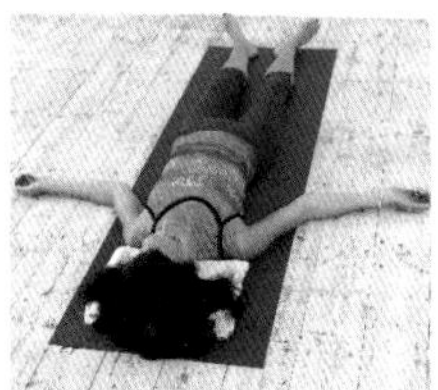

15 **Savasana**

Sequence 5 – Quiet, Calming Practice

This routine focuses on postures with the head supported and the chest lifted. If one is feeling tired or out of sorts, this quietening practice will help. Try to hold the postures for as long as possible in order to experience their calming effects. Keep the face relaxed throughout and the breathing normal, but be aware of the change of depth and rhythm of the breath as one relaxes. In Adho Mukha Svanasana, keep the spine ascending to the ceiling even though the head is down. Move the shoulders towards the front of the chest in order to broaden and create space in the chest cavity.

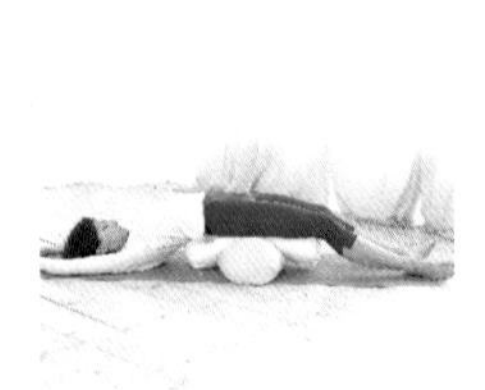
1 **Cross Bolsters**

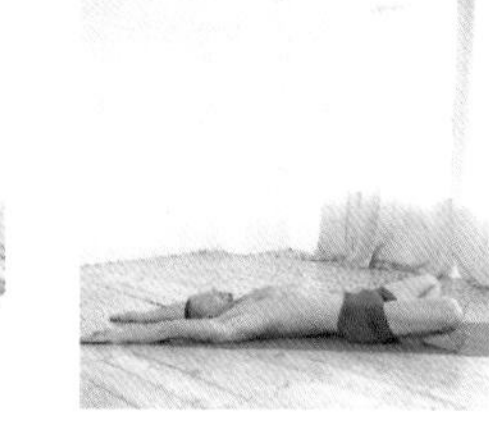
2 **Matsyasana**

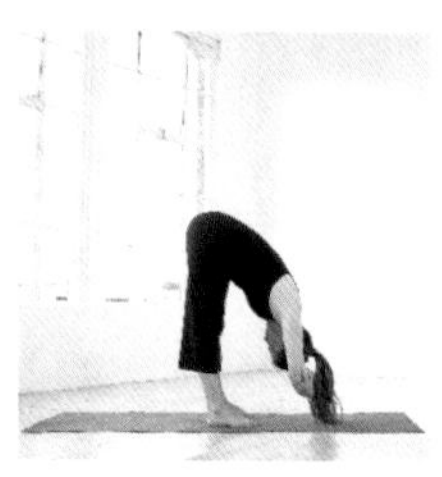
3 **Uttanasana I**

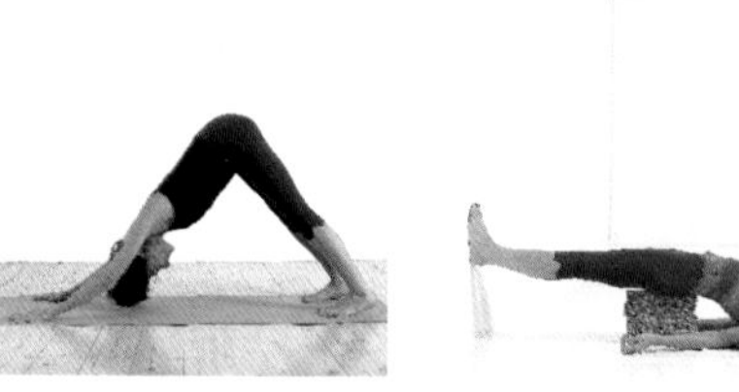
4 **Adho Mukha Svanasana**

5 **Setu Bandha Sarvangasana**

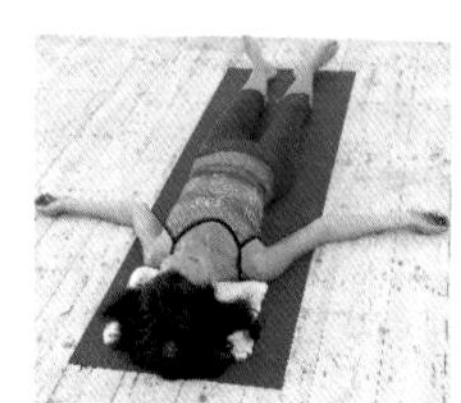
6 **Savasana**

Sequence 6 – Hamstring-stretching Poses

In these standing postures, pay attention to the feet by ensuring the soles of the feet make maximum contact with the floor. Stretch all five toes of each foot into and along the floor, and extend the legs strongly up from the ankles to the hips. In Utthita Hasta Padangusthasana (I & II), ensure the front of the trunk is lengthening up towards the ceiling, and the sides extending. In Prasarita Padottanasana, extend and lengthen the spine forwards before taking the head towards the floor. Pay attention to the feet in this posture. If they roll on to the little toe side, extreme discomfort will be felt on the side of the shin-bones, so ensure that all four corners of the feet are pressing equally into the floor.

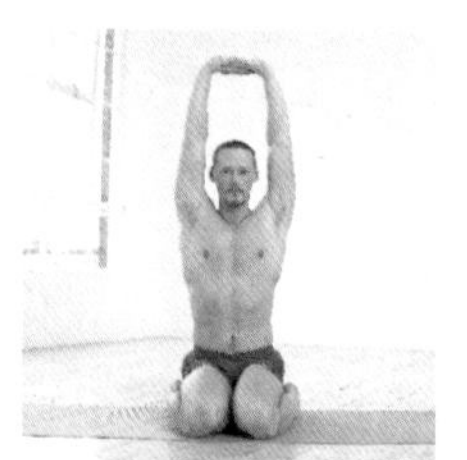
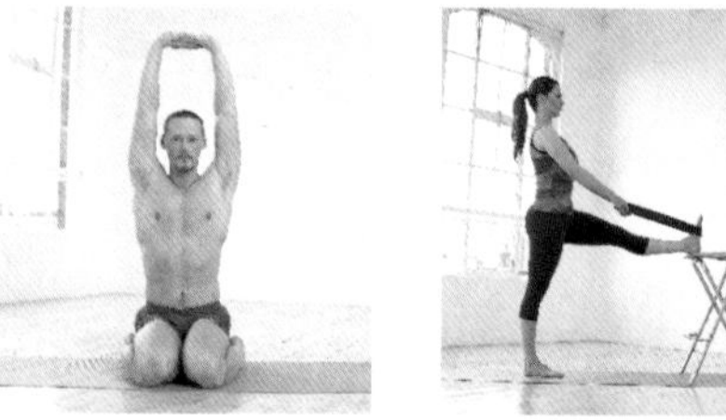
1 **Virasana with Parvatasana**

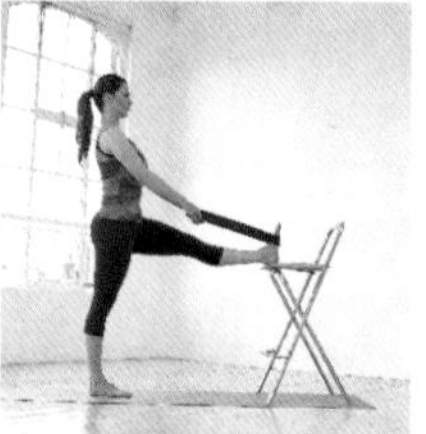
2 **Utthita Hasta Padangusthasana I** (s)

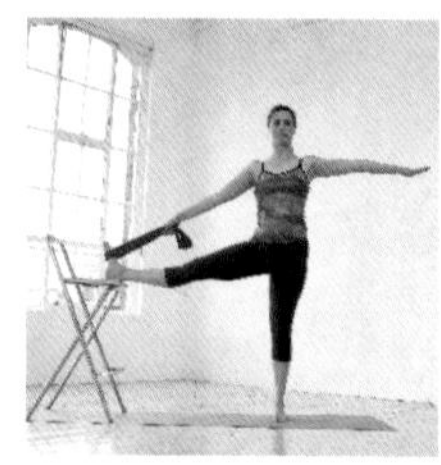
3 **Utthita Hasta Padangusthasana II** (s)

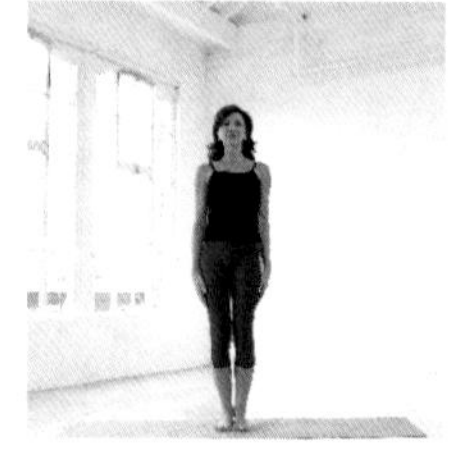
4 **Tadasana**

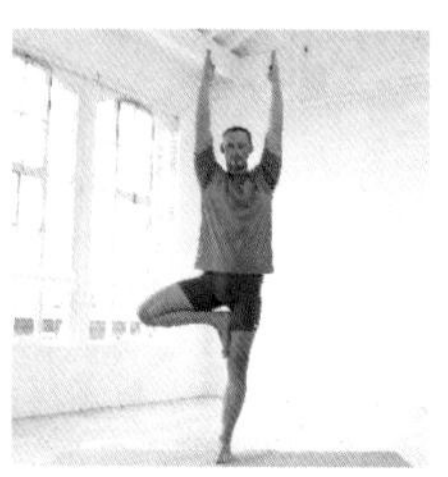
5 **Vrksasana**

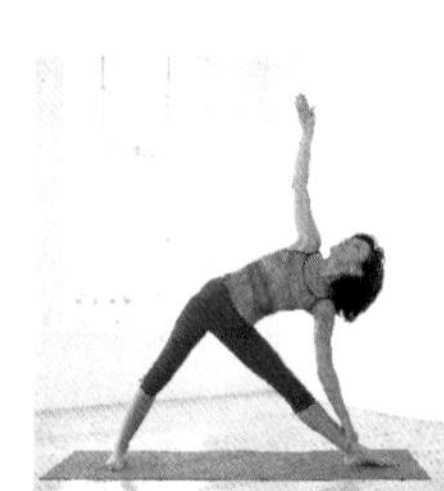
6 **Utthita Trikon.**

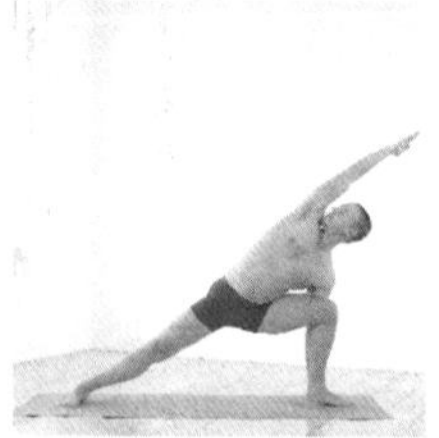
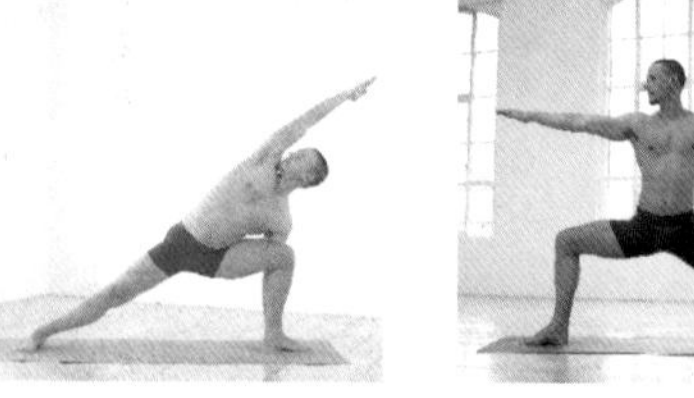
7 **Utthita Parsvakon.**

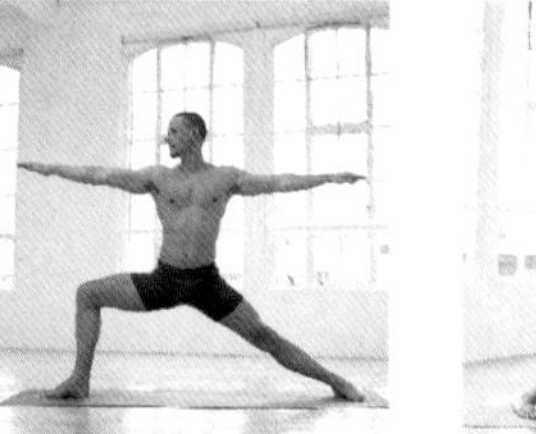
8 **Virabhadrasana II**

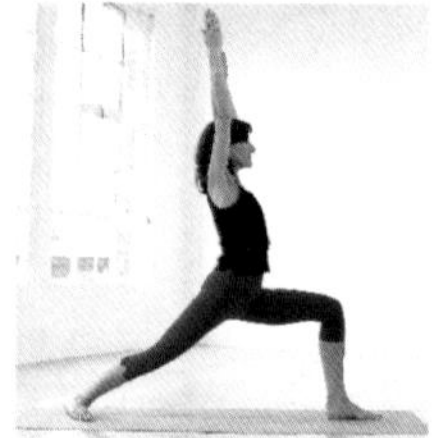
9 **Virabhadrasana I**

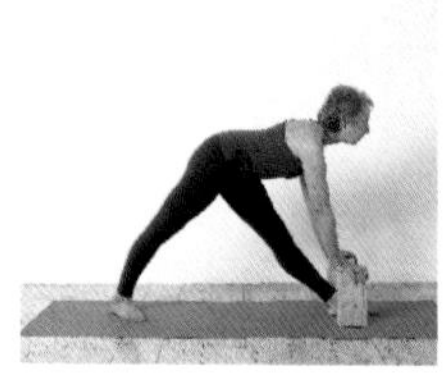
10 **Parsvottan.** (s)

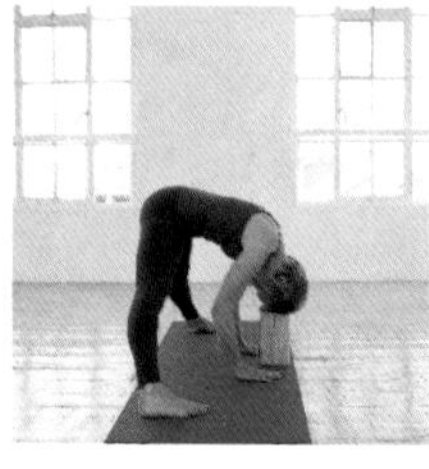
11 **Prasarita Pad.** (s)

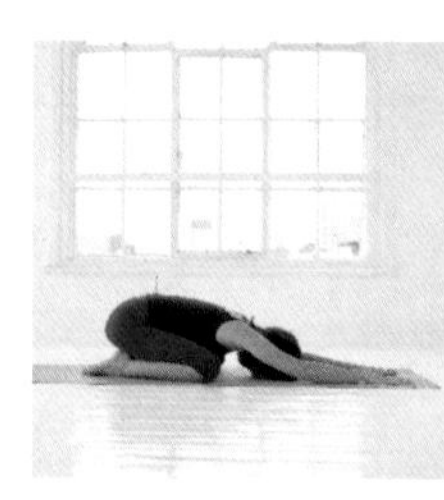
12 **Adho Mukha Vir.**

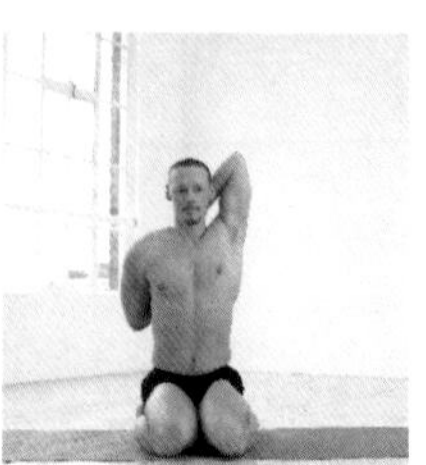
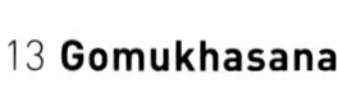
13 **Gomukhasana**

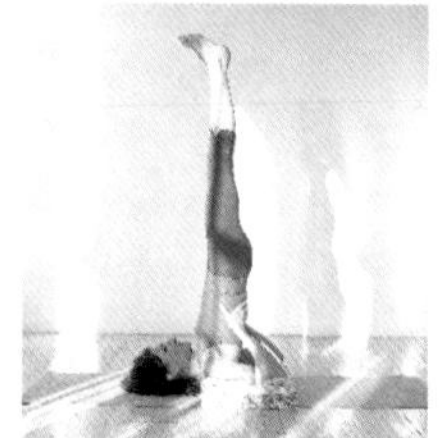
14 **Salamba Sarvang.**

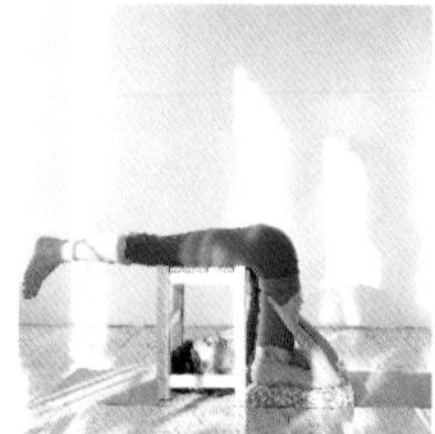
15 **Ardha Halasana**

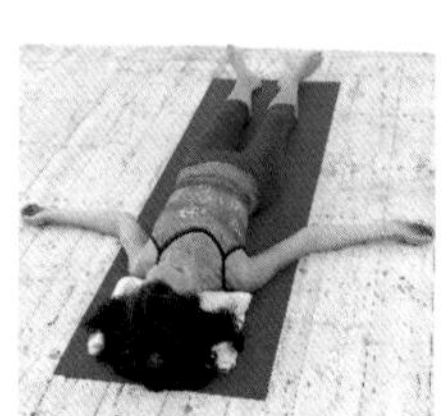
16 **Savasana**

Focus

- Repeat the Sequences 1–5 over a 2–3 week period to consolidate the postures, then continue with Sequences 6–10. Ultimately one's discrimination should be used with regard to the length of time and which postures to practice.

Sequence 7 – Sitting Postures with Simple Twists

In the twisting postures, the spine must first be extended and lengthened, and then turned. Move the whole trunk around when you turn, keep the shoulders moving away from the ears and turn your head without tensing the neck. In Virasana with Parvatasana, ensure that the shoulders move away from the ears so the neck can lengthen and extend.

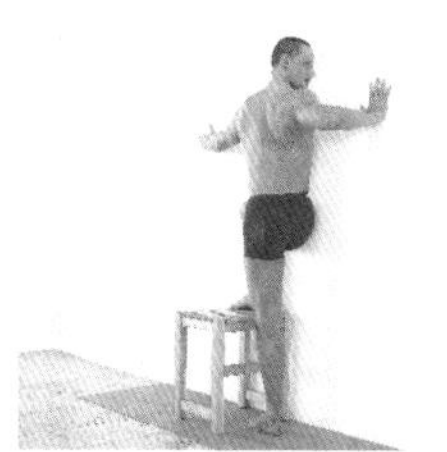
1 **Standing Maricyasana**

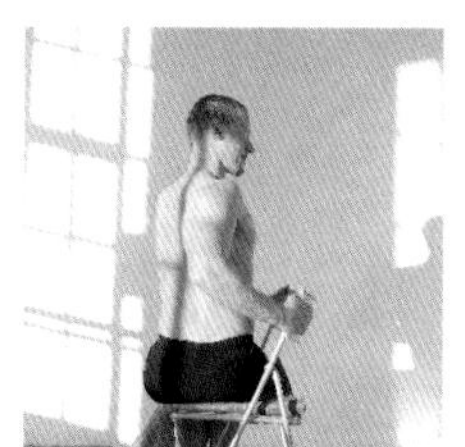
2 **Bharadvajasana**

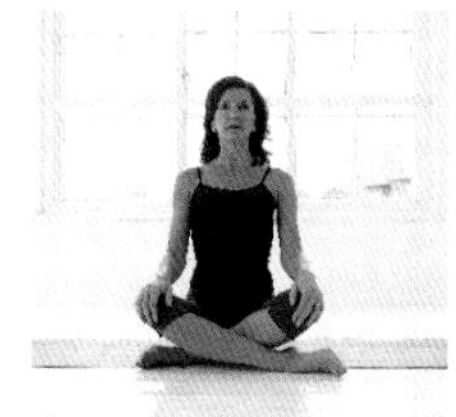
3 **Sukhasana**

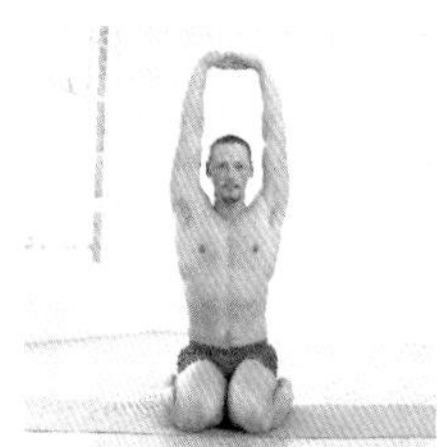
4 **Virasana with Parvatasana**

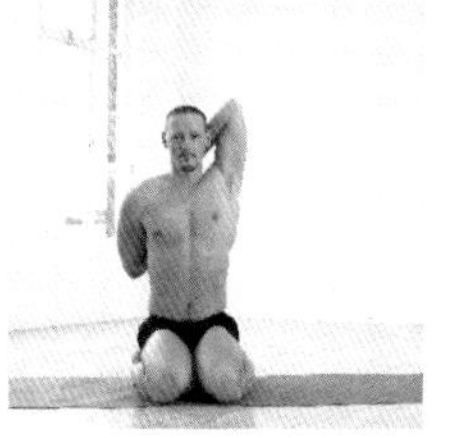
5 **Gomukhasana**

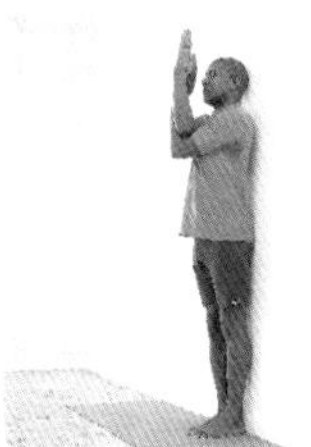
6 **Garudasana** (s)

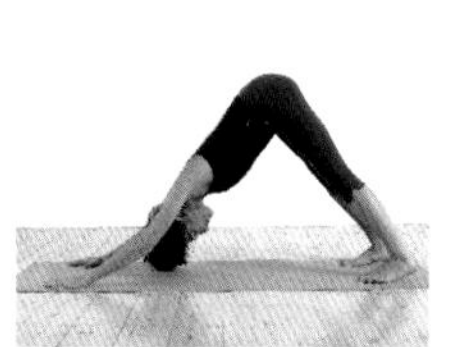
7 **Adho Mukha Svan.**

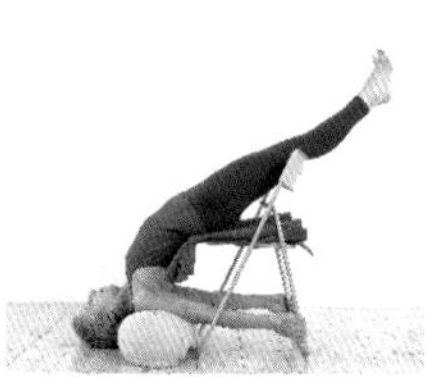
8 **Chair Sarvang.**

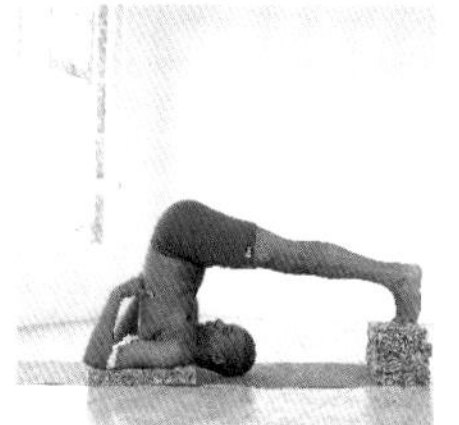
9 **Halasana**

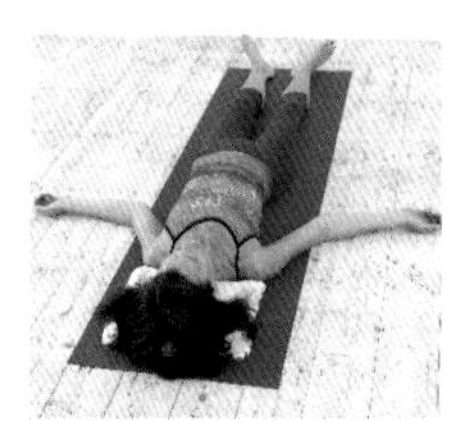
10 **Savasana**

Focus

- Halasana is introduced without a stool for support. If the back aches or the neck becomes painful, use a support (Ardha Halasana) until the discomfort goes away.

Sequence 8 – Introduction of Utkatasana and Garudasana

When the arms are extended, ensure that they stretch from the tops of the shoulders to the tips of the fingers, and keep the palms of the hands broad. Virabhadrasana I can be attempted, but if this causes backache, put the hands on the hips. Garudasana may be done standing in Tadasana, but gradually work towards doing the full posture.

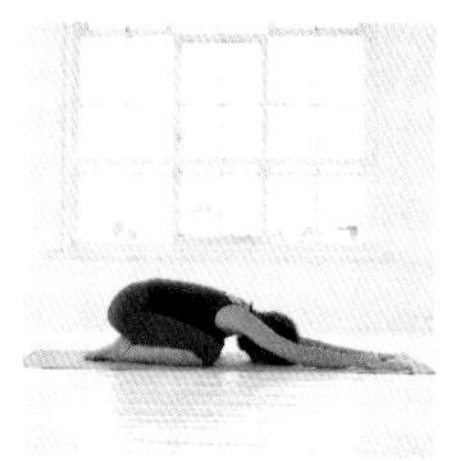
1 **Adho Mukha Vir**

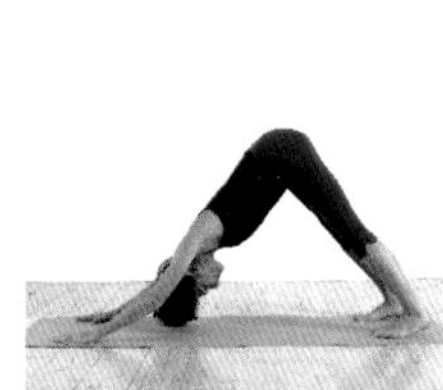
2 **Adho Mukha Svan.**

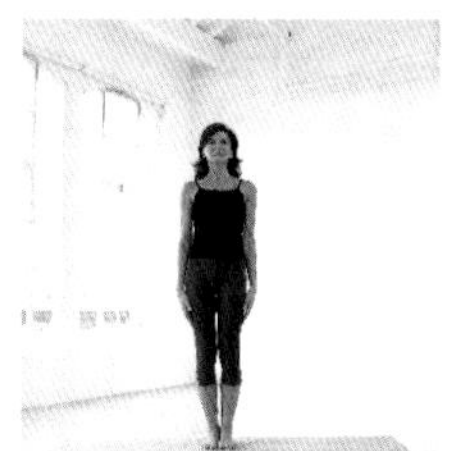
3 **Tadasana**

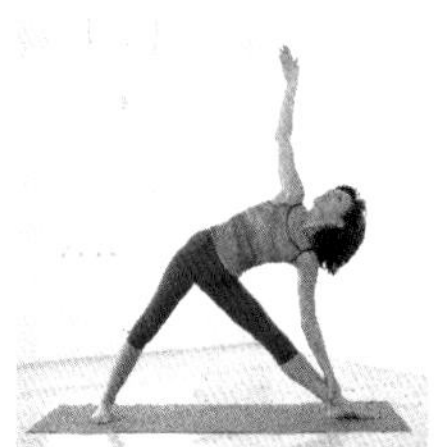
4 **Utthita Trikon.**

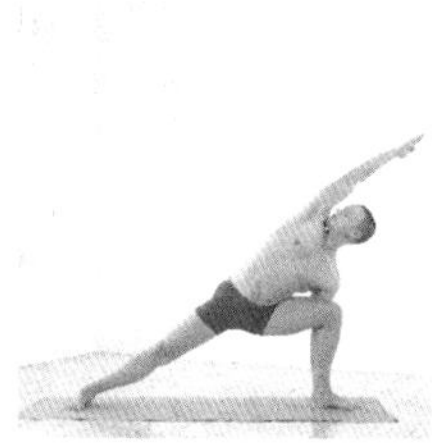
5 **Utthita Parsvakon.**

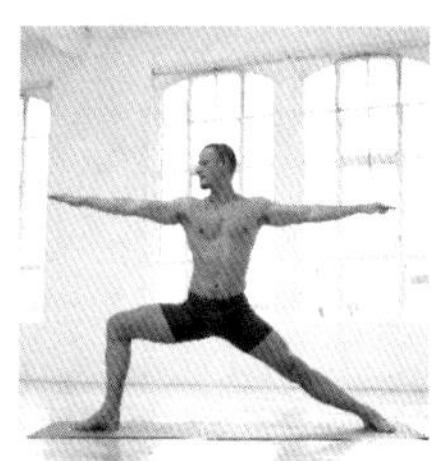
6 **Virabhadrasana II**

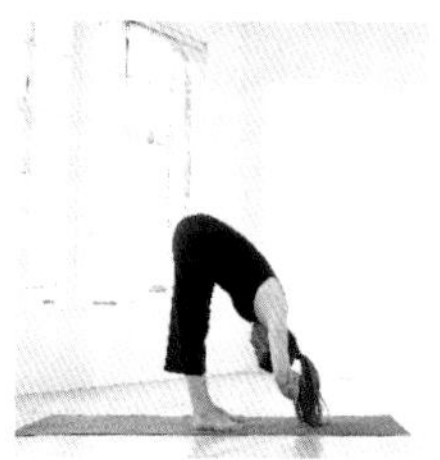
7 **Uttanasana I**

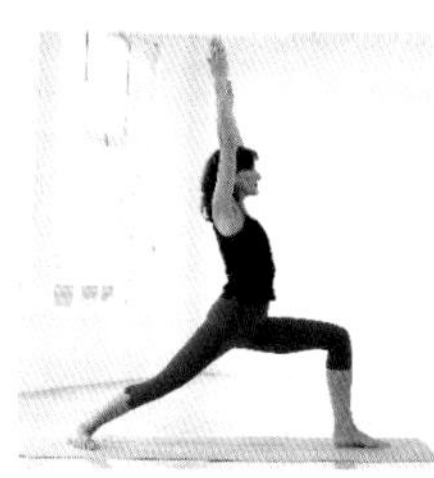
8 **Virabhadrasana I**

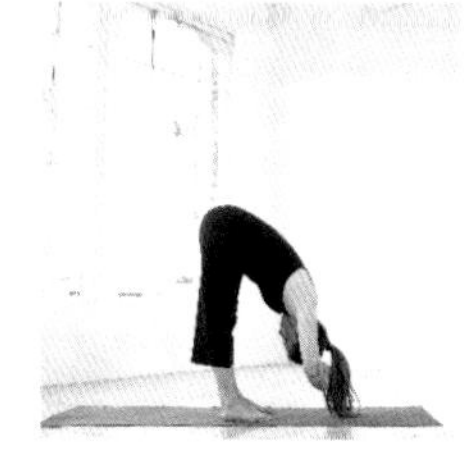
9 **Uttanasana I**

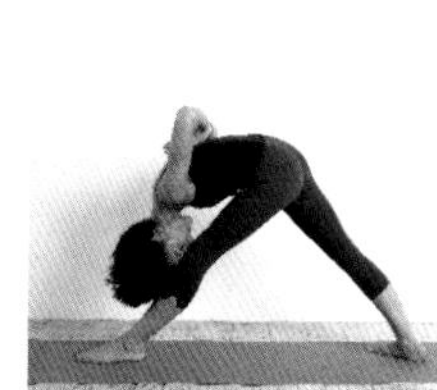
10 **Parsvottanasana**

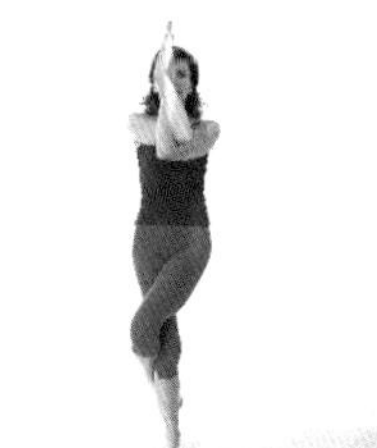
11 **Garudasana**

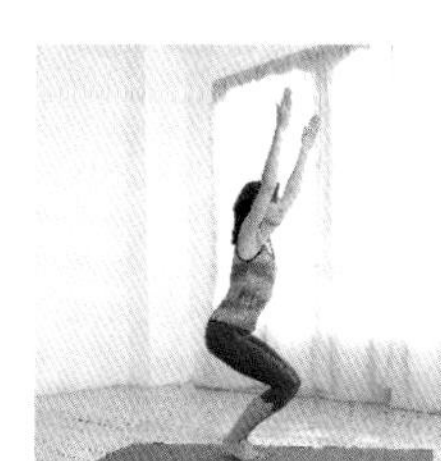
12 **Utkatasana**

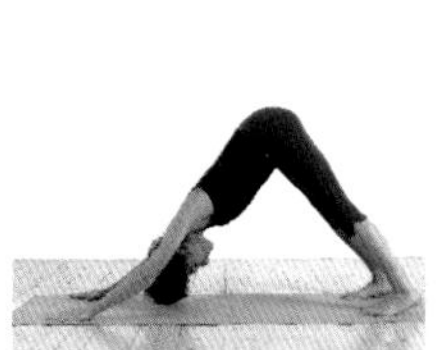
13 **Adho Mukha Svan.**

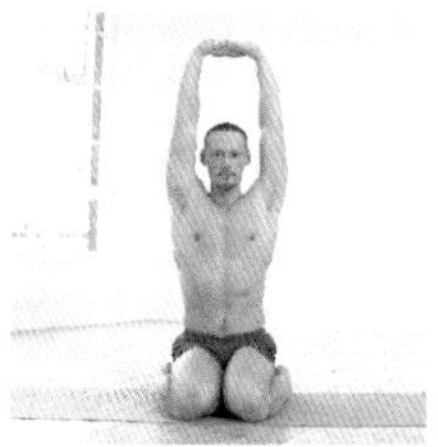
14 **Virasana/Parvat.**

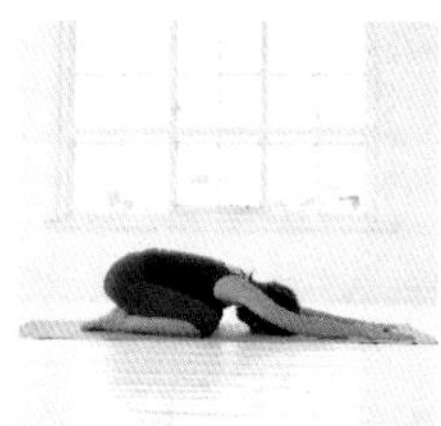
15 **Adho Mukha Vir.**

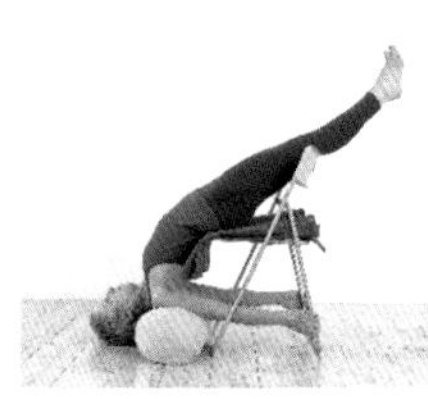
16 **Chair Sarvang.**

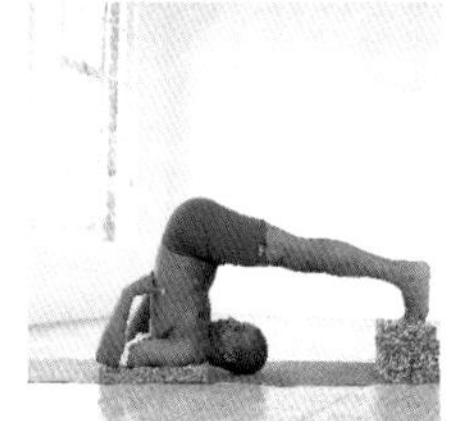
17 **Halasana** (s)

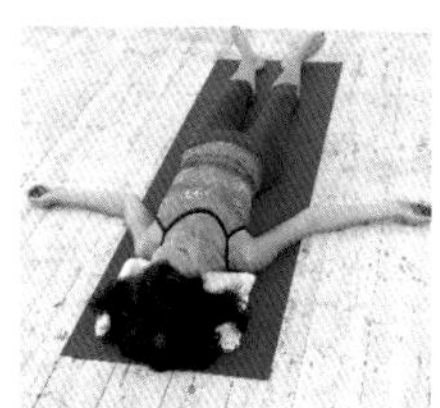
18 **Savasana**

Sequence 9 – Relaxation Practice

Ensure that the chest is lifted and open in these postures. The brain should remain passive and the mind quietly focusing on the breath throughout the poses. These postures can be held for 3–5 minutes to gain maximum benefit. If the muscles of the groin are painful in Supta Baddhakonasana, place foam blocks under each thigh to lessen the stretch. If the back and/or knees hurt in Supta Virasana, add as much support as is needed to relieve the discomfort. To eliminate visual distractions, close your eyes and keep them still, focusing on the breath.

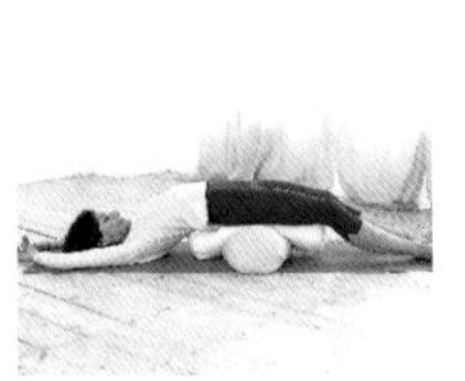

1 **Cross Bolsters**

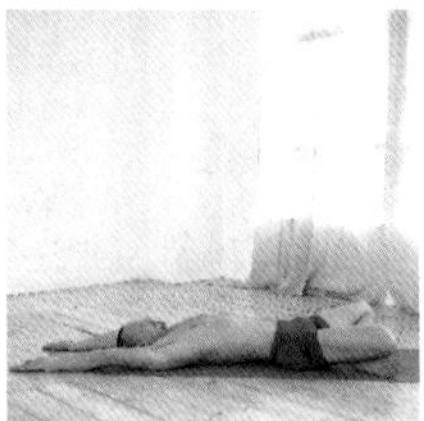

2 **Matsyasana**

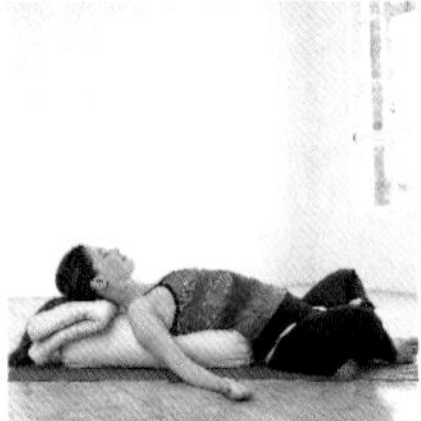

3 **Supta Baddhkonasana**

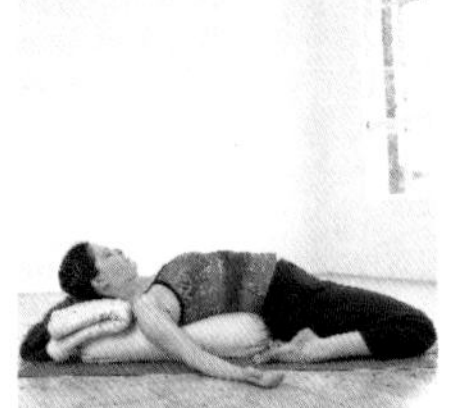

4 **Supta Virasana**

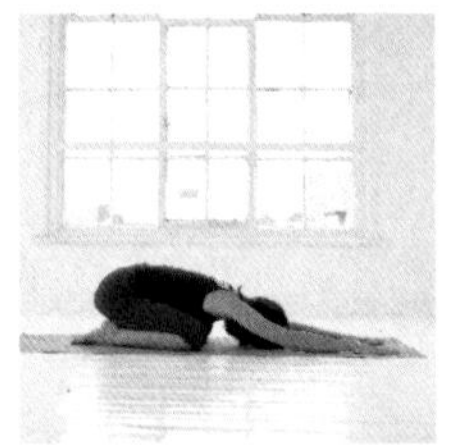

5 **Adho Mukha Virasana**

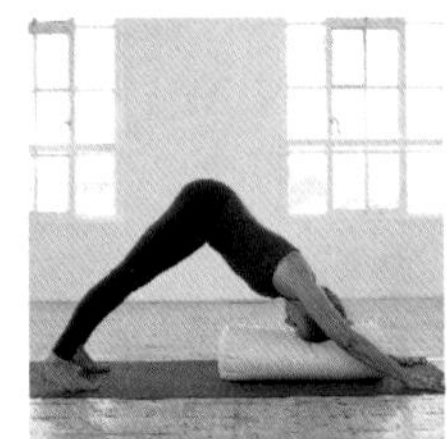

6 **Adho Mukha Svanasana**

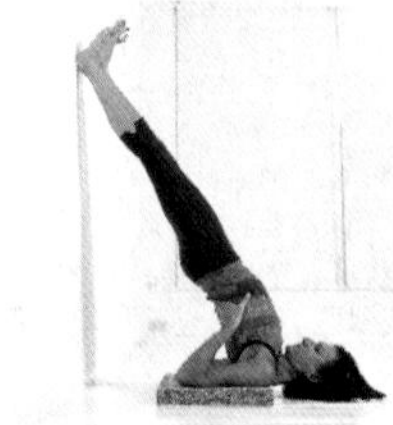

7 **Salamba Sarv.** (w)

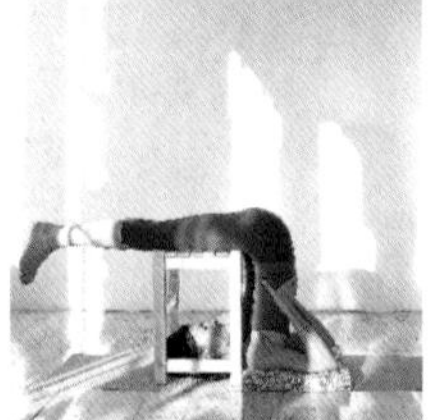

8 **Ardha Halasana**

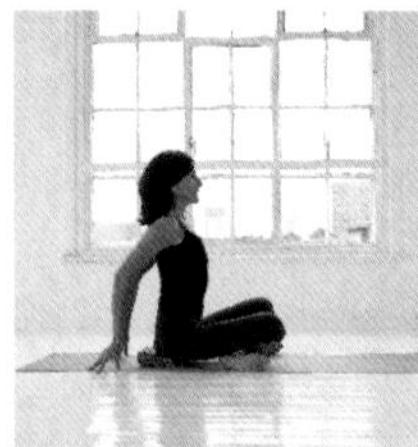

9 **Sukhasana**

Focus

- Practise Sequences 6–10 by repeating them over several weeks and learn to increase timings before proceeding to the next five.

Sequence 10 – Introduction to Seated Forward Bends

Sit on a support for these seated postures to help lift the spine. The forward bends are done with a concave back, an action achieved by lifting and opening the chest, moving the shoulders away from the ears and moving the shoulder blades towards the front of the body. If the back hurts, hold a strap caught around the foot, so the angle between the trunk and the leg lessens and the backache is relieved. Keep the arms straight when holding the strap. In Urdhva Prasarita Padasana, the entire back of both legs (from buttock bones to heels) should be against the wall.

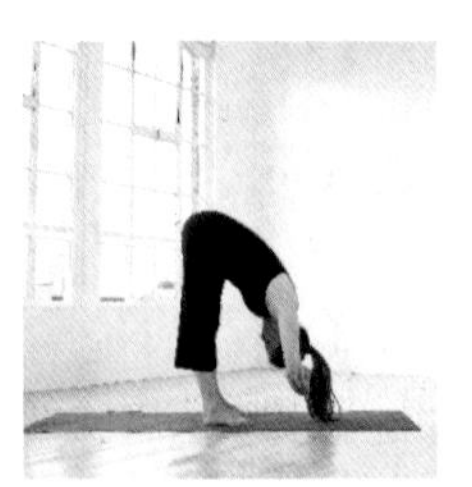

1 **Uttanasana I**

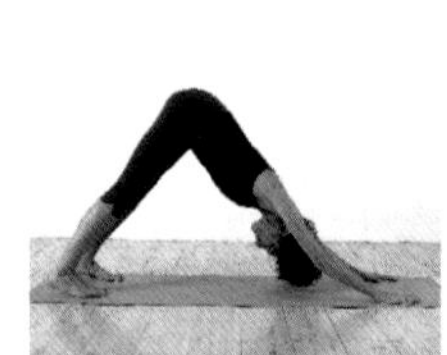

2 **Adho Mukha Svanasana**

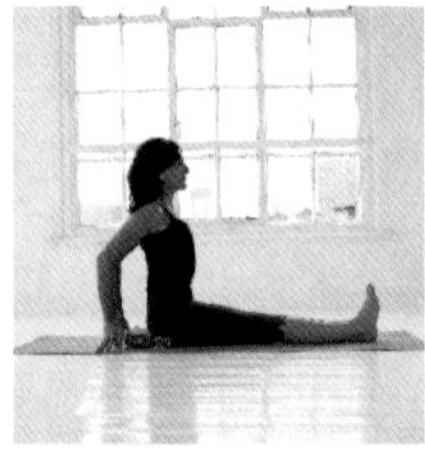

3 **Dandasana**

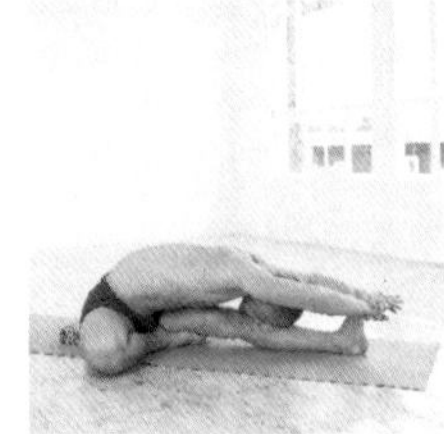

4 **Janusirsasana**

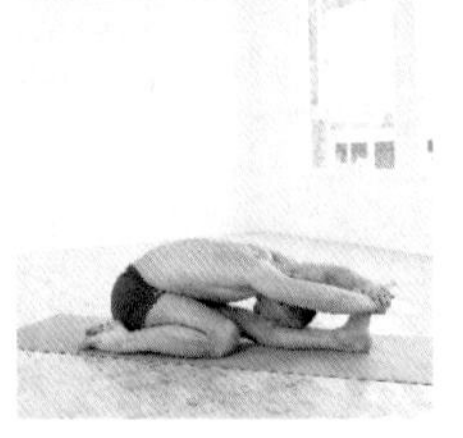

5 **Trianga Mukha. Pascimottanasana**

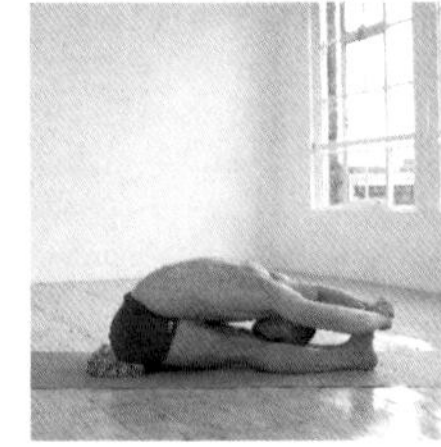

6 **Pascimottanasana**

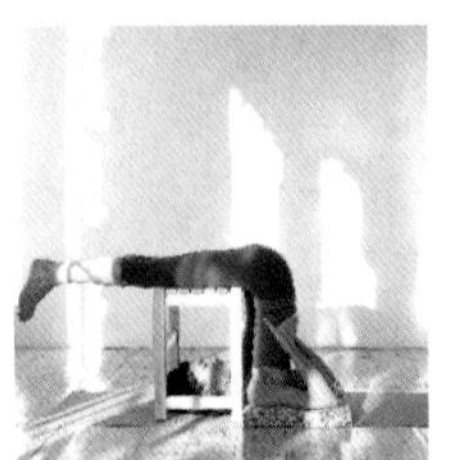

7 **Ardha Halasana**

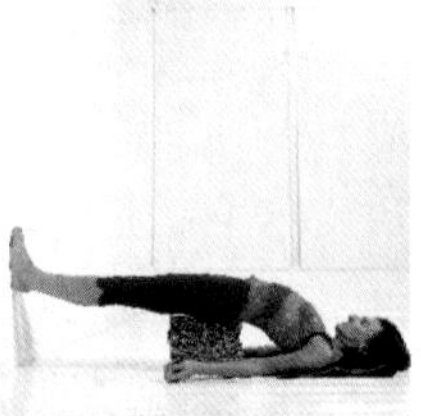

8 **Setu Bandha Sarvangasana**

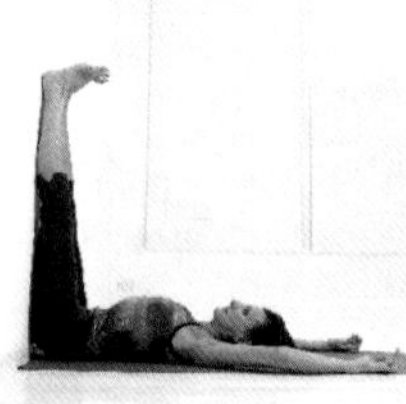

9 **Urdhva Prasarita Padasana**

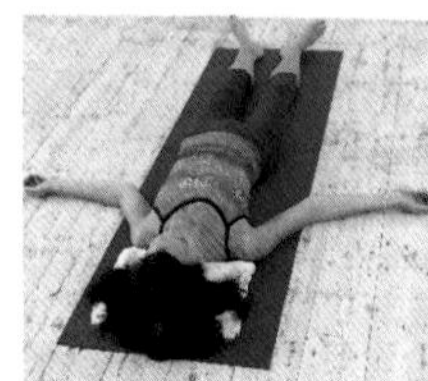

10 **Savasana**

Sequence 11 - Standing Poses Held for Longer

This sequence consolidates the standing postures and should be done with more awareness and attention to detail. If discomfort is experienced, try to locate it, think about what has caused it and, by understanding the technique of the pose, try to remove it. Try to hold each posture for a little longer than you have done previously.

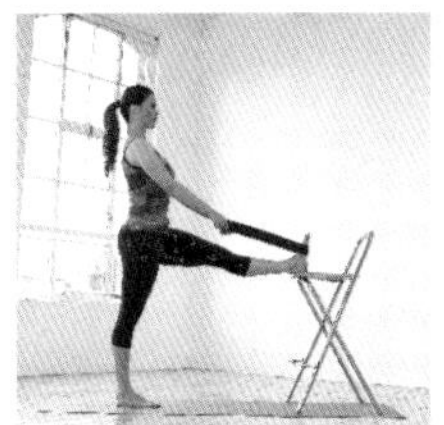

1 **Utthita Hasta Padangusthasana I** (s)

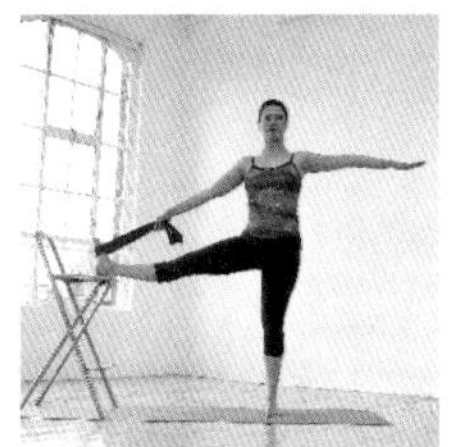

2 **Utthita Hasta Padangusthasana II** (s)

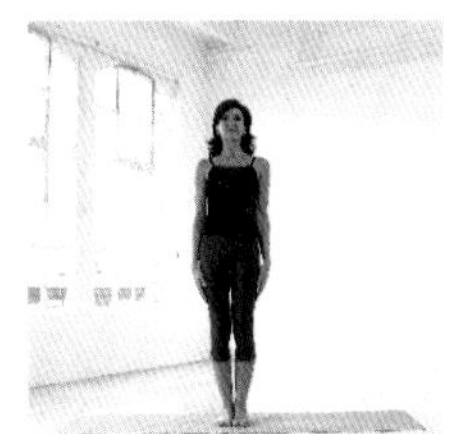

3 **Tadasana**

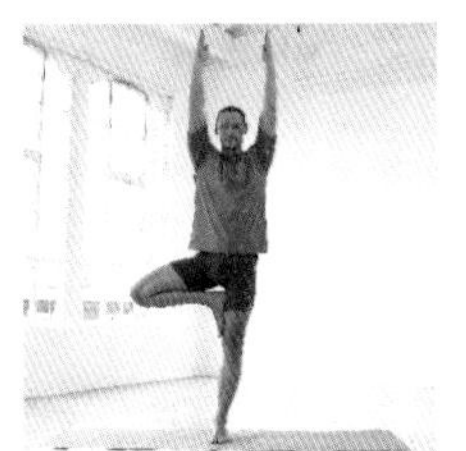

4 **Vrksasana**

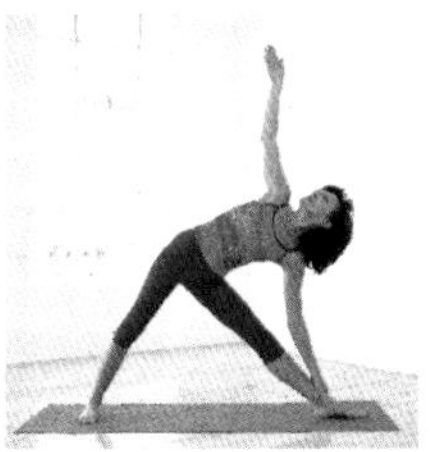

5 **Utthita Trikonasana**

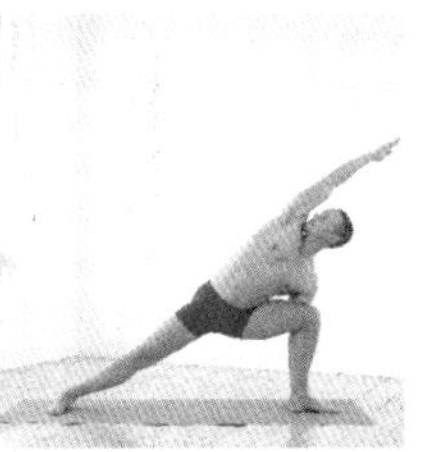

6 **Utthita Parsvakonasana**

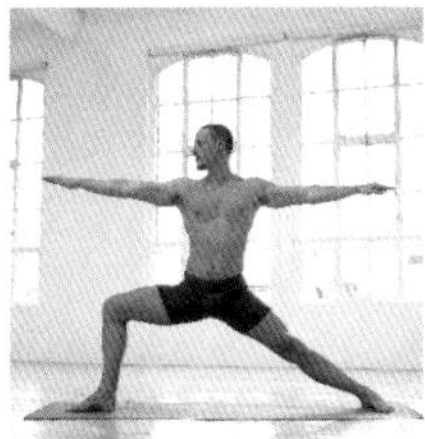

7 **Virabhadrasana II**

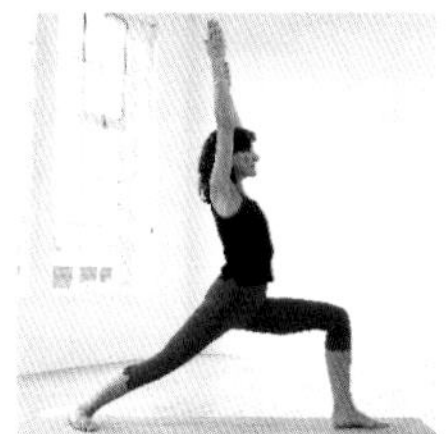

8 **Virabhadrasana I**

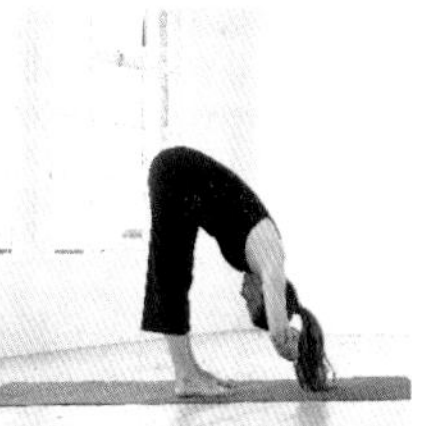

9 **Uttanasana I**

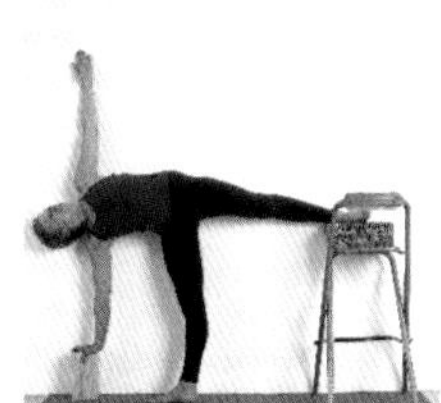

10 **Ardha Chandr.** (s)

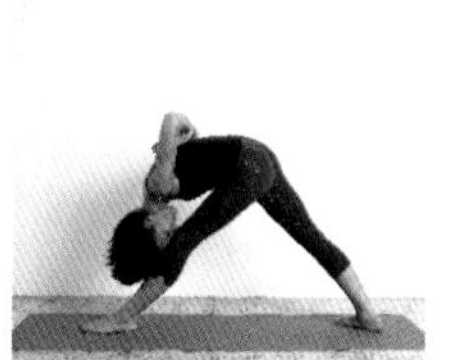

11 **Parsvottanasana**

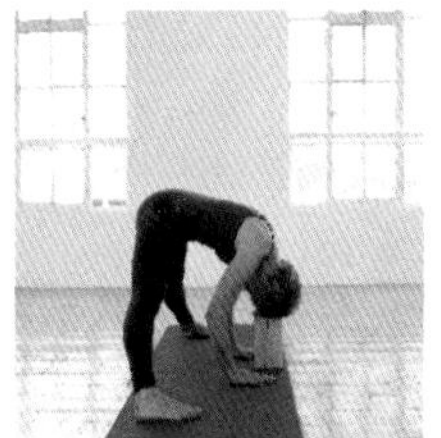

12 **Prasarita Pad.** (s)

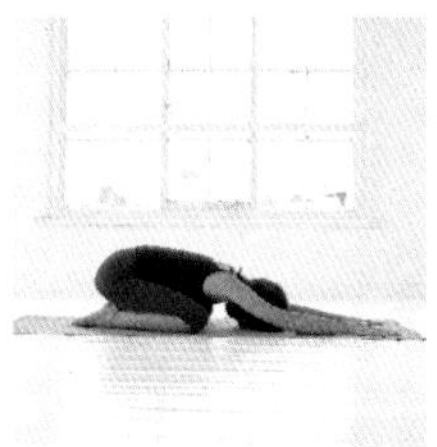

13 **Adho Mukha Vir.**

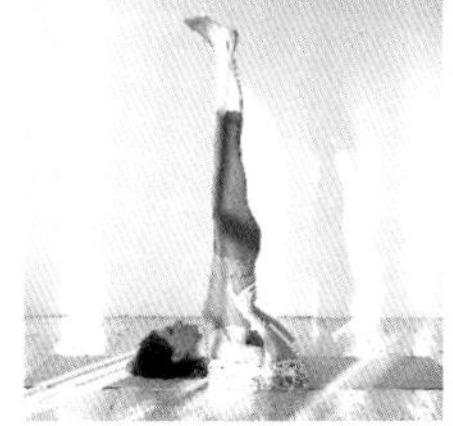

14 **Salamba Sarvang.**

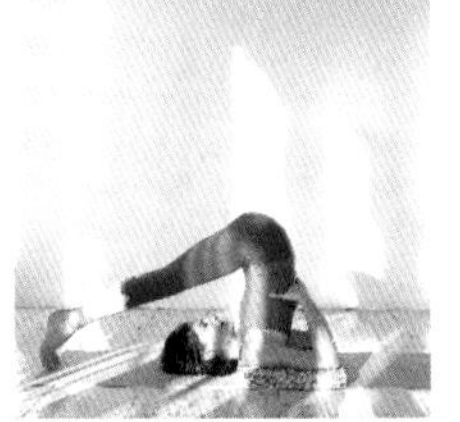

15 **Halasana**

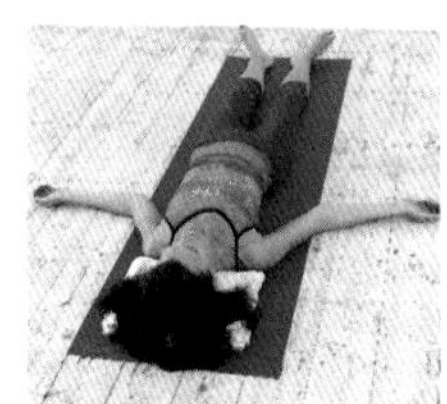

16 **Savasana**

Focus

- This sequence should take longer than the others so far, as the timing of each posture is increased.

Sequence 12 – Increased Timings in Seated Forward Bends with Concave Back

Doing the forward bends with a concave back improves the elasticity of the spine and helps to open the chest. The whole trunk must be lengthened. When looking up, be careful not to compress the back of the neck.

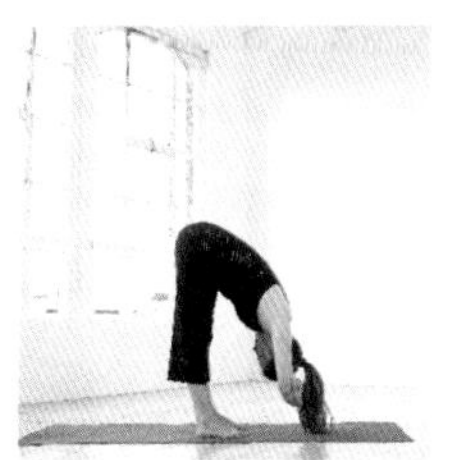

1 **Uttanasana I**

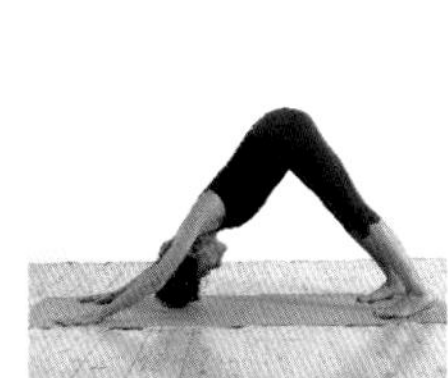

2 **Adho Mukha Svanasana**

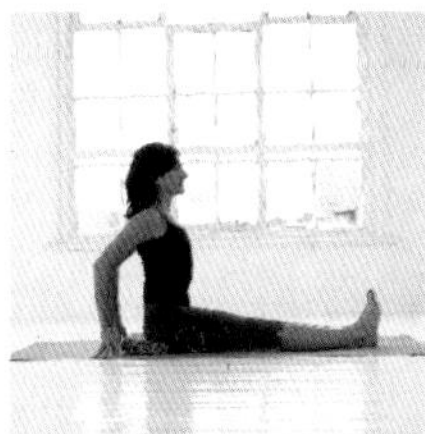

3 **Dandasana**

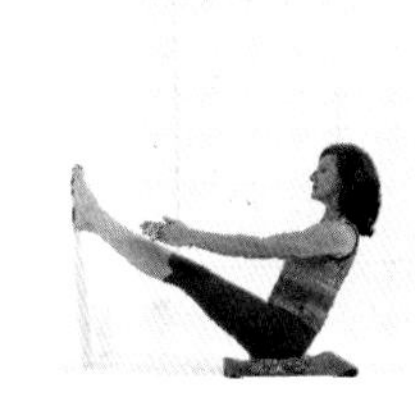

4 **Paripurna Navasana** (s)

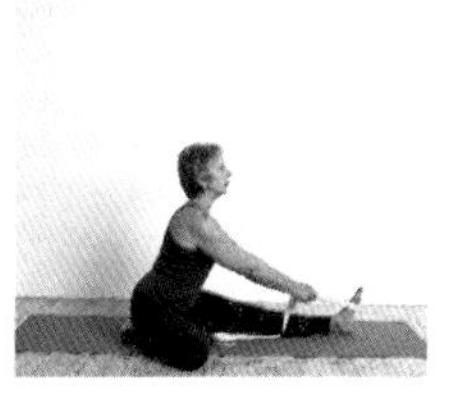

5 **Janusirsasana** (s)

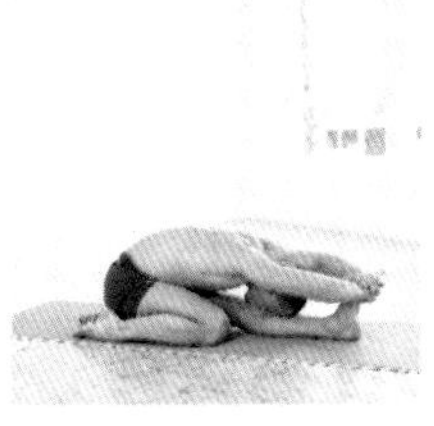

6 **Trianga Mukha. Pascimottanasana**

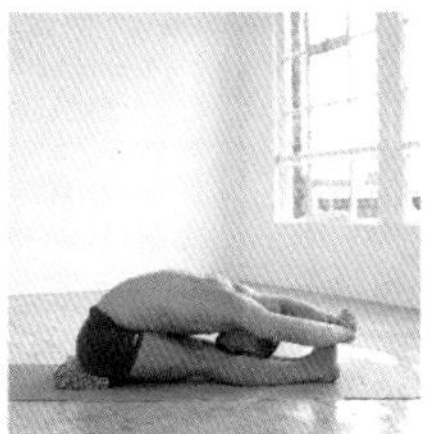

7 **Pascimottanasana**

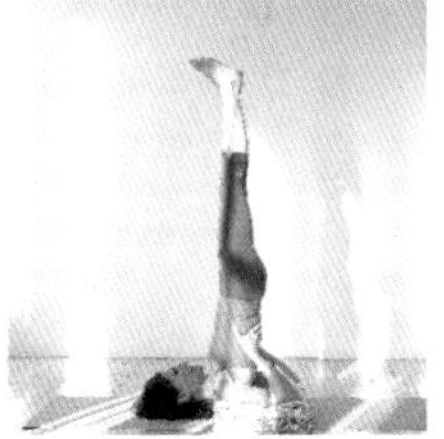

8 **Salamba Sarvang.**

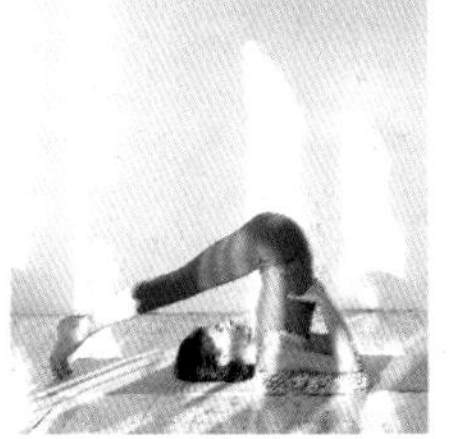

9 **Halasana**

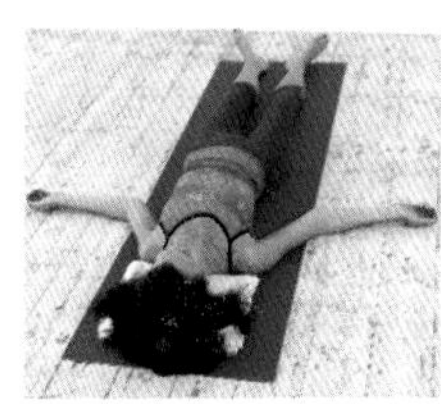

10 **Savasana**

Focus

- In Paripurna Navasana, lift the trunk upwards. If the lower back becomes painful, do the posture with the fingertips on the floor.

Sequence 13 – Basic Standing Postures and Introducing Seated Postures

Try to practise the standing postures with less strain and more composure. By now the technicalities of the poses should be physically ingrained, so try to just "be" in the posture and allow the psychological effects to emerge.

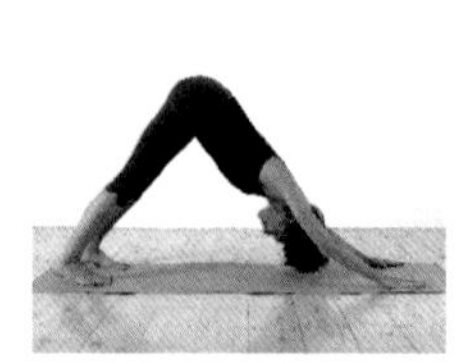
1 **Adho Mukha Svan.**

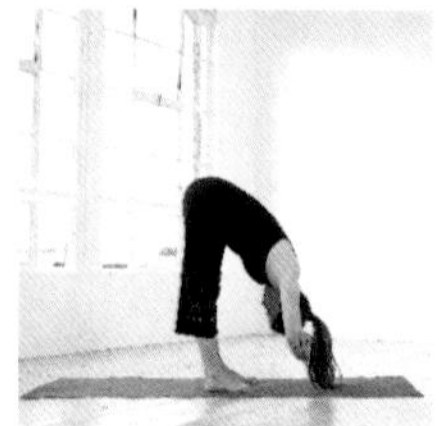
2 **Uttanasana I**

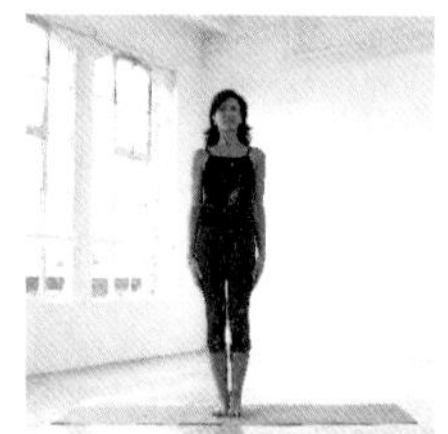
3 **Tadasana**

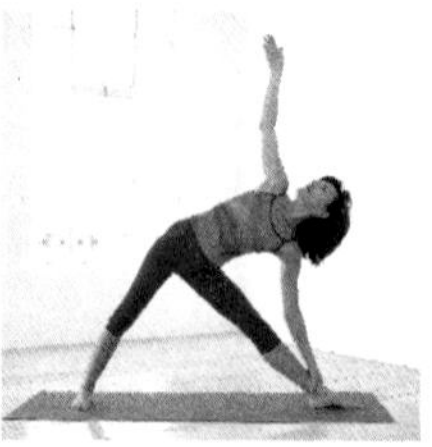
4 **Utthita Trikonasana**

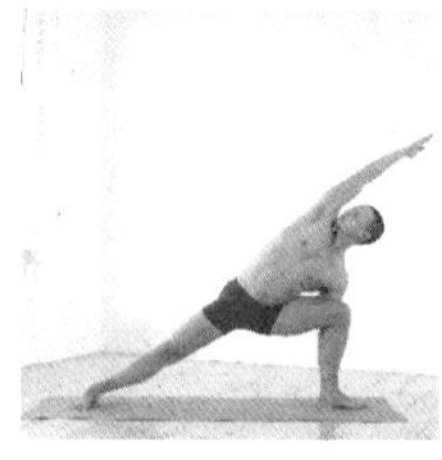
5 **Utthita Parsvakon.**

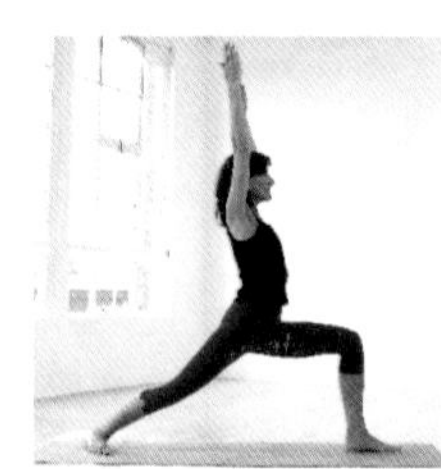
6 **Virabhadrasana I**

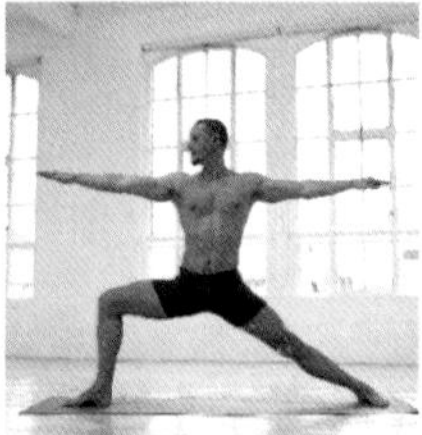
7 **Virabhadrasana II**

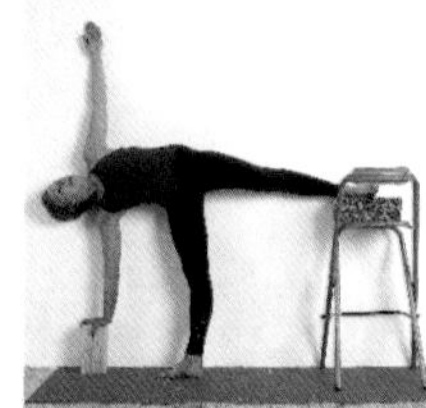
8 **Ardha Chandr.** (s)

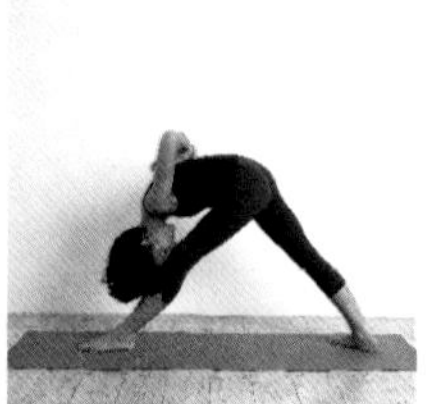
9 **Parsvottansana**

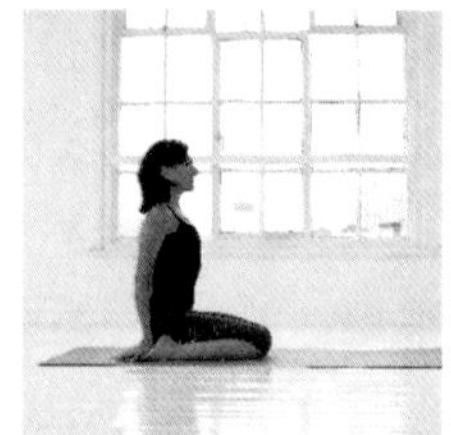
10 **Virasana**

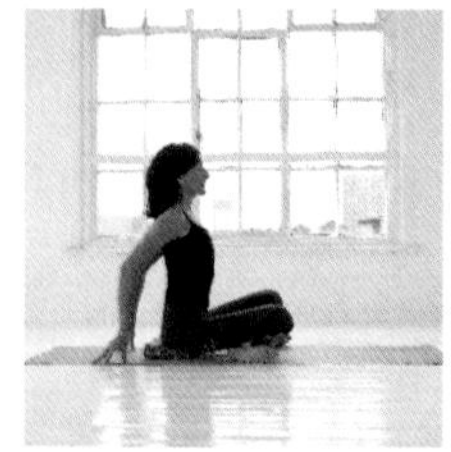
11 **Sukhasana**

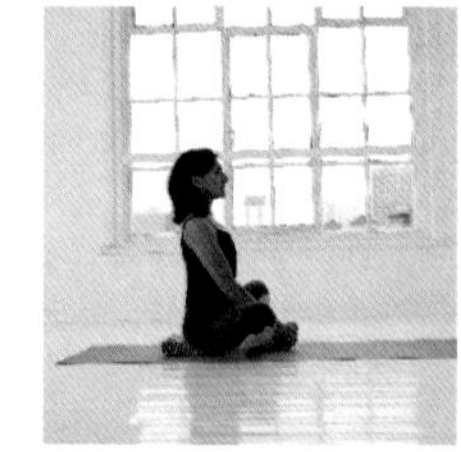
12 **Baddhakonasana**

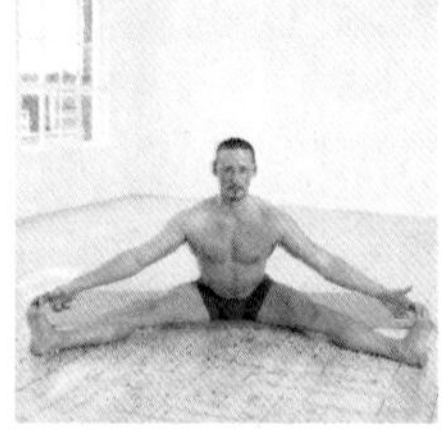
13 **Upavistakonasana**

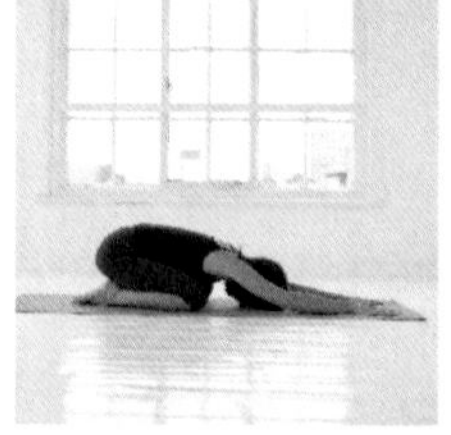
14 **Adho Mukha Vir.**

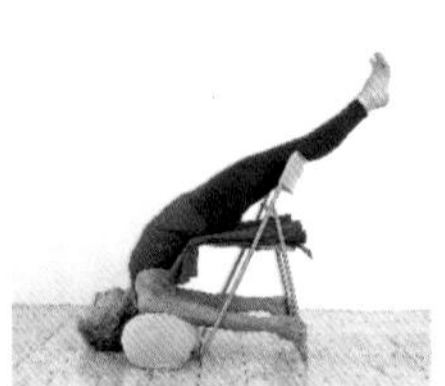
15 **Chair Sarvang.**

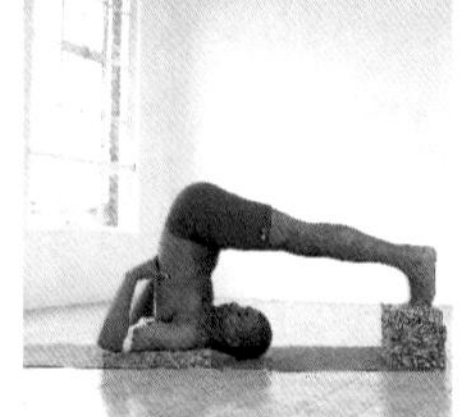
16 **Halasana** (s)

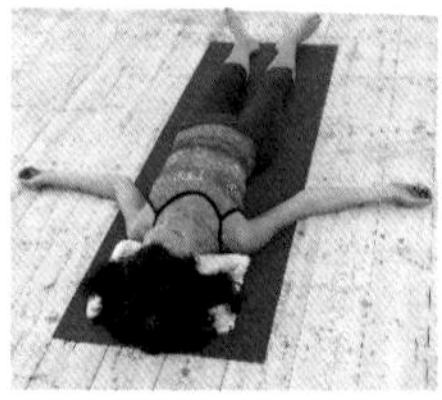
17 **Savasana**

Sequence 14 – Twists and Seated Forward Bends

After doing the first two twists, which allow the spine to extend and rotate, the forward bends become easier. In this sequence, full forward bend poses are done, where the trunk is extended and, if possible, the foot of this leg is caught with the hands. If you cannot reach the foot or the lower back is painful, catch a strap around the foot.

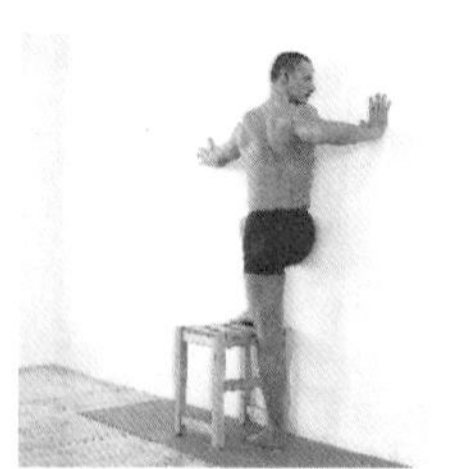
1 **Standing Maricyasana**

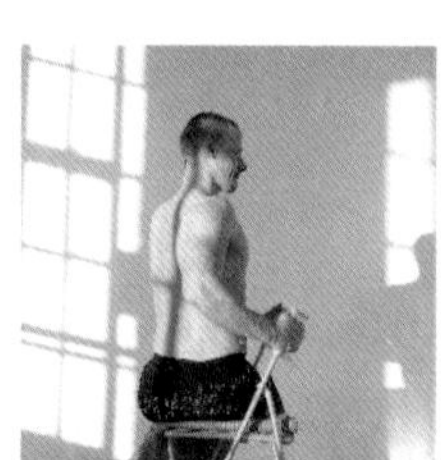
2 **Bharadvajasana (chair)**

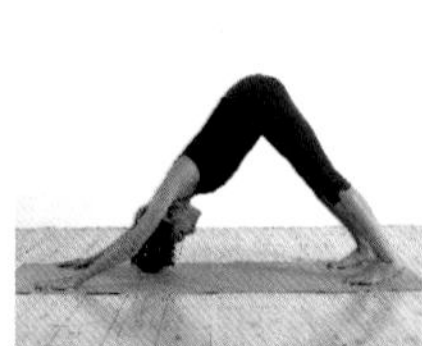
3 **Adho Mukha Svanasana**

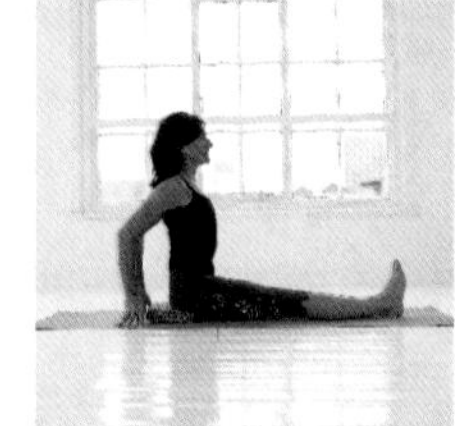
4 **Dandasana**

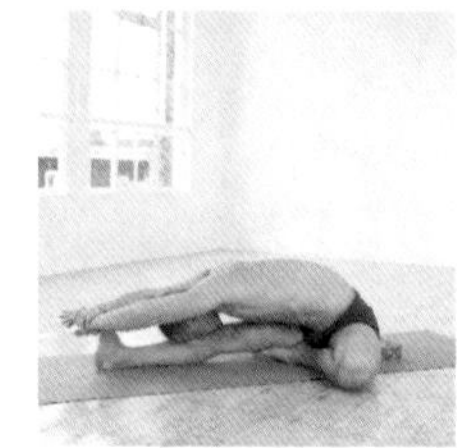
5 **Janusirasana**

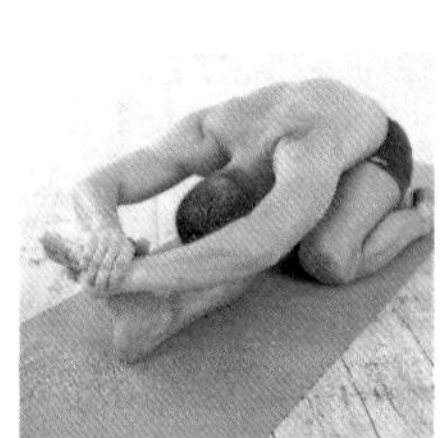
6 **Trianga Mukha. Pascimottanasana**

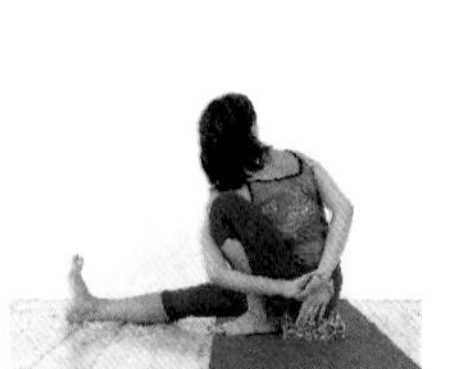
7 **Maricyasana I**

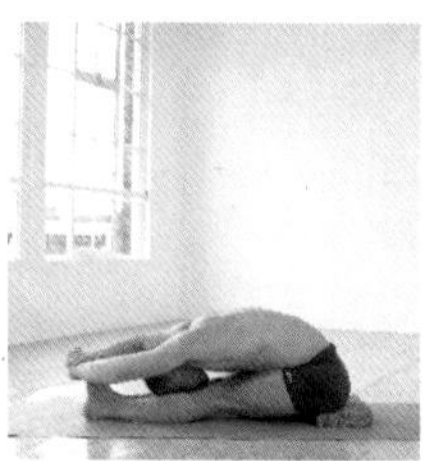
8 **Pascimottanasana**

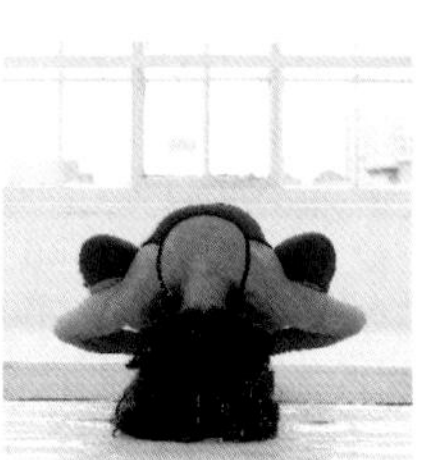
9 **Malasana**

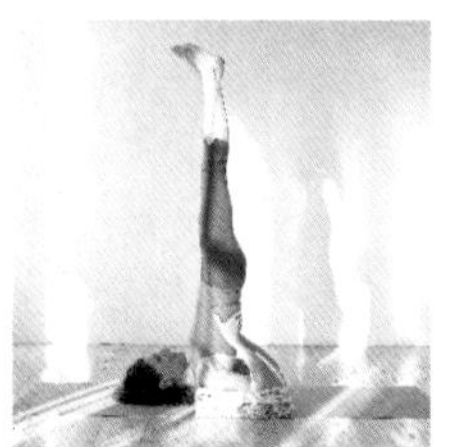
10 **Salamba Sarvang.**

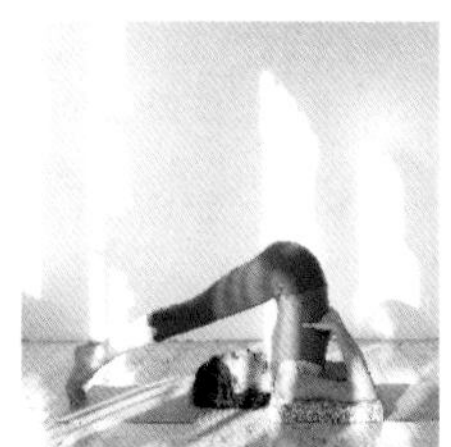
11 **Halasana**

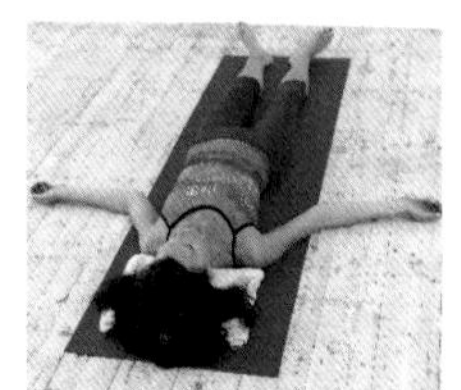
12 **Savasana**

Sequence 15 – Relaxing and Recuperative Postures

This sequence should not be rushed and the postures can be safely held for up to 5 minutes. The chest should be lifted and open, the eyes soft and closed, the facial features relaxed and the brain calm and focused on the breathing. Do not fall asleep, just relax and breathe. The back should feel comfortable in all the poses, so use support if necessary.

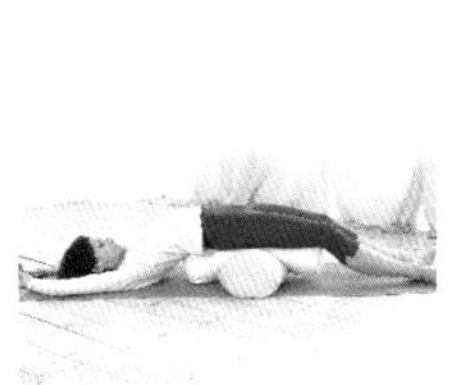
1 **Cross Bolsters**

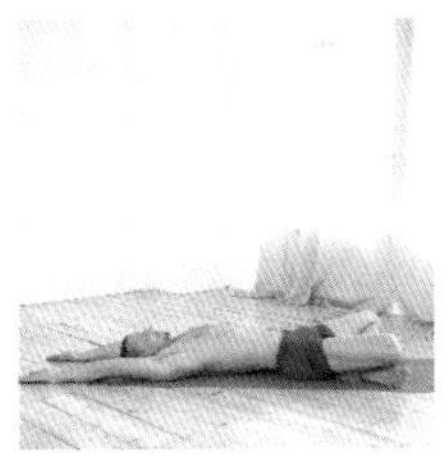
2 **Matsyasana**

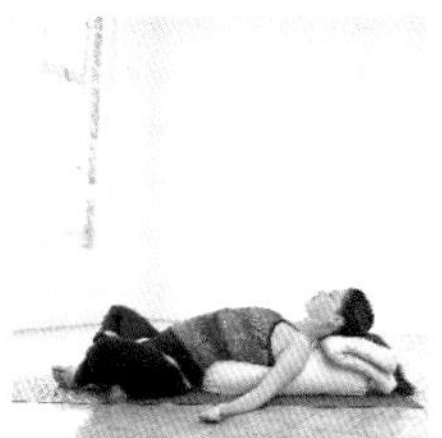
3 **Supta Baddhakon.**

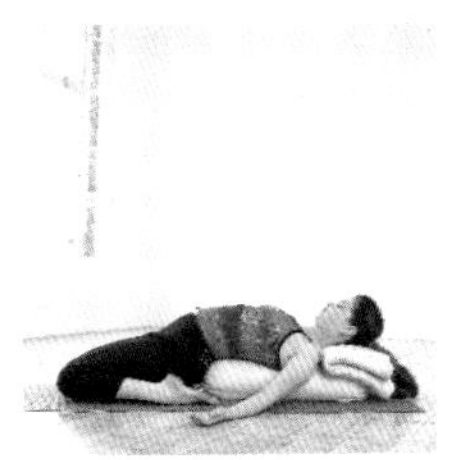
4 **Supta Virasana**

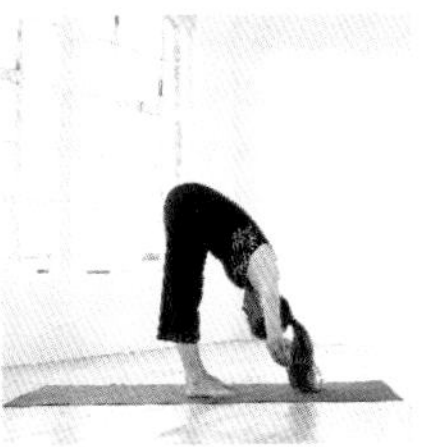
5 **Uttanasana I**

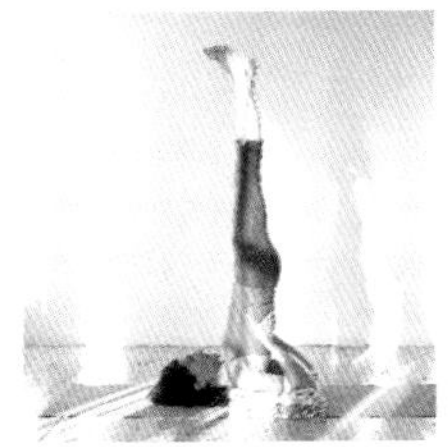
6 **Salamba Sarvangasana**

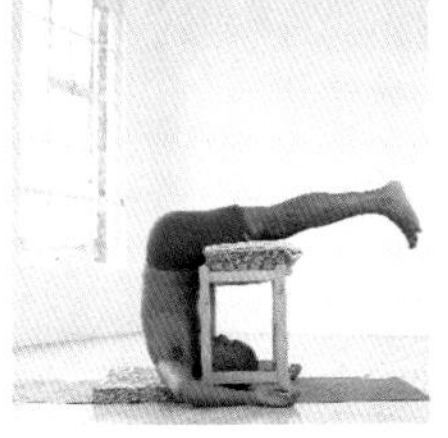
7 **Ardha Halasana** (s)

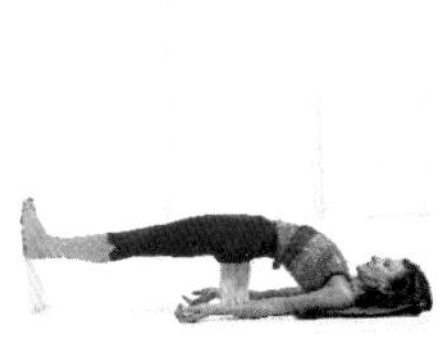
8 **Setu Bandha Sarv.**

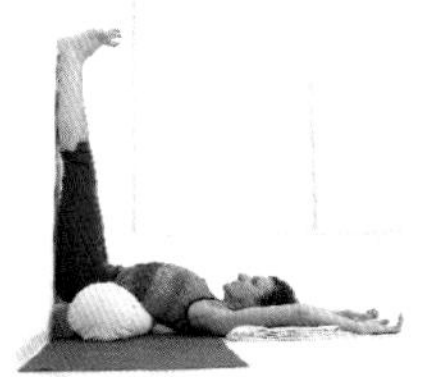
9 **Viparita Karani**

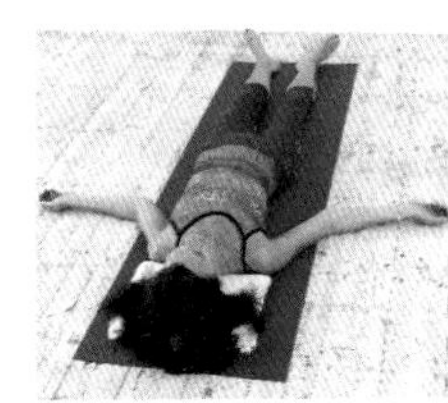
10 **Savasana**

Focus

- Consolidate these postures, going back to ones which you may find more difficult and practising them again until they feel easier.

Sequence 16 – Standing Postures and Standing Forward Bends

This routine can take up to 2 hours to complete, and if fatigue is experienced, do Uttanasana I in between to rest the brain and allow the body to recover. Increase timings in the postures, especially Salamba Sarvangasana and Halasana.

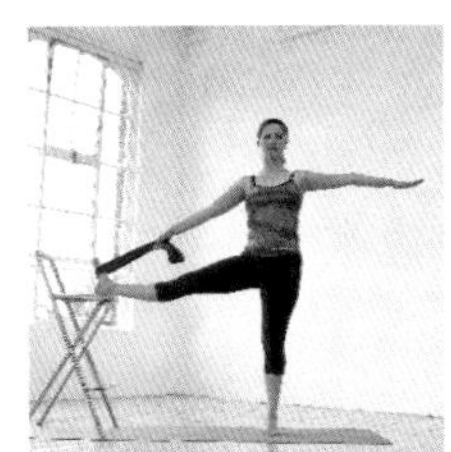
1 **Utthita Hasta Pad. I & II** (s)

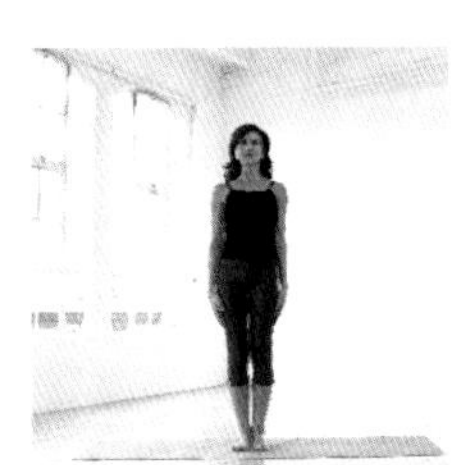
2 **Tadasana**

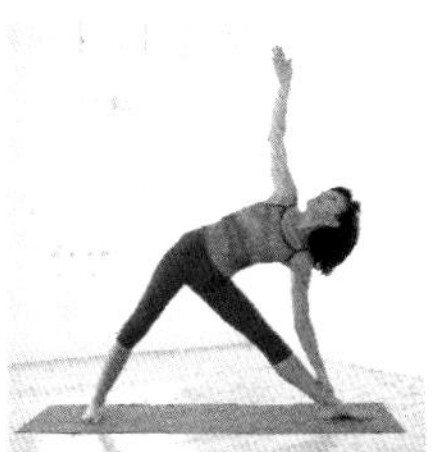
3 **Utthita Trikonasana**

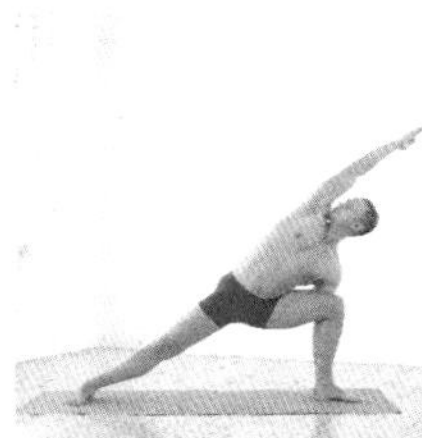
4 **Utthita Parsvakonasana**

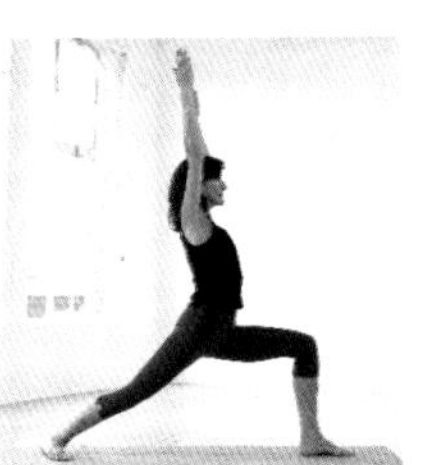
5 **Virabhadrasana I**

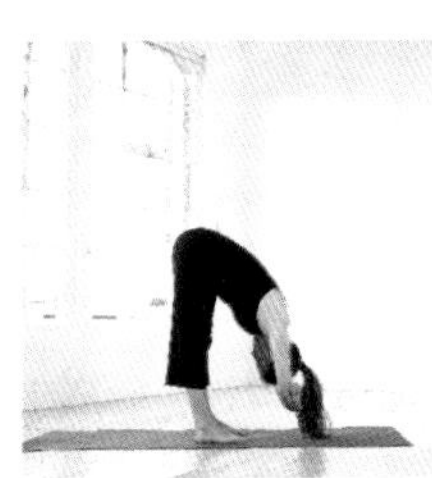
6 **Uttanasana I**

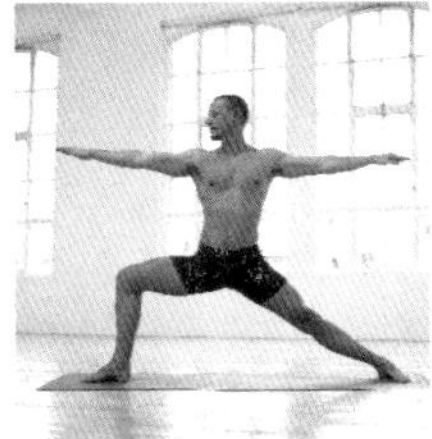
7 **Virabhadrasana II**

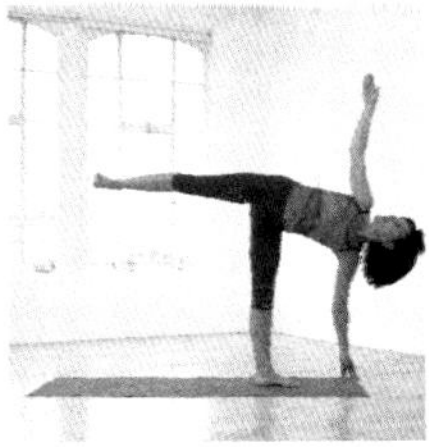
8 **Ardha Chandrasana**

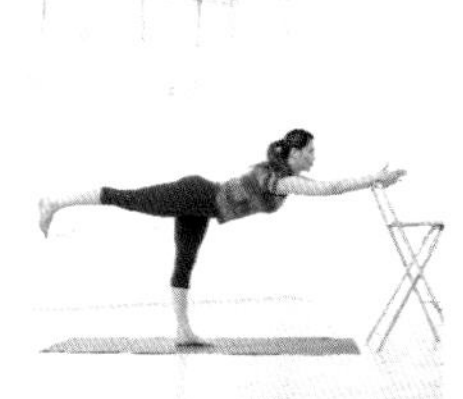
9 **Virabhadrasana III** (s)

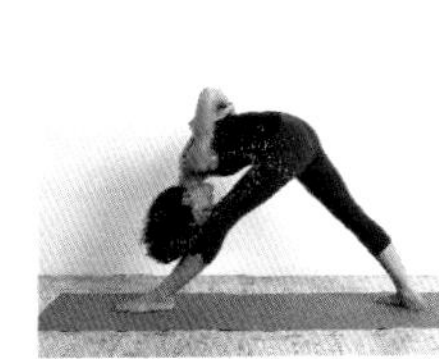
10 **Parsvottanasana**

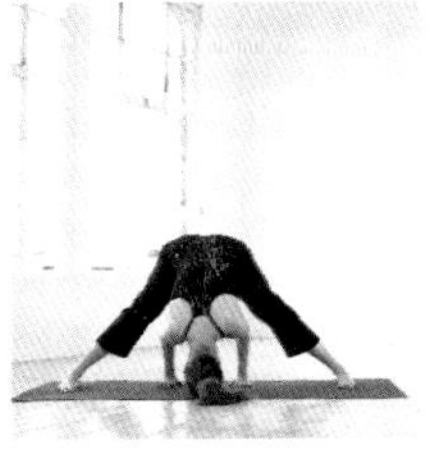
11 **Prasarita Padattonasana**

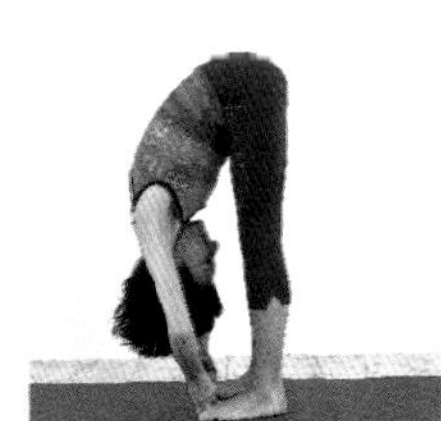
12 **Padangusthasana**

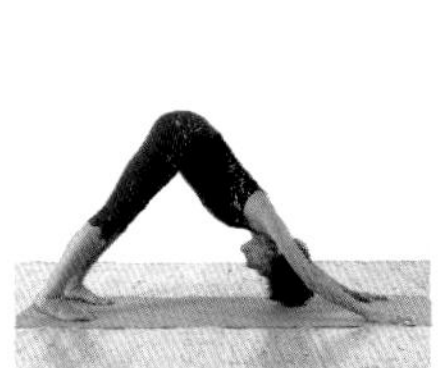
13 **Adho Mukha Svan.**

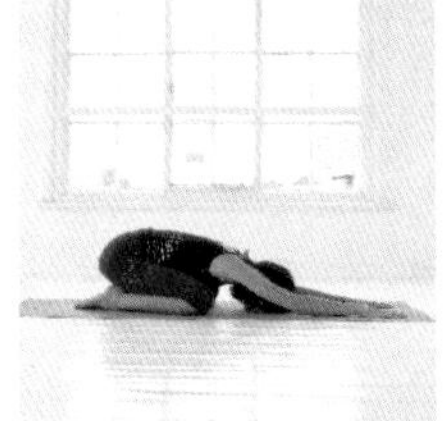
14 **Adho Mukha Vir.**

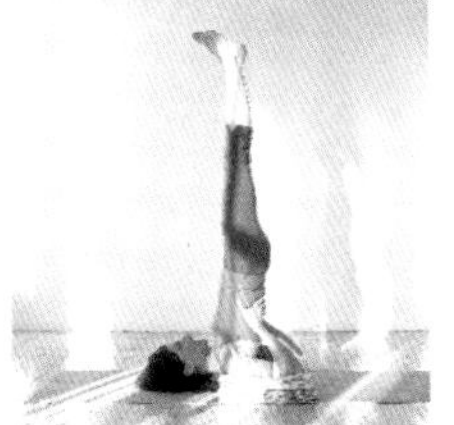
15 **Salamba Sarvang.**

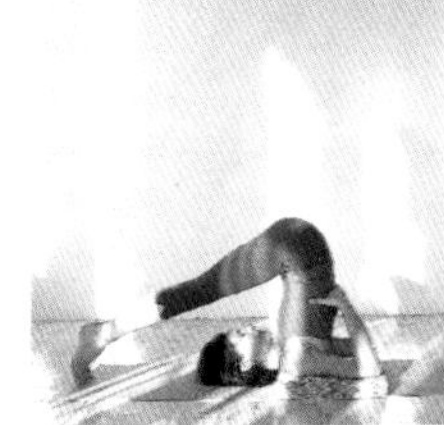
16 **Halasana**

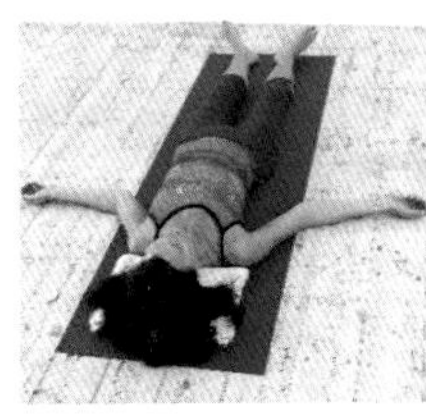
17 **Savasana**

Sequence 17 – Stronger Forward Bends and Floor Twists

Lift, open and broaden the chest in all these seated poses. Sit on a support to help with the lift of the spine. While practising the twists, make sure the spine is extended and lengthened before twisting. Both buttock bones should remain on the support in the twists. Increase the timing of the forward bends and keep the brain passive.

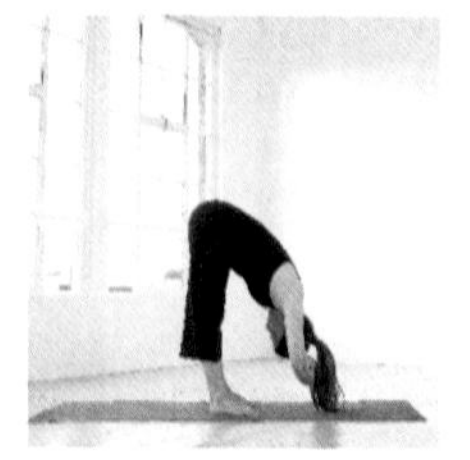
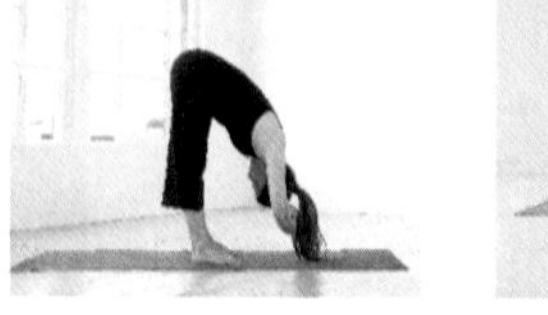

1 **Uttanasana I**

2 **Virasana**

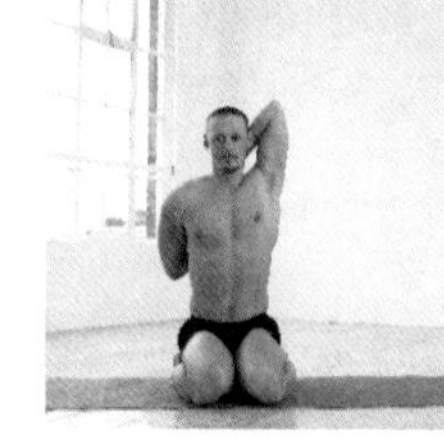

3 **Gomukhasana**

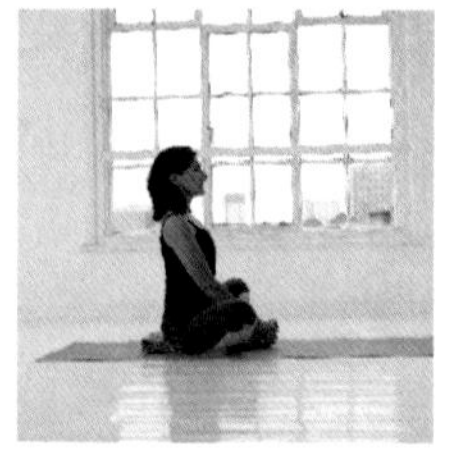

4 **Baddhakonasana**

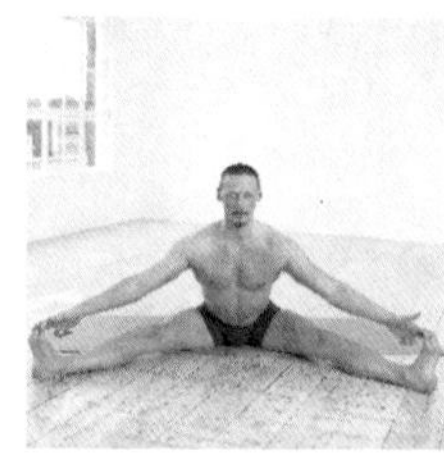

5 **Upavistakonasana**

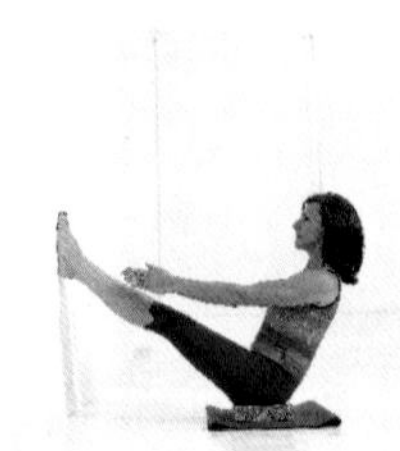

6 **Paripurna Nav.** (s)

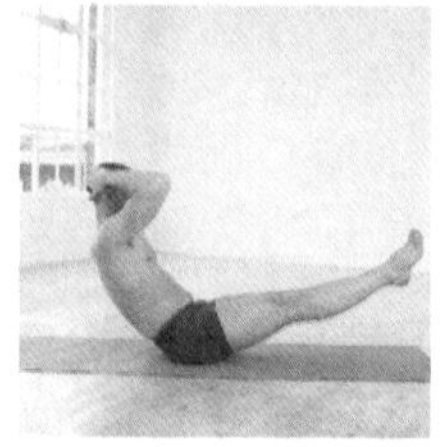
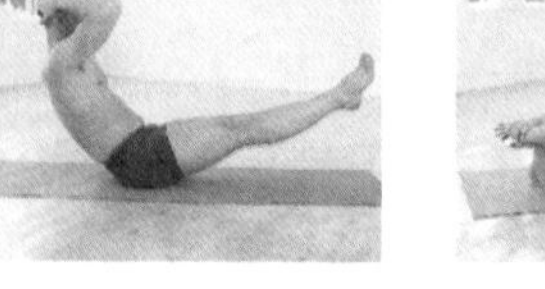

7 **Ardha Navasana**

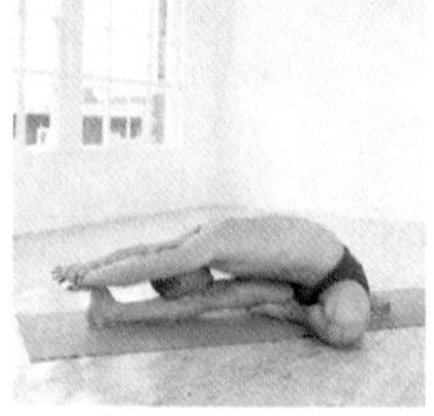

8 **Janusirsasana**

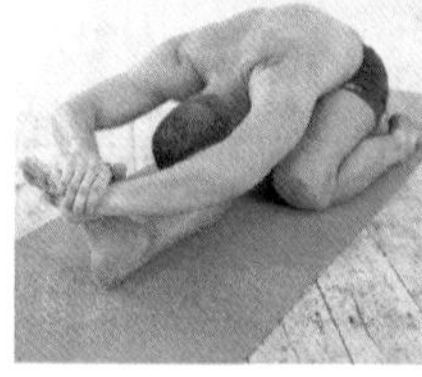

9 **Trianga Mukha.**

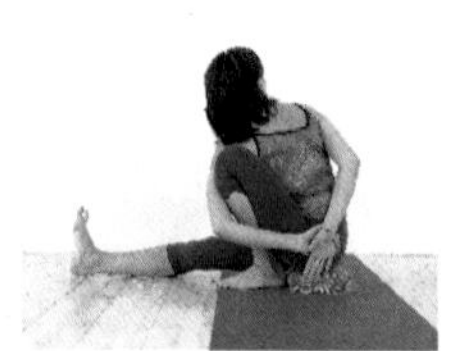

10 **Maricyasana I**

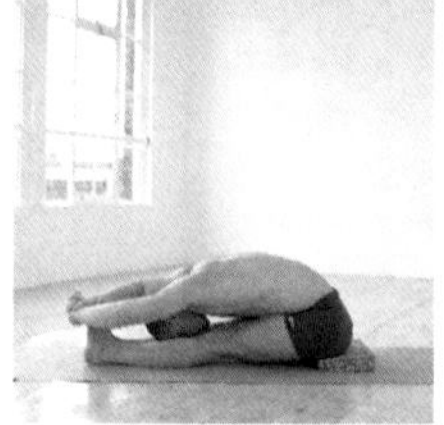

11 **Pascimottanasana**

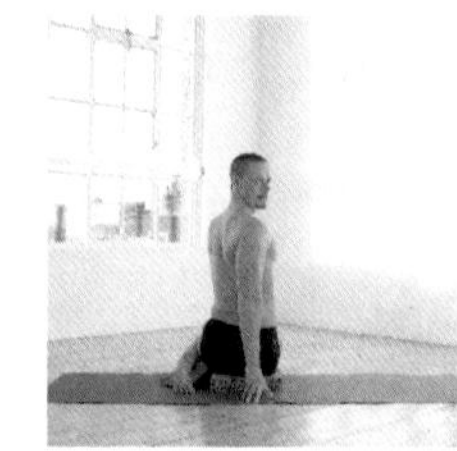

12 **Bharadvajasana I**

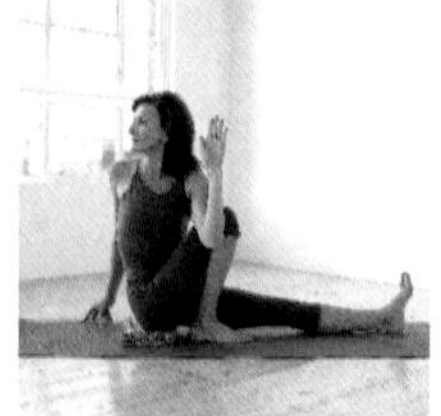
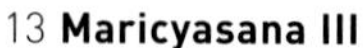

13 **Maricyasana III**

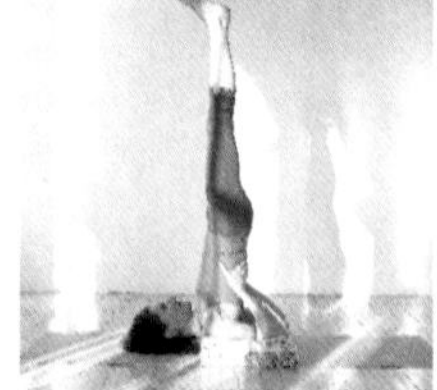

14 **Salamba Sarvang.**

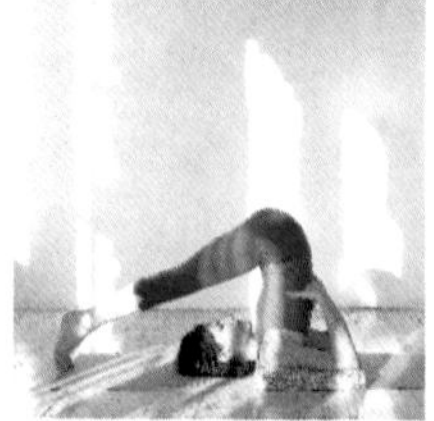

15 **Halasana**

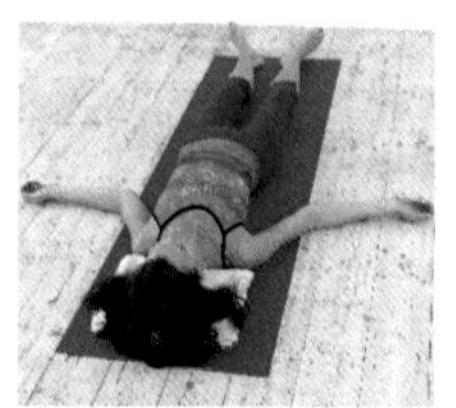

16 **Savasana**

Focus

- In Paripurna Navasana and Ardha Navasana, try to straighten the legs. If the back hurts, practice these postures with bent knees.

Sequence 18 – Progressively More Difficult Postures

At this stage of practice, one's stamina, endurance and flexibility should have improved, so this sequence of postures should be challenging but manageable. Practise Virabhadrasana III with only the hands supported, and fully extend the back (lifted) leg away from the head while the arms stretch strongly towards the fingertips.

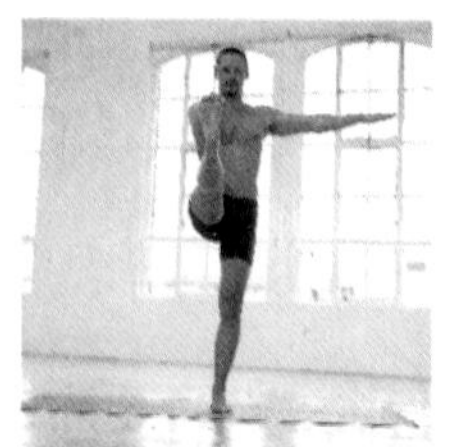

1 **Utt. Hasta Pad. I & II**

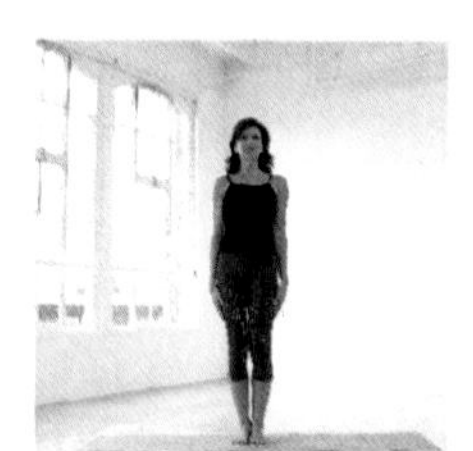

2 **Tadasana**

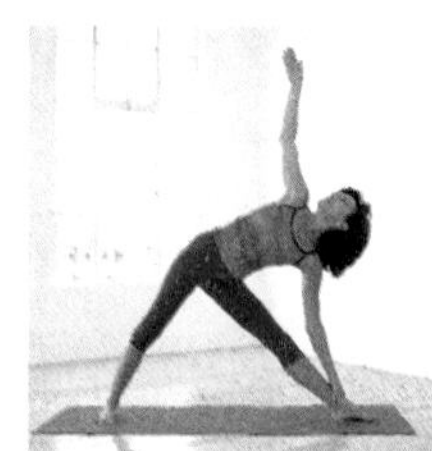

3 **Utthita Trikonasana**

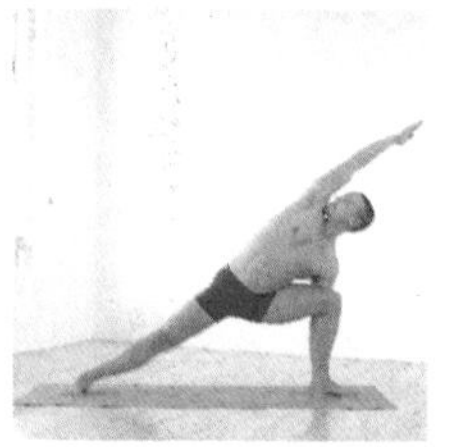

4 **Utthita Parsvakon.**

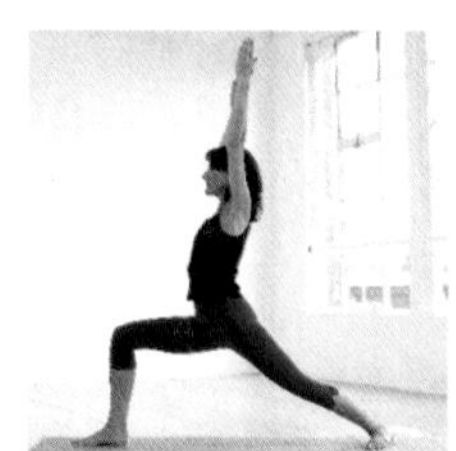

5 **Virabhadrasana I**

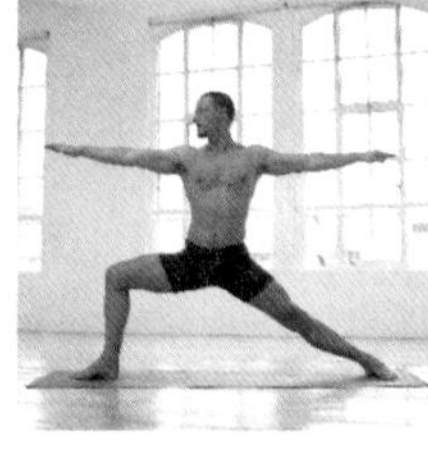

6 **Virabhadrasana II**

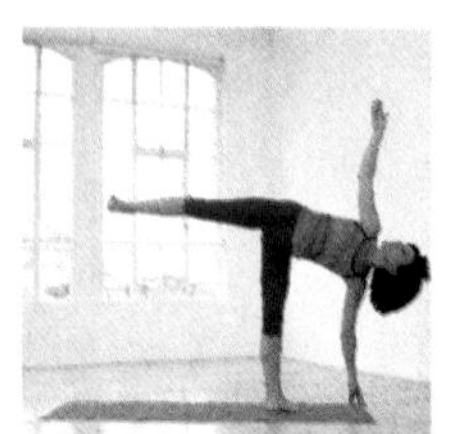

7 **Ardha Chandrasana**

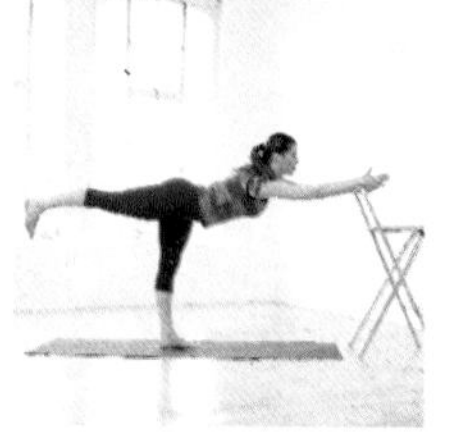

8 **Virabhadrasana III** (s)

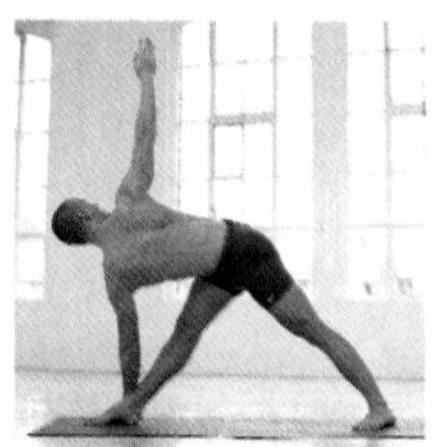

9 **Parivrtta Trikonasana**

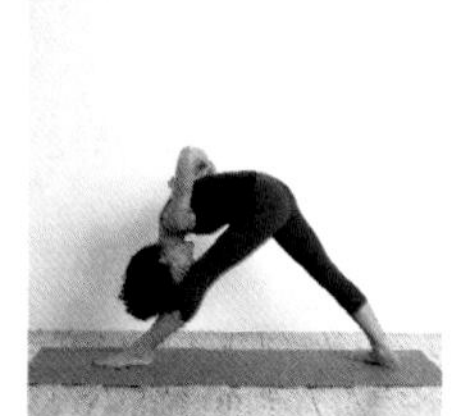

10 **Parsvottanasana**

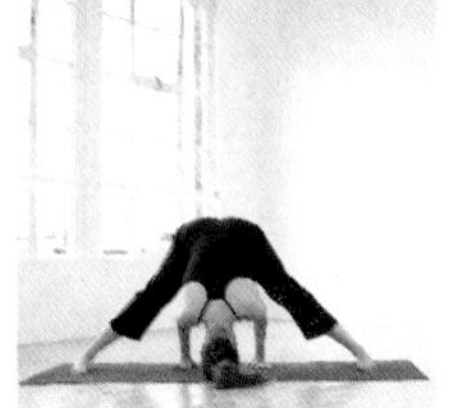

11 **Prasarita Padottanasana**

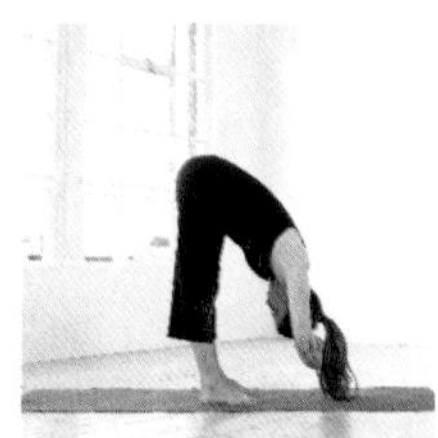

12 **Uttanasana I**
13 **Savasana**

Sequence 19 – Relaxation

In this relaxation routine, forward bends are practised with the head supported. Once the head touches the support, the brain should become calm and passive, allowing you to focus on the breath. Do not strain or create tension while practising supported forward bends, just allow the body to take on the shape of the posture and let go.

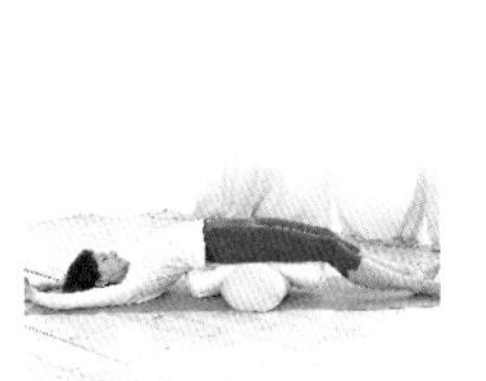
1 **Cross Bolsters**

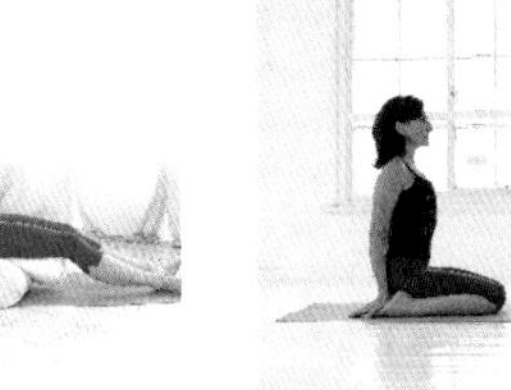
2 **Virasana**

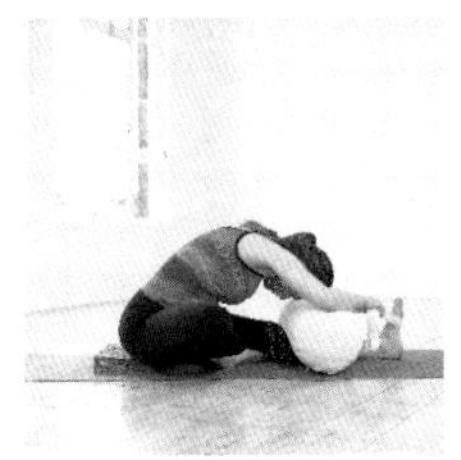
3 **Janusirsasana**

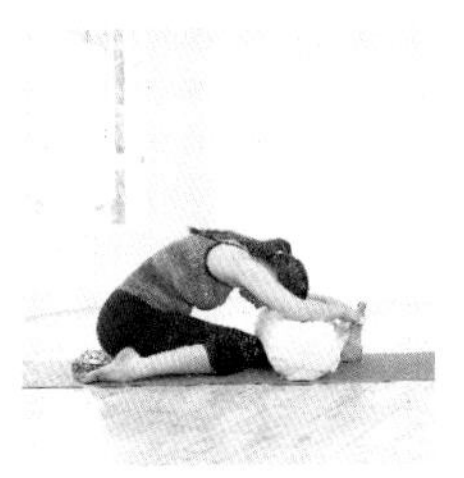
4 **Trianga Mukha.**

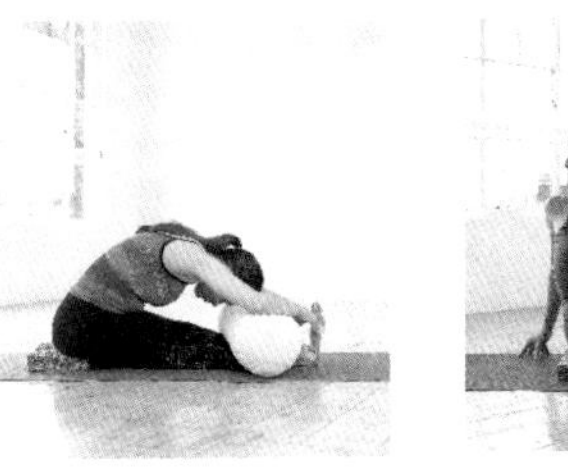
5 **Pascimottanasana**

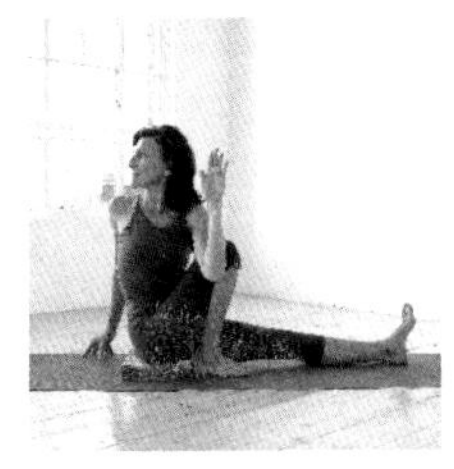
6 **Maricyasana III**

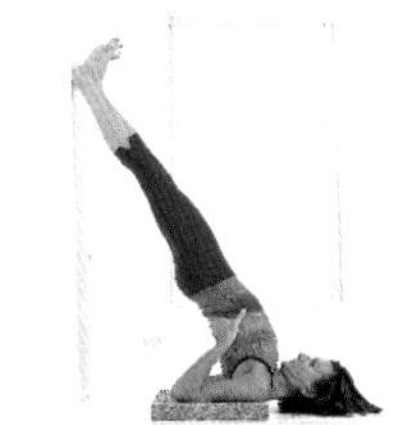
7 **Salamba Sarv.** (w)

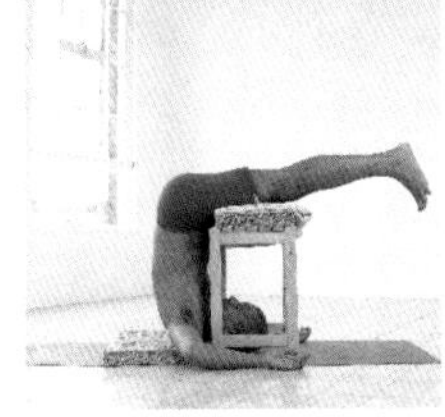
8 **Ardha Halasana** (s)

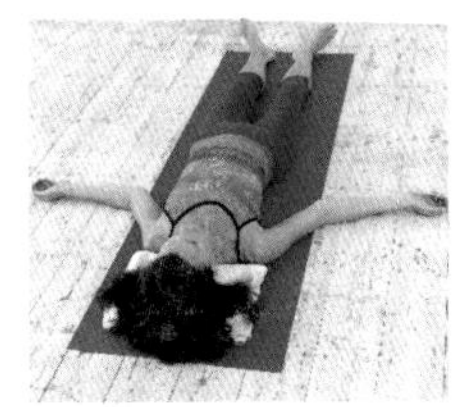
9 **Savasana**

Focus

- If the sequences are becoming too challenging, go back to Sequence 1. There is no race to get through all the sequences as quickly as possible. It is more sensible to work slowly, methodically and intelligently than to rush ahead and lay oneself open to pain and injury.

Sequence 20 – Prone Poses and Basic Standing Poses

Urdhva Mukha Svanasana is one of the preparatory postures for backbend work. In this posture the centre of the tops of the feet should be on the floor, the inner legs should lift up towards the ceiling, and the elbows and knees should be locked. If difficulty is experienced with lifting the body off the floor, use blocks under the hands and tuck the toes under.

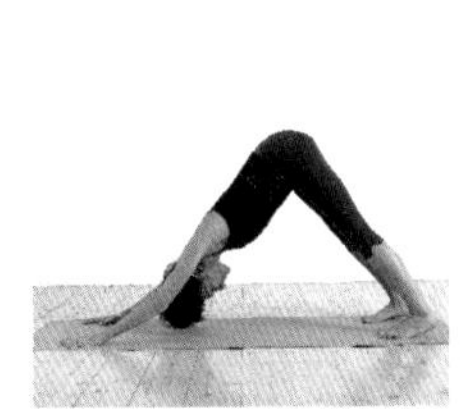
1 **Adho Mukha Svan.**

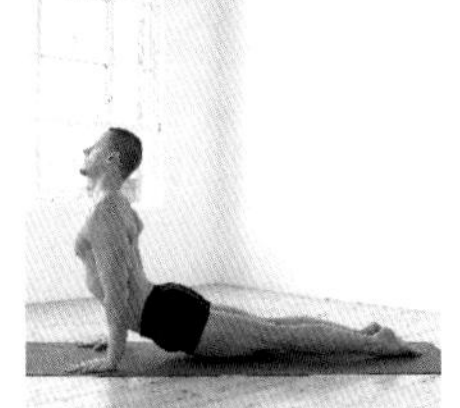
2 **Urdhva Mukha Sv.**

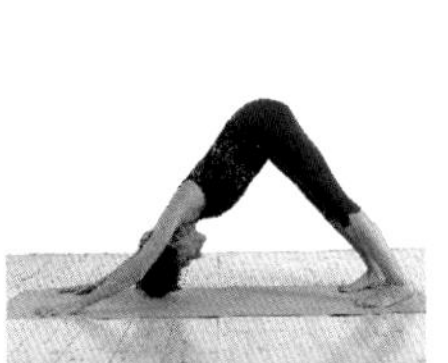
3 **Adho Mukha Svan.**

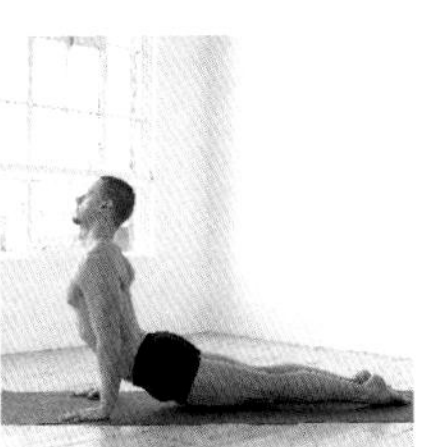
4 **Urdhva Mukha Sv.**

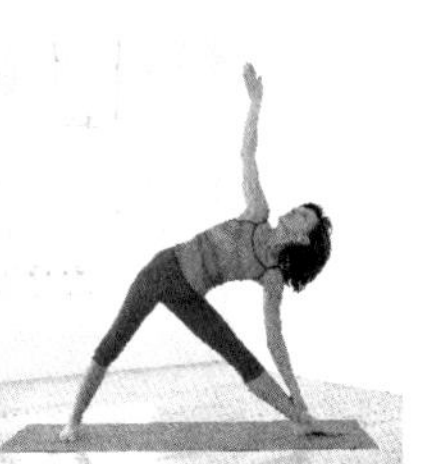
5 **Utthita Trikonasana**

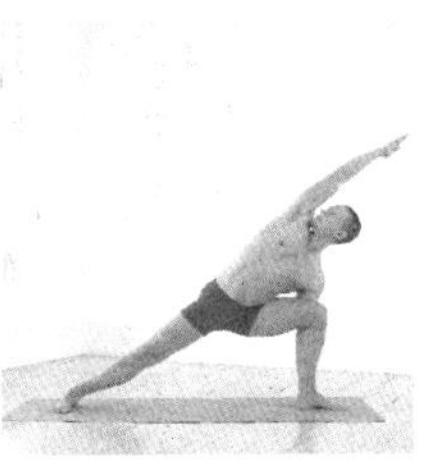
6 **Utthita Parsvakon.**

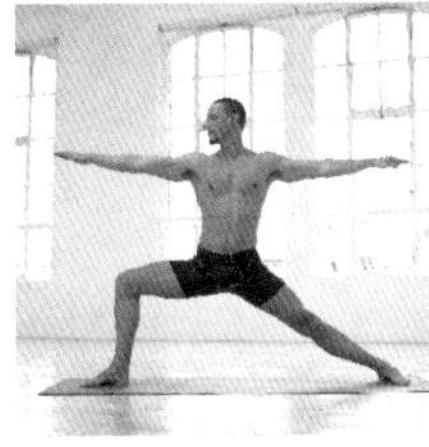
7 **Virabhadrasana II**

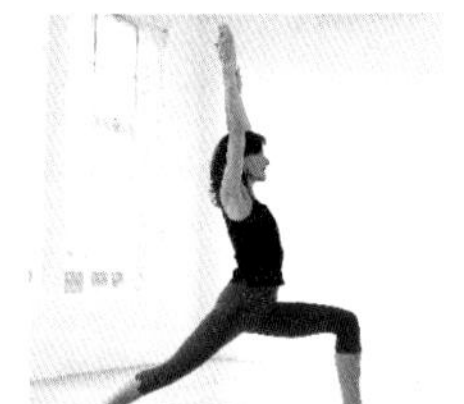
8 **Virabhadrasana I**

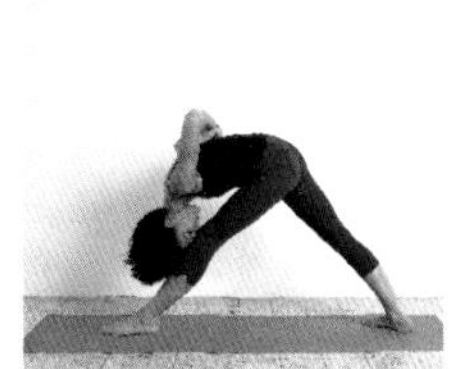
9 **Parsvottanasana**

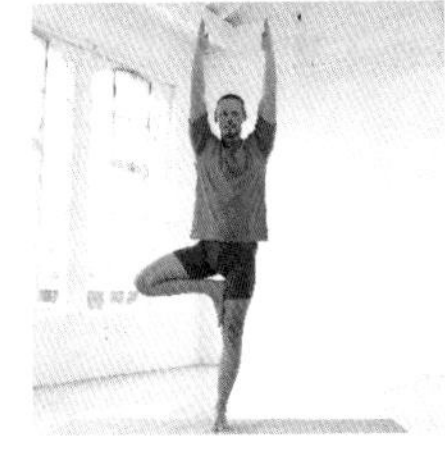
10 **Vrksasana**

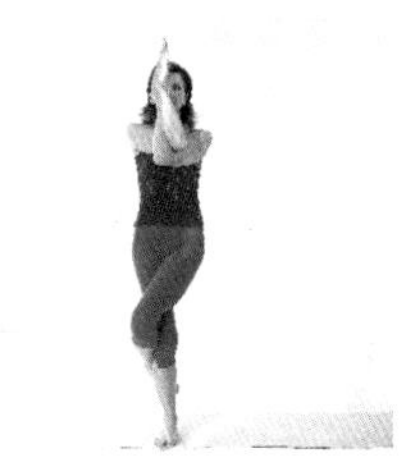
11 **Garudasana**

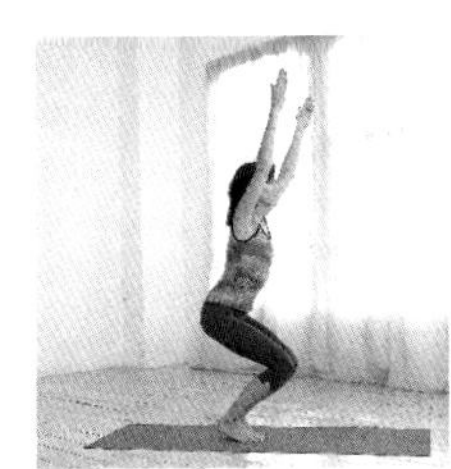
12 **Utkatasana**

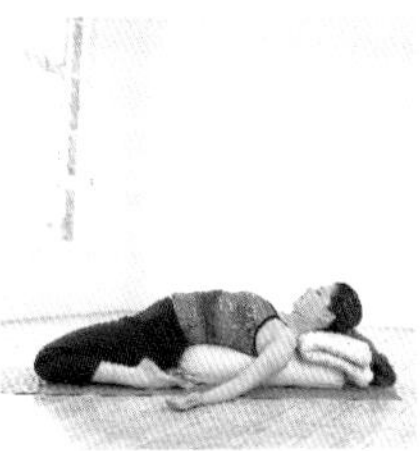
13 **Supta Virasana**

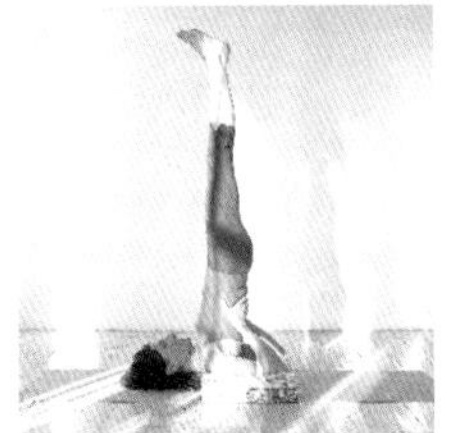
14 **Salamba Sarvang.**

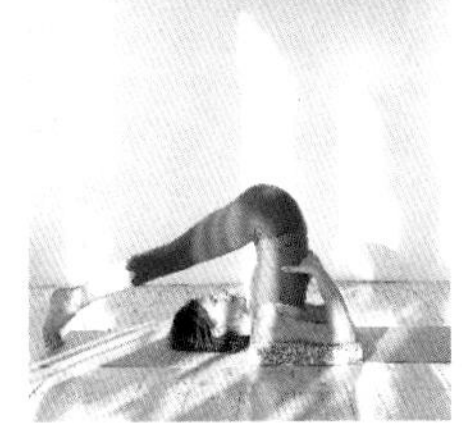
15 **Halasana**

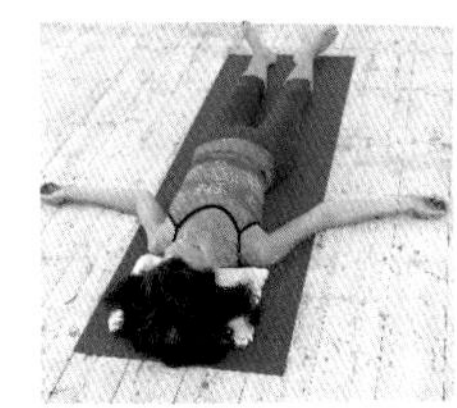
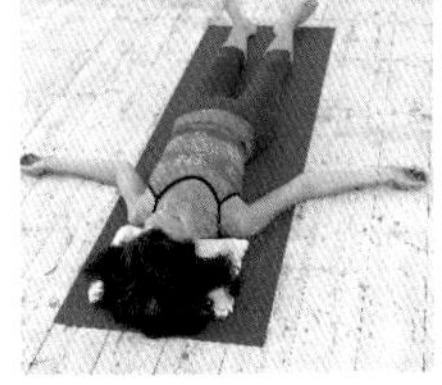
16 **Savasana**

Focus

- As a result of opening the chest and extending the spine upwards, the standing postures require less effort and are improved.

Sequence 21 – Seated Postures and Knee Work

Practising Padmasana incorrectly may result in severe knee problems, so never force the knee. Practise Sukhasana a few times prior to Padmasana in order to "lubricate" the hip and knee joints, and then practise Padmasana with one leg in Sukhasana – be patient, consolidate your practice and, with courage and determination, your goal will be achieved.

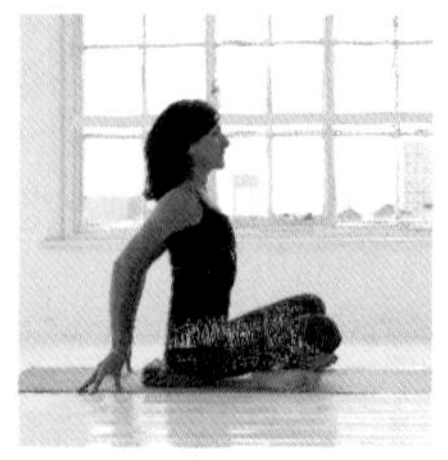
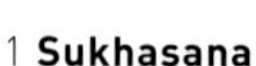

1 **Sukhasana**

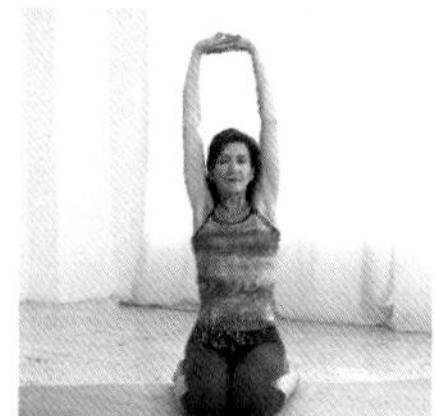

2 **Virasana with Parv.**

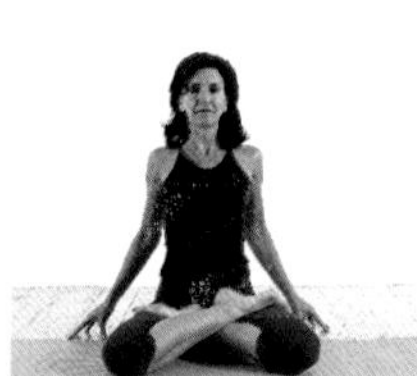

3 **Padmasana**

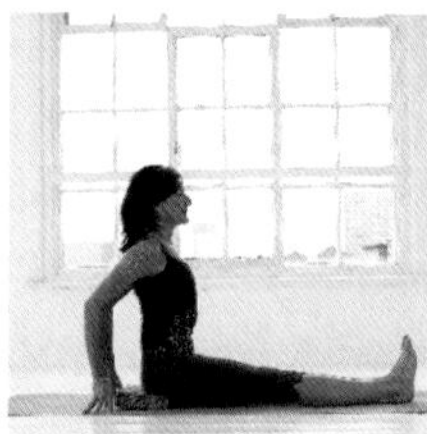

4 **Dandasana**

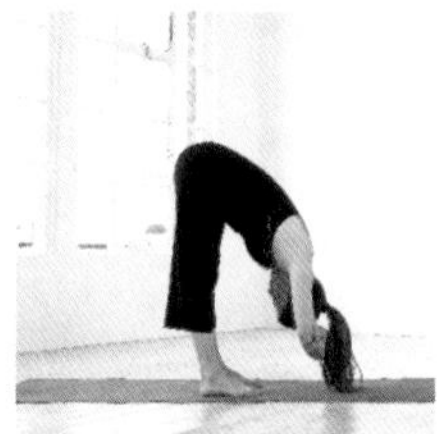

5 **Uttanasana I**

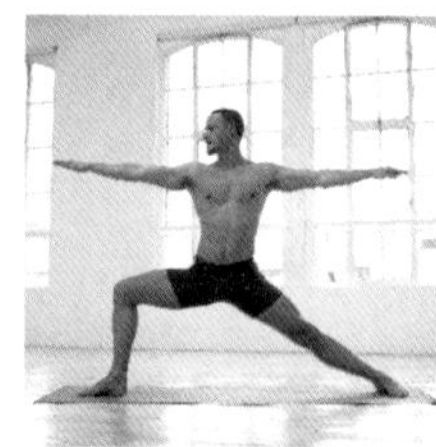

6 **Virabhadrasana II**

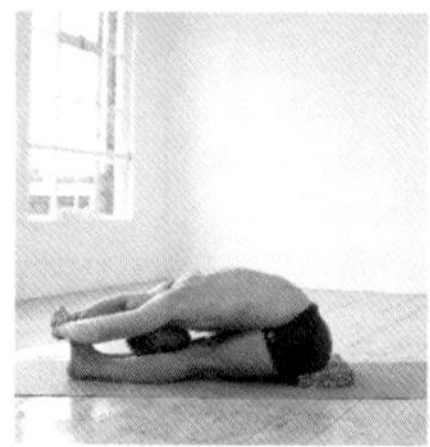

7 **Pascimottanasana**

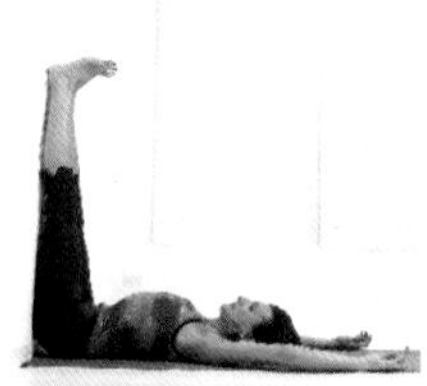

8 **Urdhva Pras. Pad.**

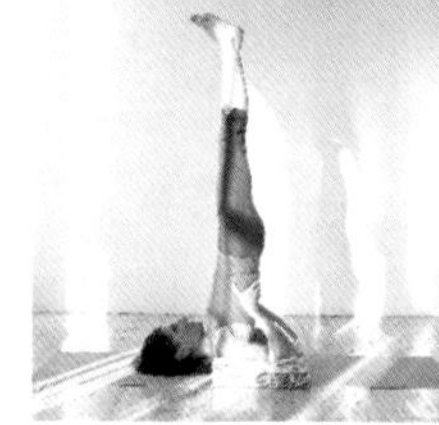

9 **Salamba Sarvang.**

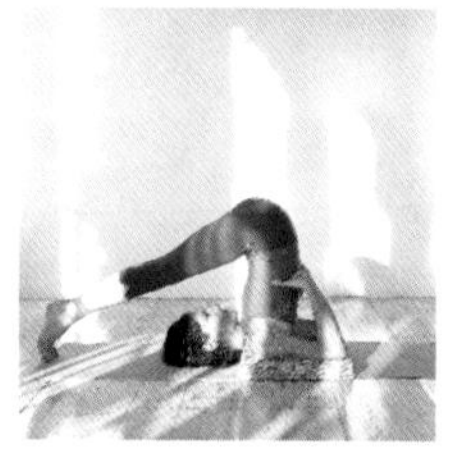

10 **Halasana**

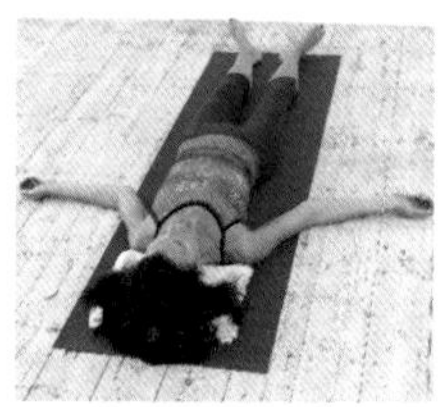

11 **Savasana**

Sequence 22 – Standing, Reverse Standing and Seated Posures

This group of mixed postures requires stamina, strength and flexibility and should be practised with care. Rest in Uttanasana I between the standing postures if necessary. You should set aside at least 2 hours to do this practice, doing the directional postures twice on each side, and at the end of the sequence practise Savasana for 10 minutes.

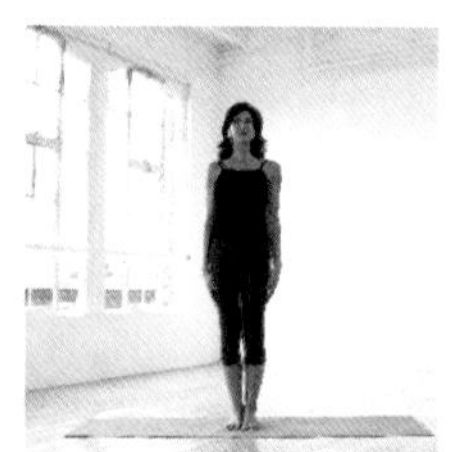

1 **Tadasana**

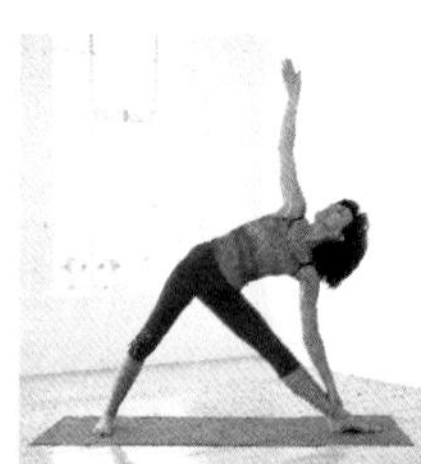

2 **Utthita Trikonasana**

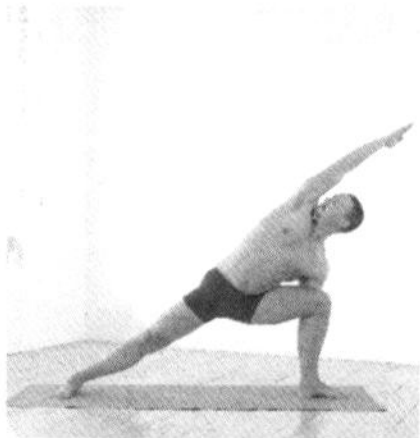

3 **Utthita Parsvakon.**

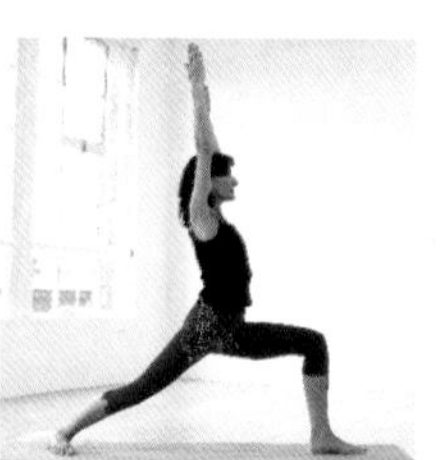

4 **Virabhadrasana I**

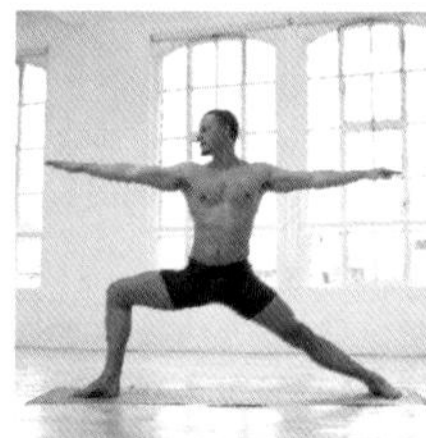

5 **Virabhadrasana II**

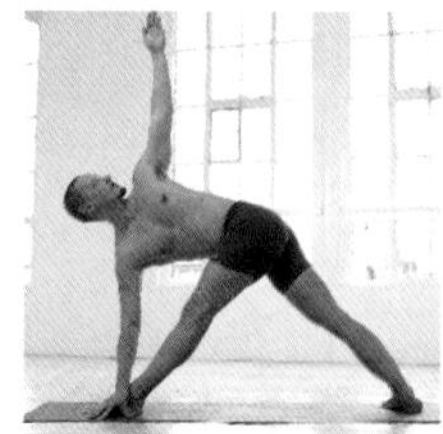

6 **Parivrtta Trikon.**

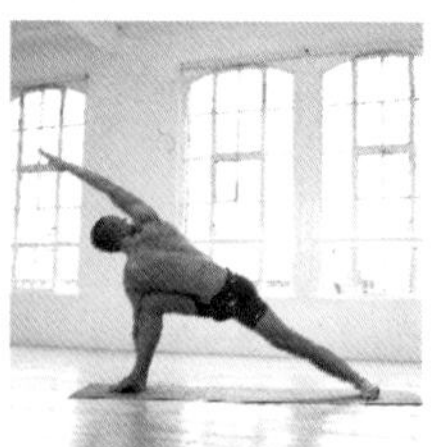

7 **Parivrtta Pars.**

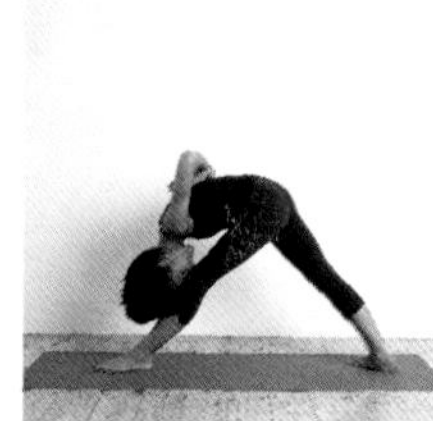

8 **Parsvottanasana**

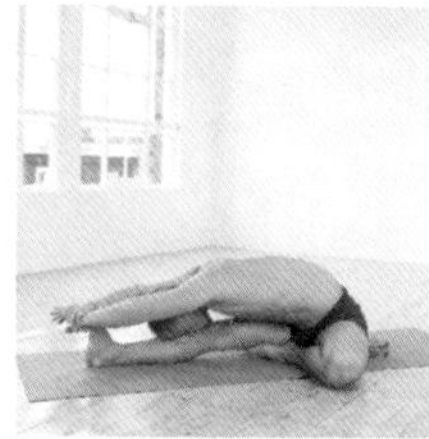

9 **Janusirsasana**

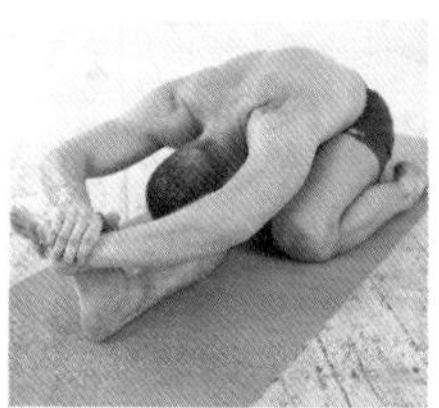

10 **Trianga Mukha.**

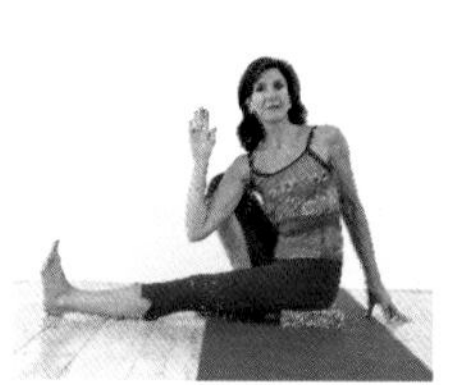

11 **Maricyasana I**

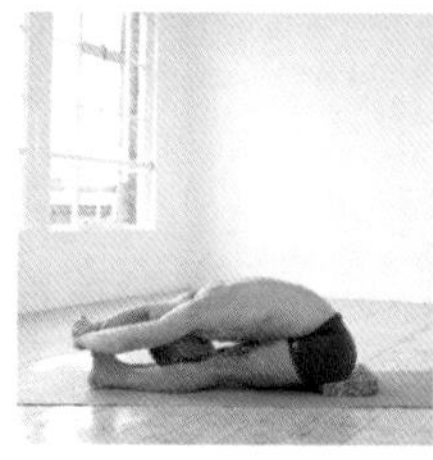

12 **Pascimottanasana**

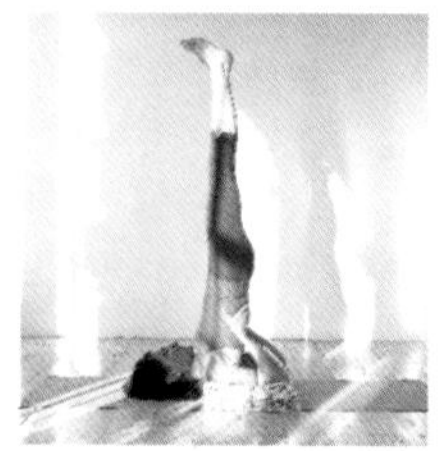

13 **Salamba Sarvang.**

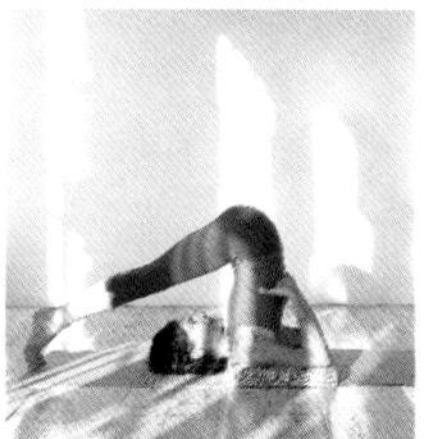

14 **Halasana**

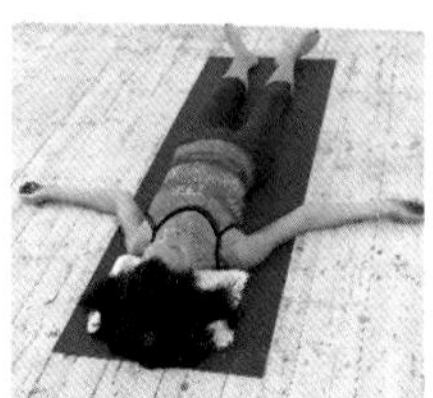

15 **Savasana**

Sequence 23 – Relaxation and Pranayama (Breathing)

Increase the timings in this group in order to open the chest more and deepen relaxation. Never strain the lungs or become agitated in Pranayama – both inhalation and exhalation must be smooth, calm and flowing. The quality of your Pranayama is more important than the quantity. If you feel uncomfortable and tense, return to normal breathing.

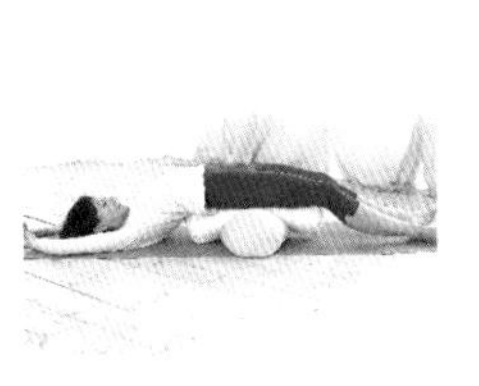
1 **Cross Bolsters**

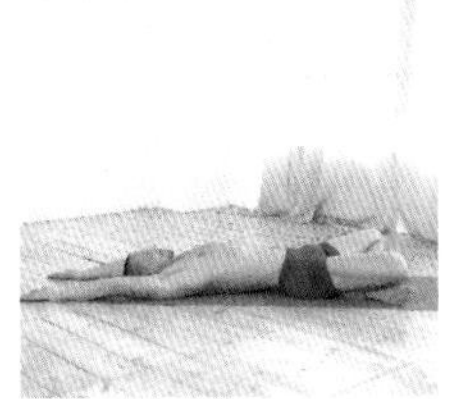
2 **Matsyasana**

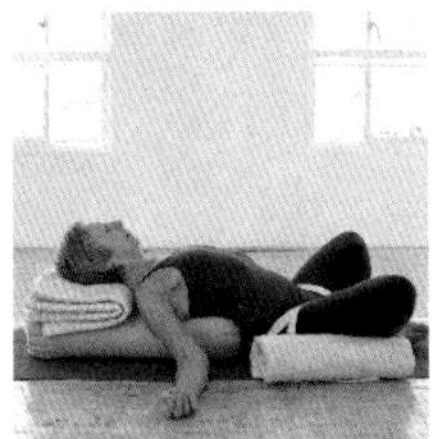
3 **Supta Baddha.** (s)

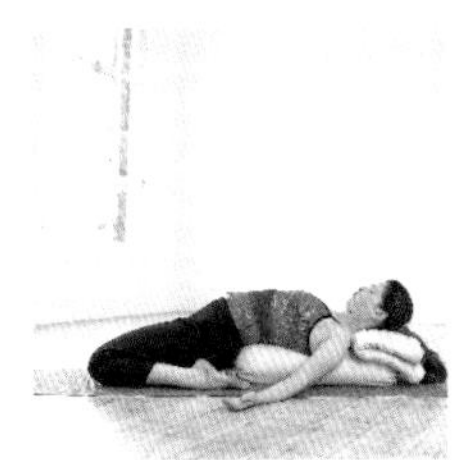
4 **Supta Virasana**

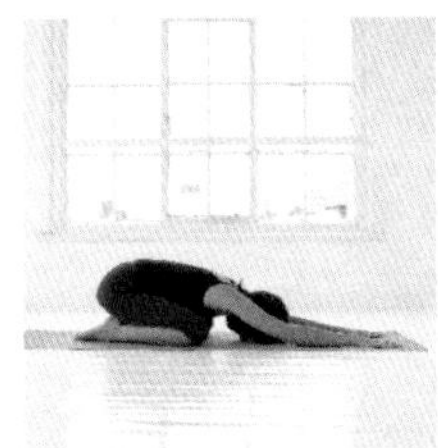
5 **Adho Mukha Vir.**

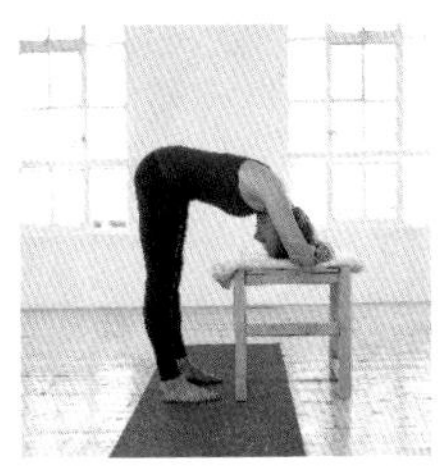
6 **Uttanasana I** (s)

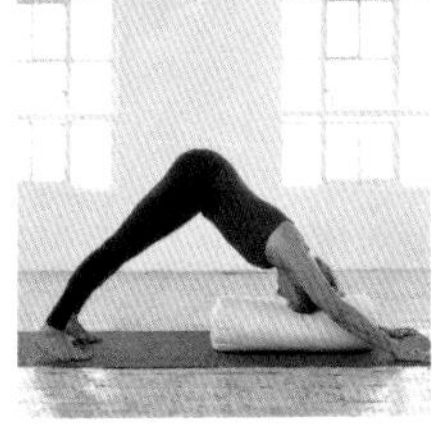
7 **Adho Mukha Svanasana** (s)

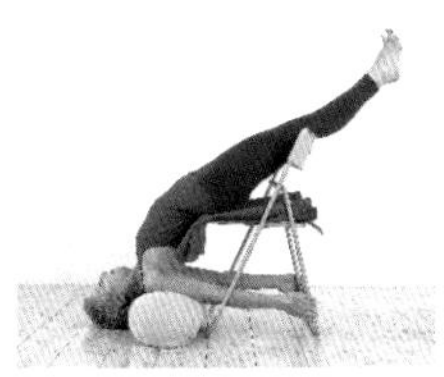
8 **Chair Sarvangasana**

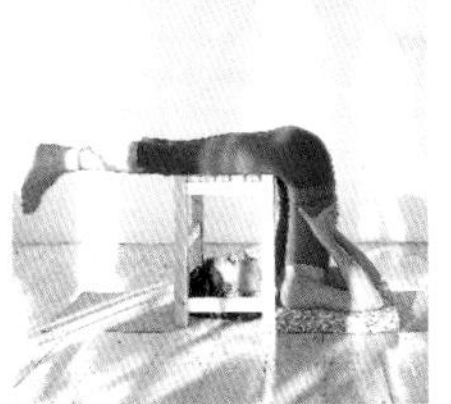
9 **Ardha Halasana**

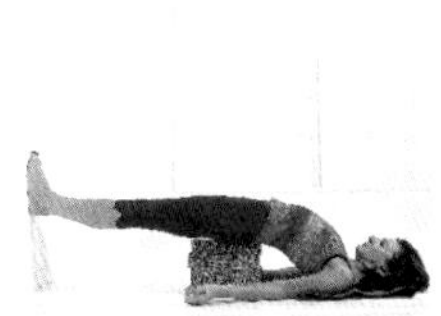
10 **Setu Bandha Sarvangasana**

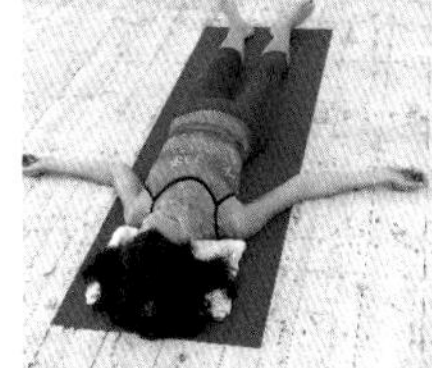
11 **Savasana**

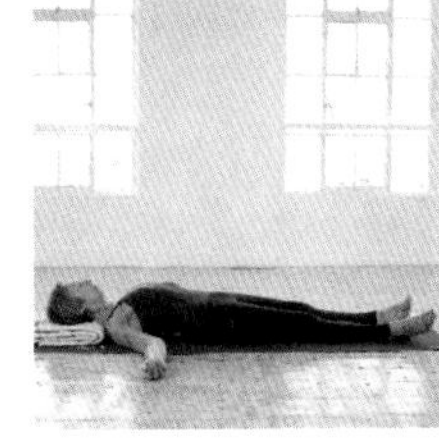
12 **Pranayama**

Sequence 24 – Standing Postures to Consolidate your Practice

In this sequence, focus on fully stretching the backs of both legs. Spend time in Tadasana, analysing and correcting the posture from the feet to the head. Repeat each standing posture twice using the "information" acquired from Tadasana to deepen your understanding and execution of the poses. Extend timings in Salamba Sarvangasana and Halasana.

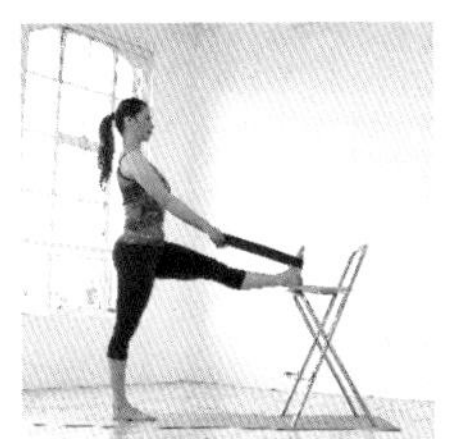
1 **Utt. Hasta Pad. I** (s)

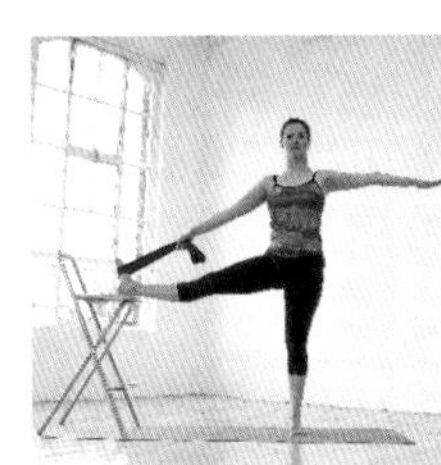
2 **Utt. Hasta Pad. II** (s)

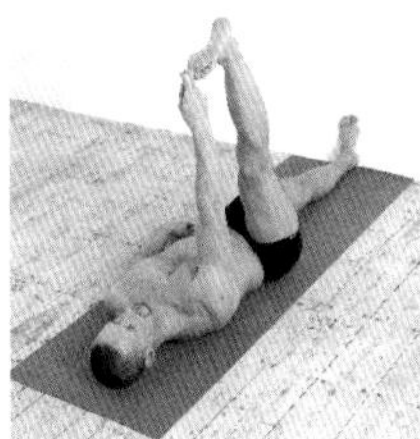
3 **Supta Pad. I**

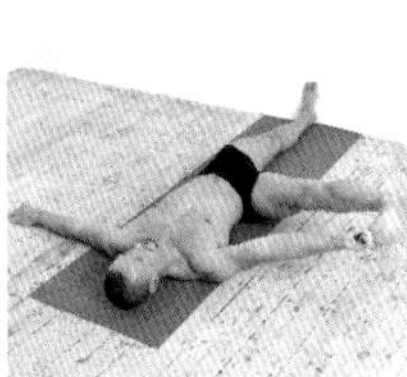
4 **Supta Pad. II**

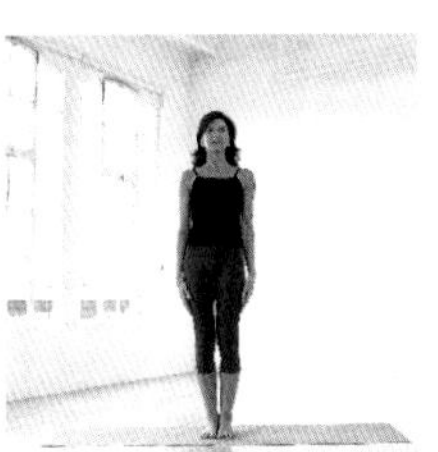
5 **Tadasana**

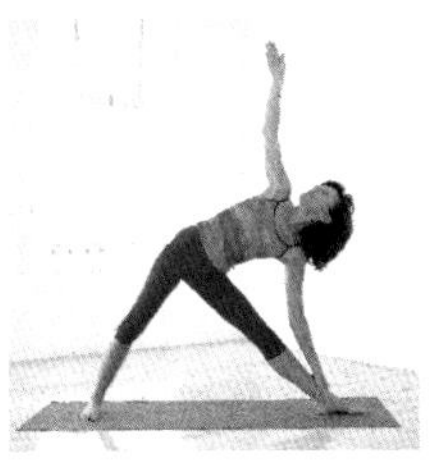
6 **Utthita Trikonasana**

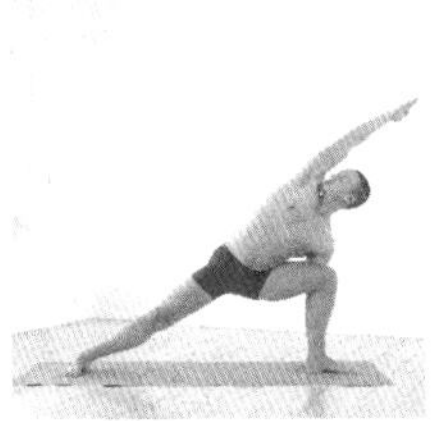
7 **Utthita Parsvakon.**

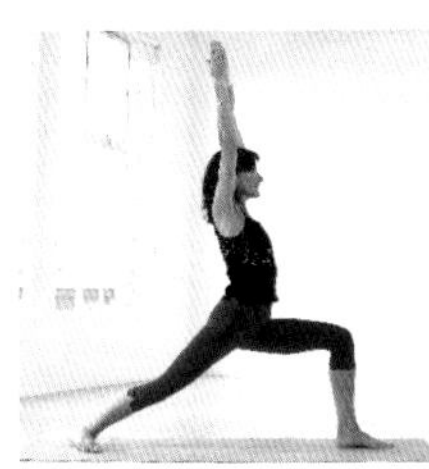
8 **Virabhadrasana I**

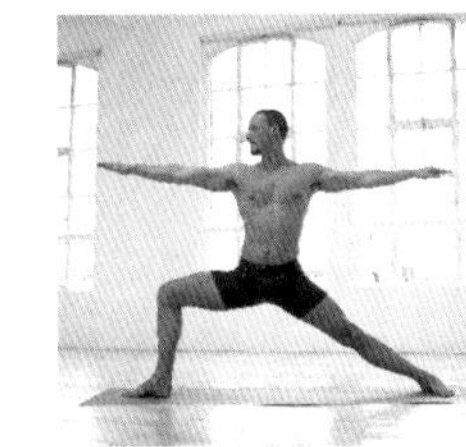
9 **Virabhadrasana II**

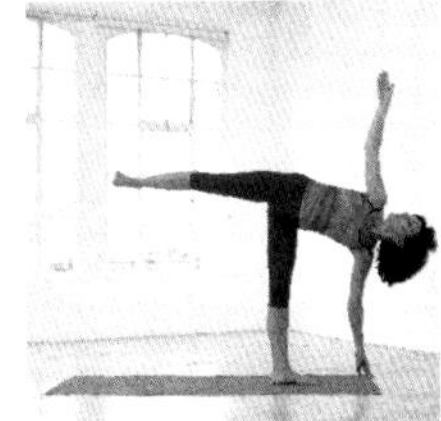
10 **Ardha Chandr.**

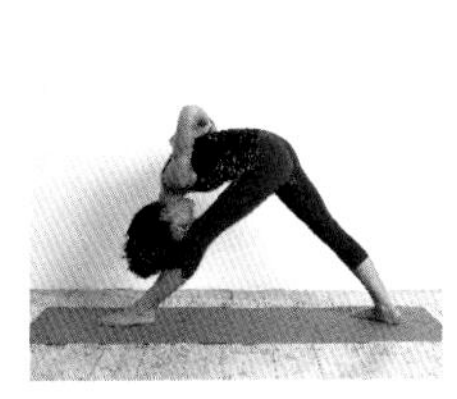
11 **Parvottanasana**

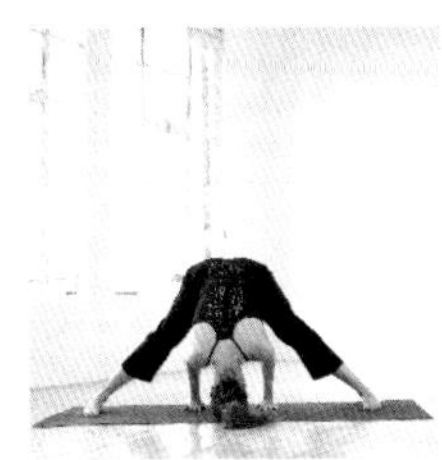
12 **Prasarita Pad.**

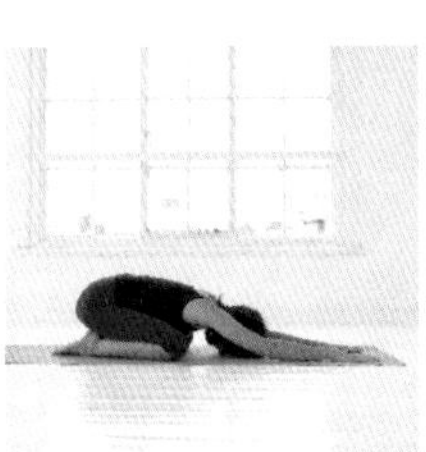
13 **Adho Mukha Vir.**

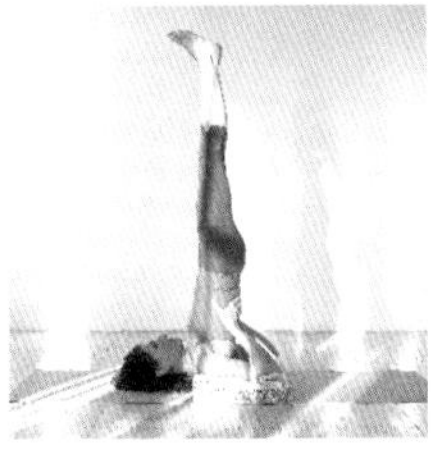
14 **Salamba Sarvang.**

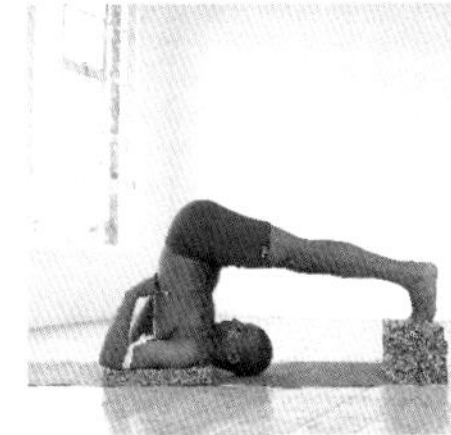
15 **Halasana** (s)

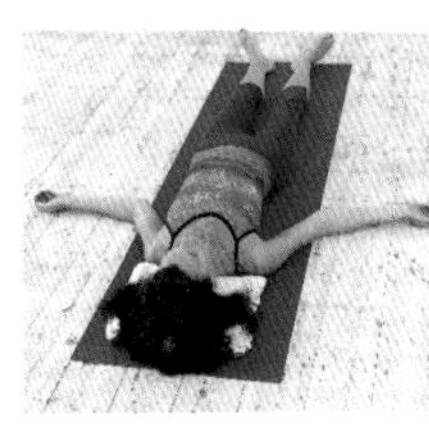
16 **Savasana**

Sequence 25 – Seated Postures

Practise Adho Mukha Svanasana and Urdhva Mukha Svanasana three times, opening the chest and lengthening the spine progressively. In Urdhva Mukha Svanasana, look up without compressing the back of the neck and keep the head in a comfortable position. In Dandasana, Paripurna Navasana, Ardha Navasana and Pascimottasana, fully stretch and lengthen the backs of the legs and keep the thighs and knees pressing towards the floor. In Baddhakonasana – and Upavistakonasana, keep the front of the body extending from pubis to chin and move the shoulder blades towards the front of the trunk to lift and open the chest. Twist further and breath more deeply in Bharadvajasana I.

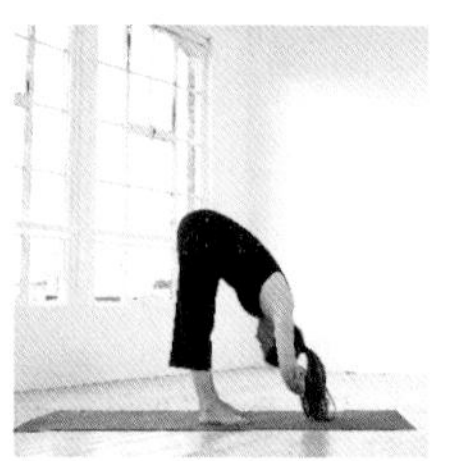
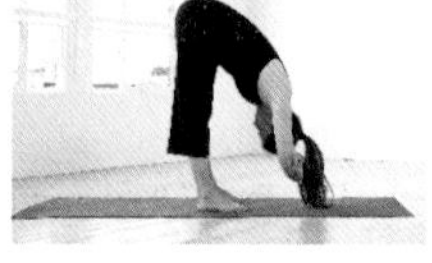

1 **Uttanasana I**

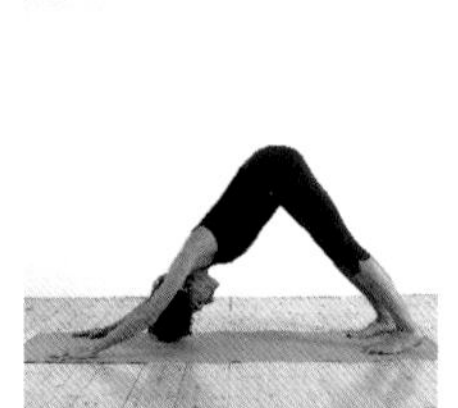

2 **Adho Mukha Svan.**

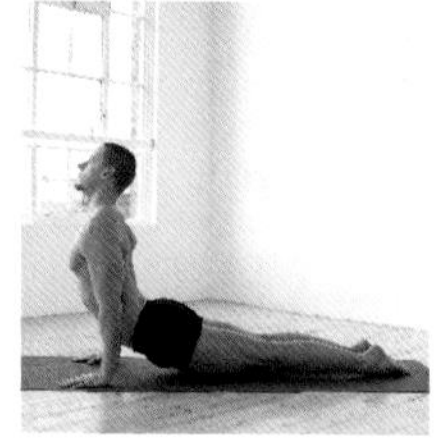

3 **Urdhva Mukha Svan.**

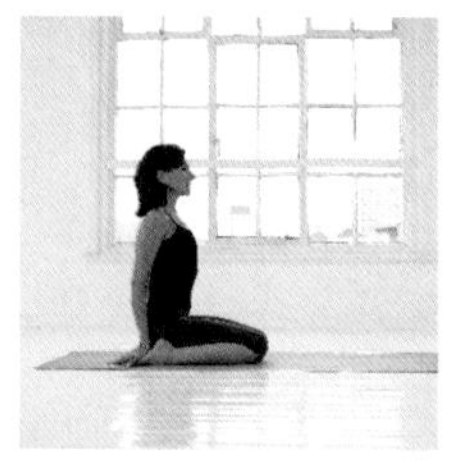

4 **Virasana**

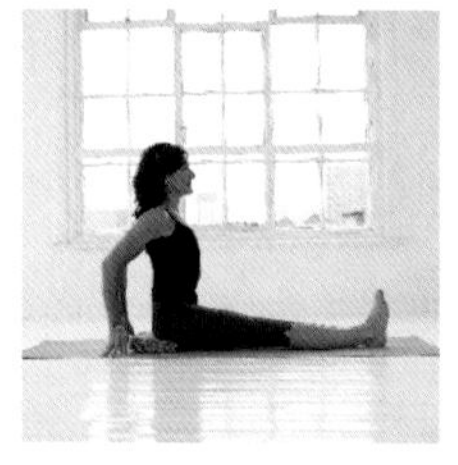

5 **Dandasana**

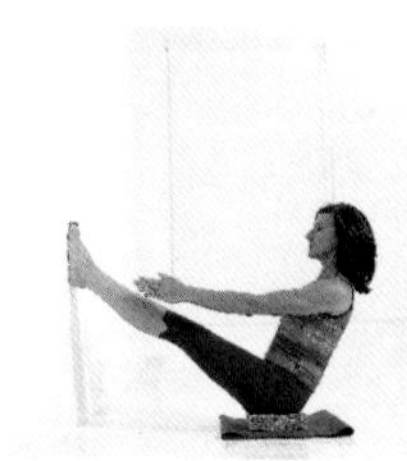

6 **Paripurna Nav.** (s)

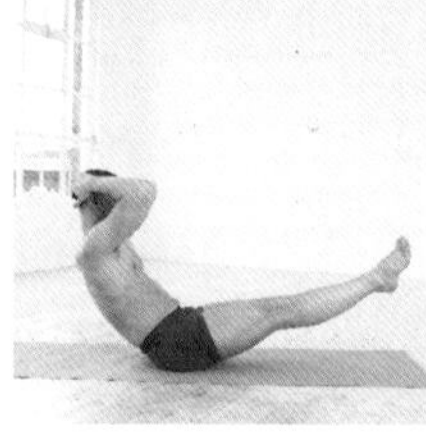

7 **Ardha Navasana**

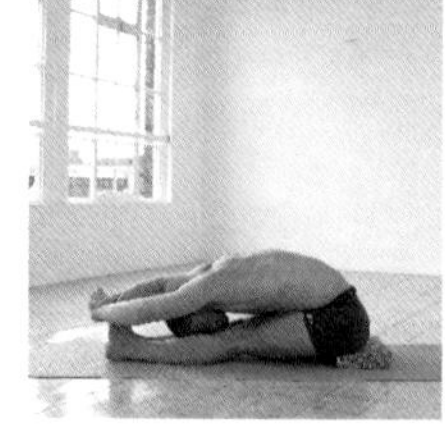

8 **Pascimottanasana**

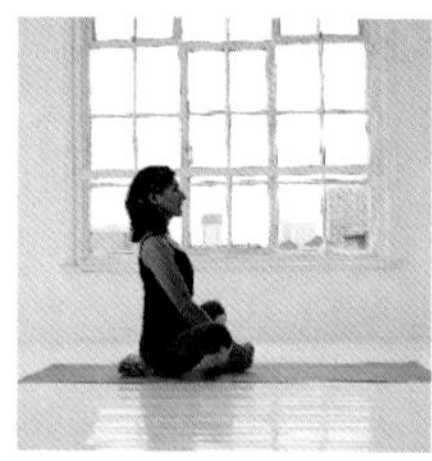

9 **Baddhakonasana**

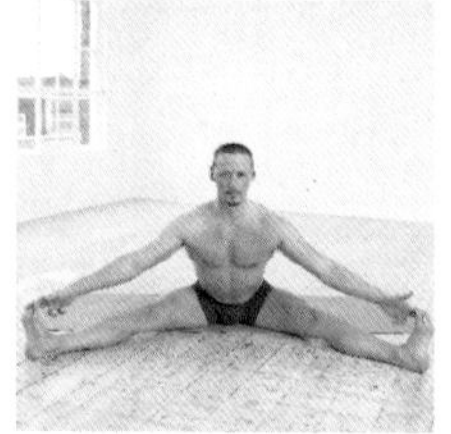

10 **Upavistakonasana**

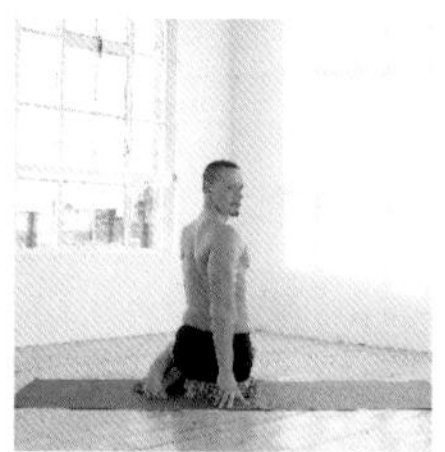

11 **Bharadvajasana I**

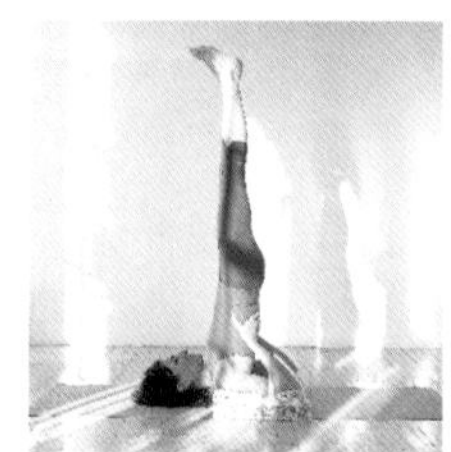

11 **Salamba Sarvang.**

Sequence 26 – Standing and Prone Postures

After the standing poses in this routine, Adho Mukha Svanasana is followed by Urdhva Mukha Svanasana,which prepares the spine for Salabhasana. In the latter two poses, the pubis and sacrum move towards the floor to avoid a painful pinching sensation in the lower back. Salabhasana should be practised with the legs together, though if the back is painful, you should separate them slightly. Extend both legs strongly towards the heels, keeping the soles of the feet long and broad. Lengthen the arms from the shoulders and stretch back towards the fingertips, keeping the palms broad and facing the ceiling. Lift and open the chest as much as possible and look straight ahead, keeping the eyes soft. After Salabhasana, practise Urdhva Mukha and Adho Mukha Svanasana quietly to release the spine gently. Ensure that the back is comfortable in Ardha Halasana. If it is sore in Savasana, rest the legs on a stool.

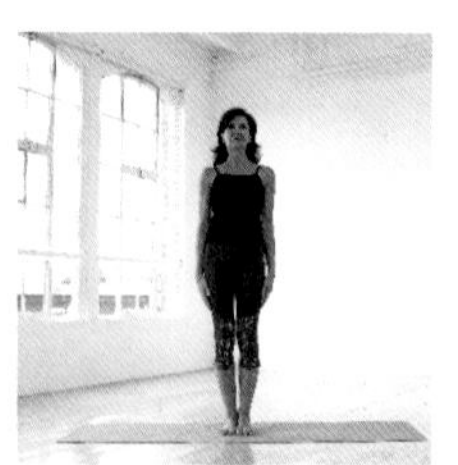
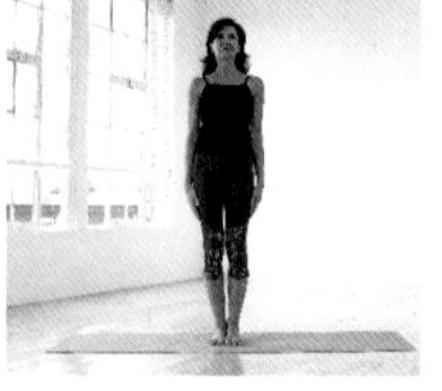

1 **Tadasana**

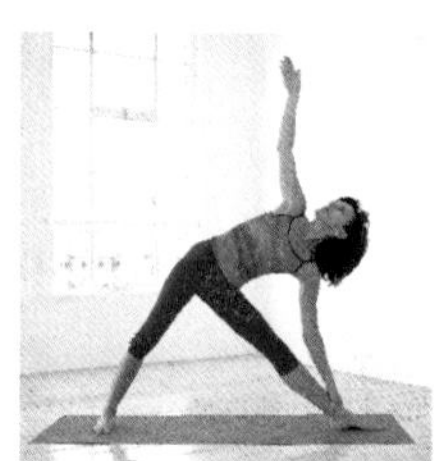

2 **Utthita Trikonasana**

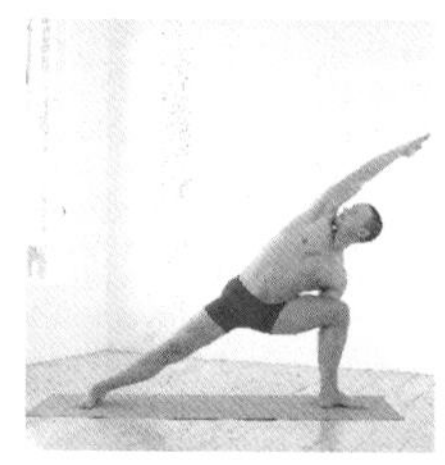

3 **Utthita Parsvakon.**

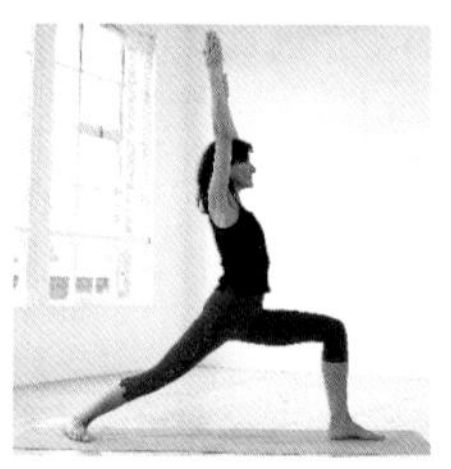

4 **Virabhadrasana I**

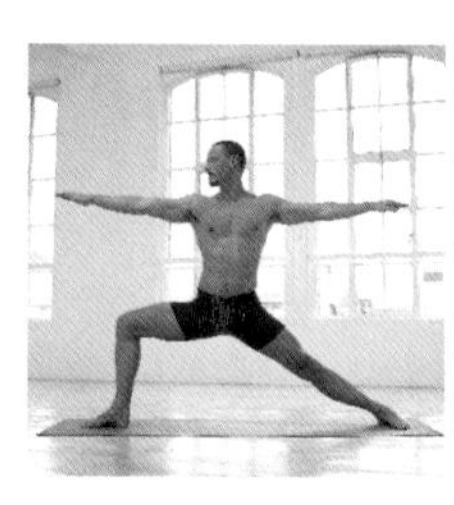

5 **Virabhadrasana II**

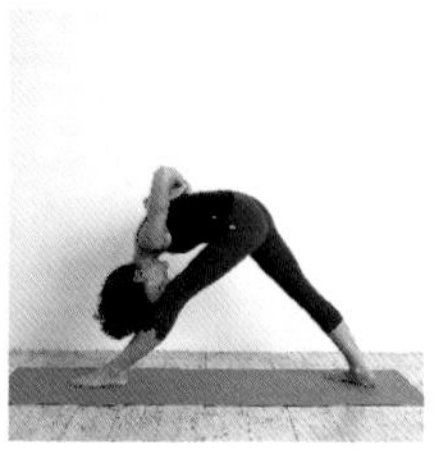

6 **Parsvottanasana**

7 **Adho Mukha Svanasana**

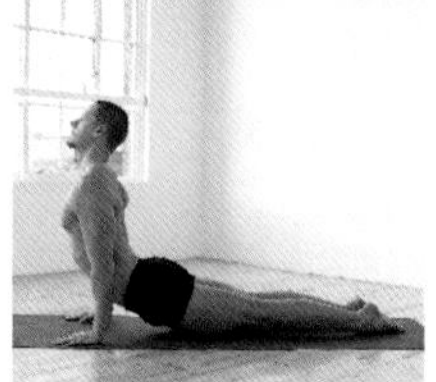

8 **Urdhva Mukha Svanasana**

9 **Salabhasana**

10 **Urdhva Mukha Svanasana**

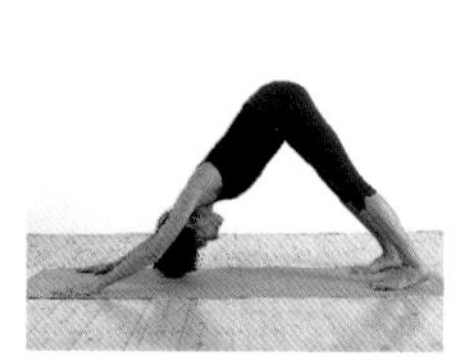
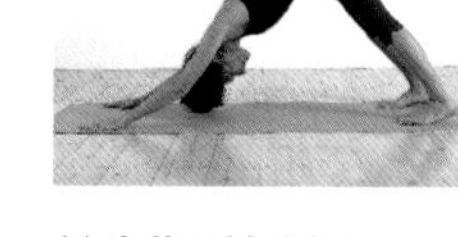

11 **Adho Mukha Svanasana**

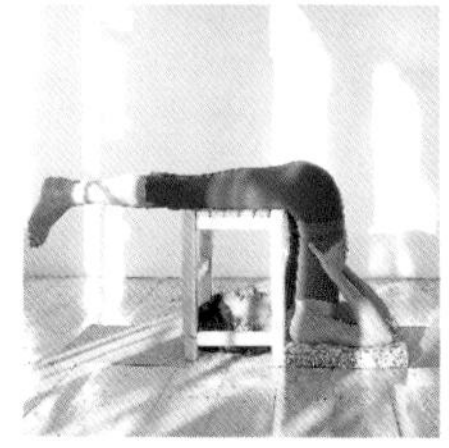

12 **Ardha Halasana**
13 **Savasana**

Sequence 27 – Relaxation

Try to let go while practising these poses. When in the posture, settle the body and focus on the breath. If the body becomes restless, the brain will follow. Once the head is resting on the support in the forward bends, soften the abdomen, relax the shoulders and back, keep the face, mouth and throat passive, and unite the breath with the mind and the mind with the breath. Extend the Pranayama practice without causing strain or tension.

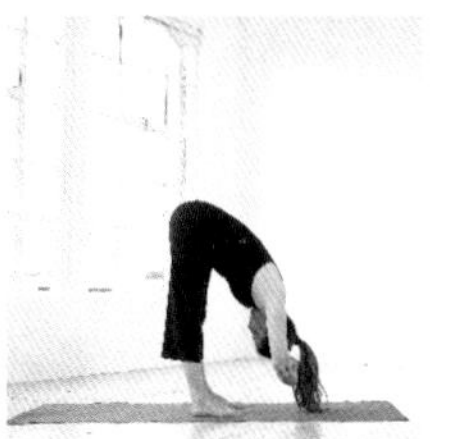
1 **Uttanasana I**

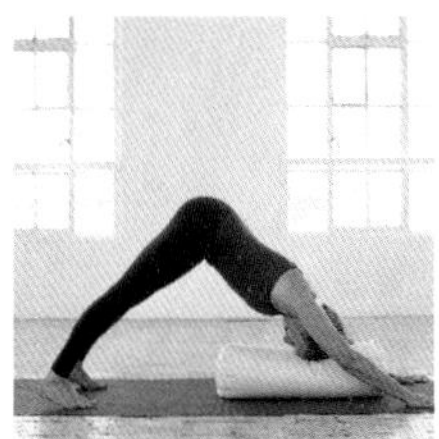
2 **Adho Mukha Svanasana** (s)

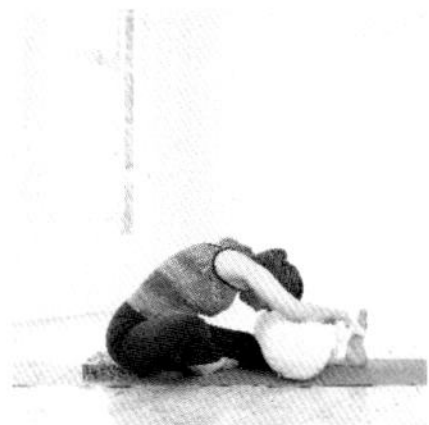
3 **Janusirsasana** (s)

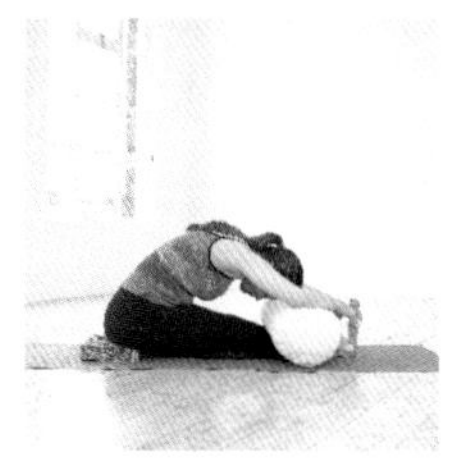
4 **Pascimottanasana** (s)

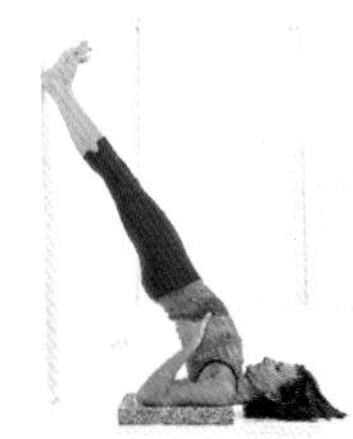
5 **Salamba Sarvangasana** (w)

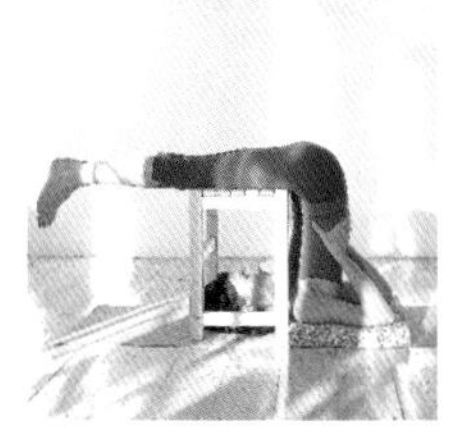
6 **Ardha Halasana**

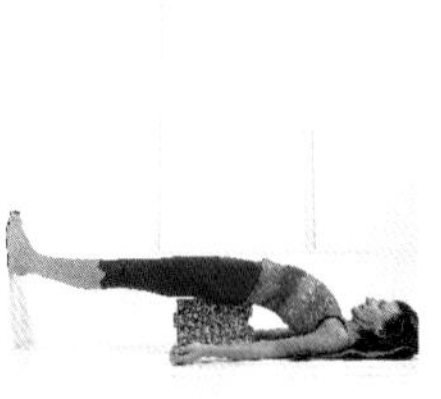
7 **Setu Bandha Sarvangasana**

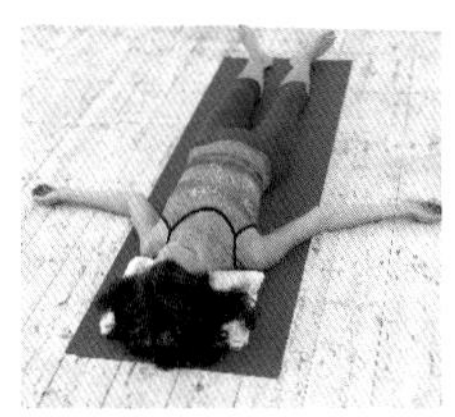
8 **Savasana**

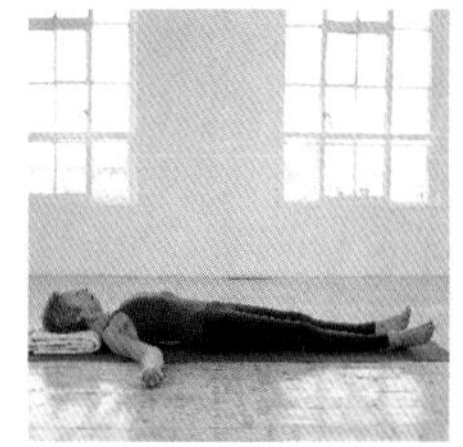
9 **Pranayama**

Surya Namaskara – Sun Salutation

In this short routine the postures are linked together in a flowing movement. It can be practised only when the individual postures have been learnt and understood, which may be after completing the previous 27 sequences. The cycle of postures can be repeated 4–12 times, depending on the time available and the energy of the practitioner.

Surya Namaskar involves quick postures and movement, with each pose held for a few breaths only. Regular practice improves mobility, alertness, agility and speed, while developing willpower and physical strength. The brain becomes active and refreshed.

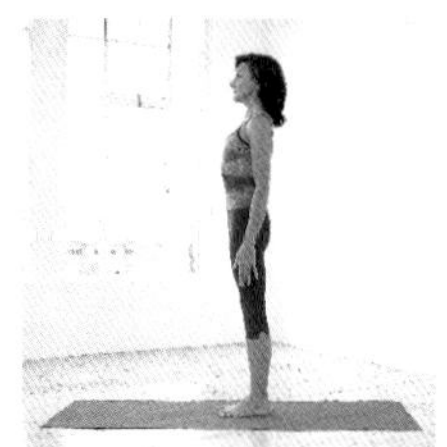
1 **Tadasana**

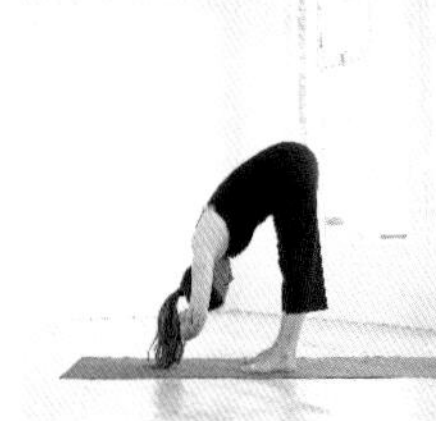
2 Exhale, extend into **Uttanasana I**

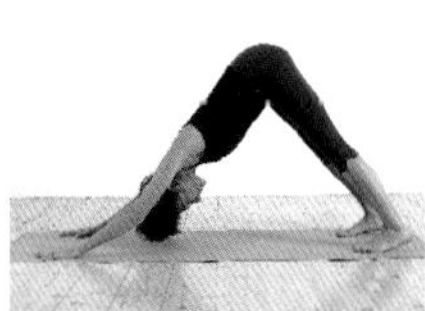
3 Step back into **Adho Mukha Svanasana**

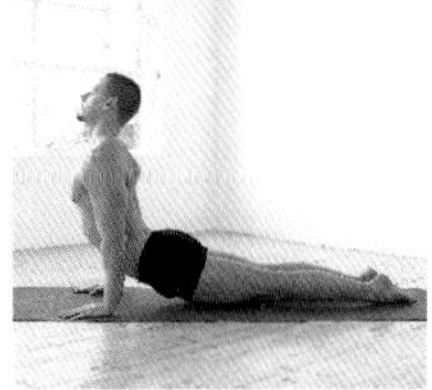
4 Inhale, roll forward into **Urdhva Mukha Svanasana**

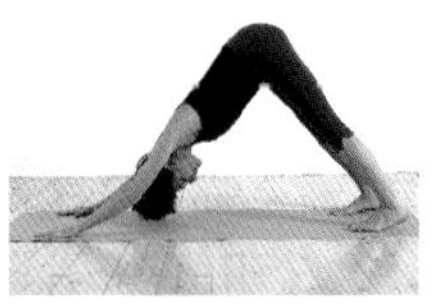
5 Exhale, come back to **Adho Mukha Svanasana**

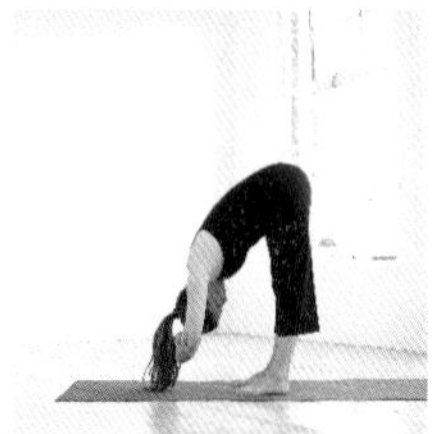
6 On the next exhale jump forwards into **Uttanasana I**

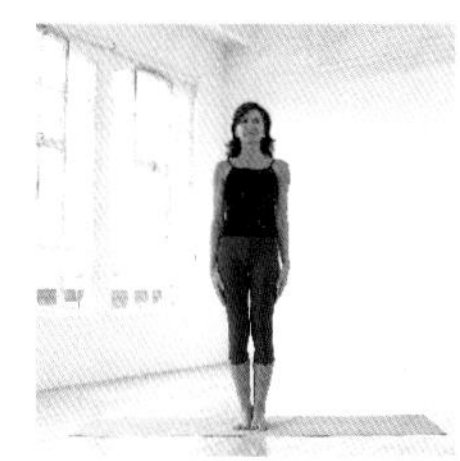
7 Exhale, release the arms and come back into **Tadasana**

Focus

- People with heart problems and women who are menstruating should not practise this routine.
- Breathe normally for 3–4 breaths before jumping or stepping into the next posture.
- Synchronize the inhalation and exhalation as you move from one position to another.
- Repeat the routine 4–12 times.
- After completion, rest in Uttanasana I to recover.

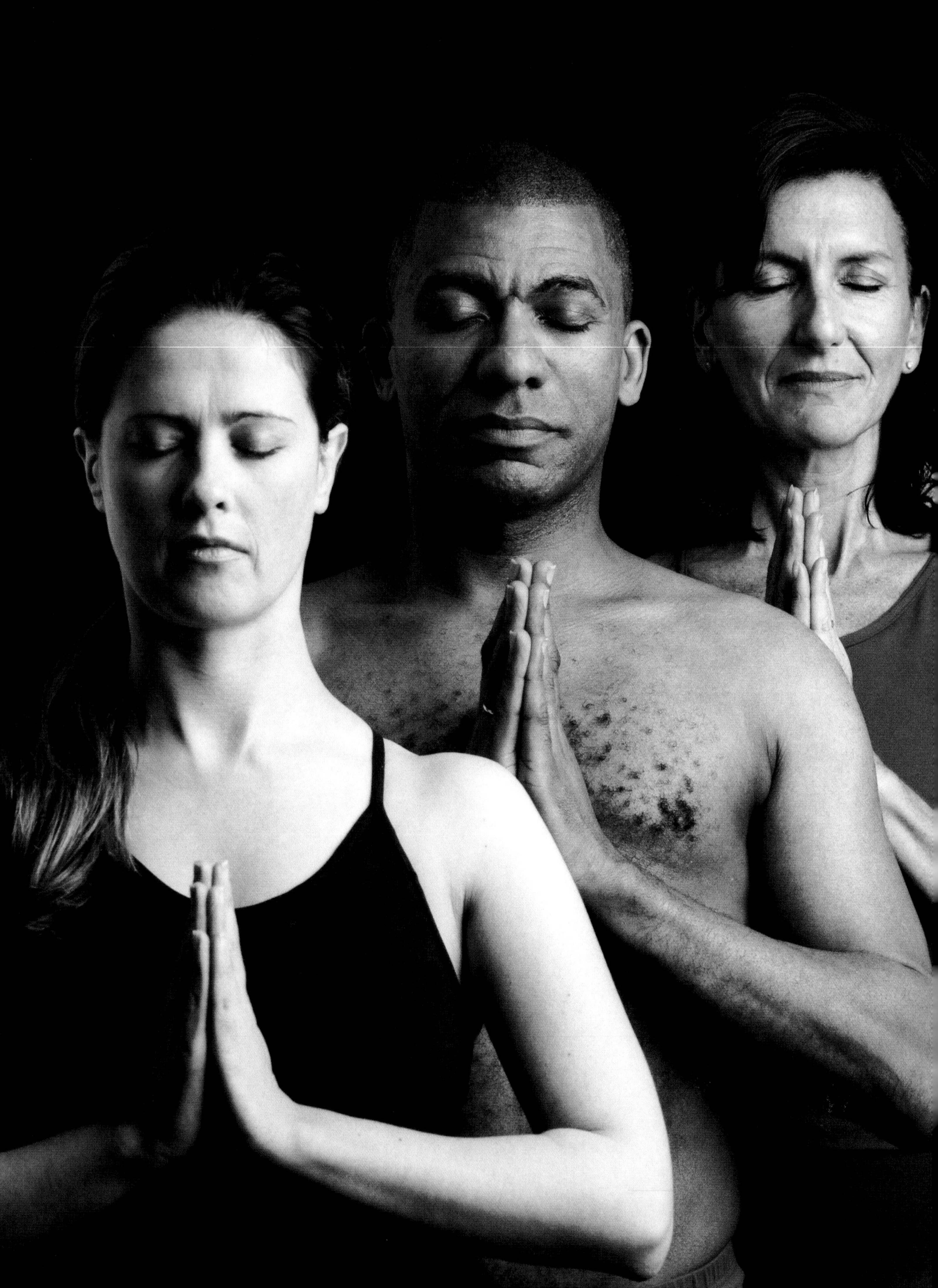

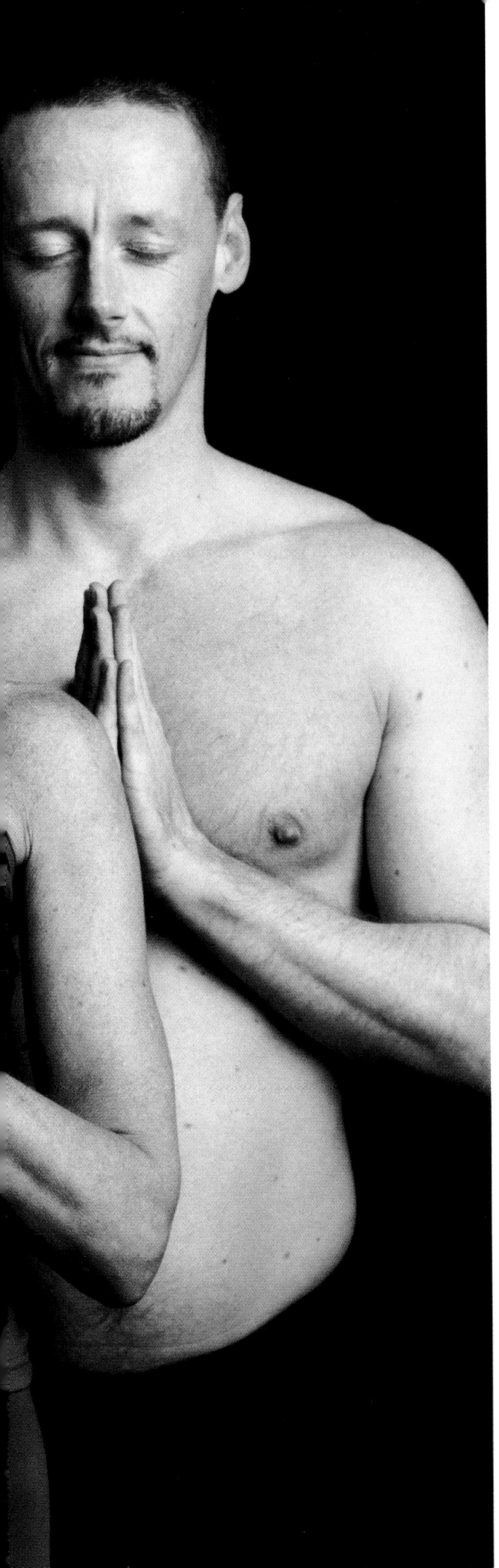

Yoga Therapy

"Yoga's system of healing is based on the premise that the body should be allowed to function as naturally as possible. Practising the recommended asanas will first rejuvenate the body, and then tackle the causes of the ailment."
B.K.S. Iyengar

Therapeutic Yoga

Yoga can help to improve and heal parts of the body that are injured, traumatized or neglected. Movement of the body in asanas stimulates injured joints, muscles or organs by increasing the flow of blood to these parts. The practice of yoga also increases one's pain threshold. This chapter on therapeutic yoga is based on the sequencing of selected postures to treat specific minor ailments. The postures are adapted by using props and are therefore accessible to all students, regardless of their complaints or the condition of their bodies.

HEALING WITH YOGA

When the body is tired and lethargic, practising with props helps to improve the posture, maintain balance and allow the student to stretch fully while experiencing a state of relaxation during practice. This feeling of peace and tranquillity is the beginning of the healing process.

In some cases, the practice of yoga will not result in a complete cure, but in most cases it will alleviate some of the suffering and discomfort associated with the condition, and boost confidence and morale. Practising the asanas with dedication and patience calms the brain and soothes the nerves. This reduces the anxiety of pain, which in itself helps to reduce the actual pain and improve one's threshold.

On my last visit to India, I was fortunate enough to work as an assistant in the Therapeutic Class run by Mr Iyengar and his daughter, Geeta. I teach in the Remedial Class at The Iyengar Institute in London, and was interested to compare the two. What struck me most was the severity of some of the medical conditions treated and the sheer determination and dedication of the practitioners. I dealt with a 76-year-old Indian lady with severe knee and lower back problems that resulted in difficulty in walking and constant pain. Using props, we worked through her sequence of postures and, although she was obviously in pain, she enthusiastically, resolutely and patiently worked through her poses. At the end of the class the change in her persona from when she arrived was remarkable. Her body was much more flexible and fluid, her walking was much improved and her pain had diminished. All this was reflected in her serene and peaceful face.

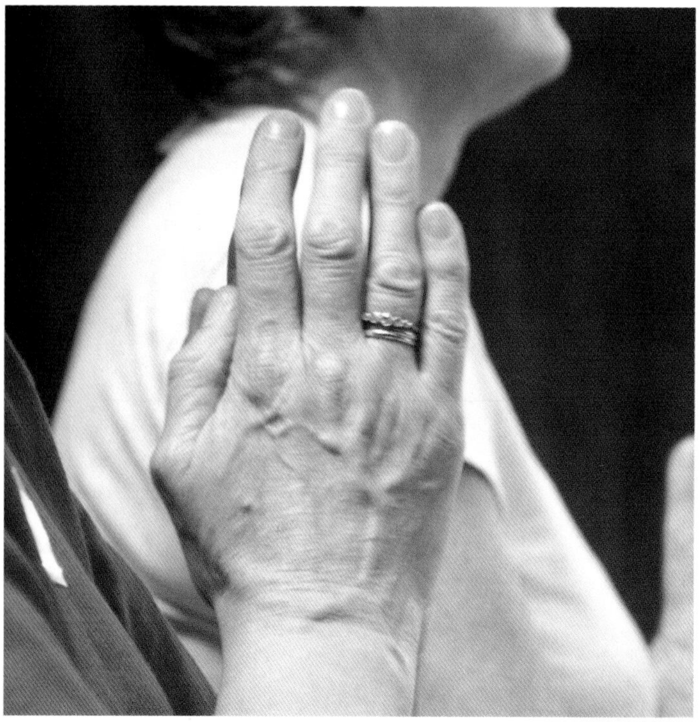

In this section of the book I have offered programmes for minor ailments and common problems. I have not included sequences for serious medical conditions, as these should be done only under the guidance and supervision of a suitably qualified Iyengar teacher. My hope is that the reader/student understands the tremendous need to include yoga in their daily life, and how it can be used effectively with conventional medicine, or alone, to improve or alleviate certain disorders.

Listed on the following pages are postures for everyday ailments. Commonsense should prevail when practising them, and the poses should be held for only as long as is comfortable. When following a sequence for a specific condition, it is best to continue with this programme until some relief is obtained. If difficulty is experienced with a programme, it is advisable to consult an experienced teacher.

Left Iyengar Yoga is a gentle and supportive system of exercise that can help to fend off illness and keep the body supple, whatever the age of the practitioner.

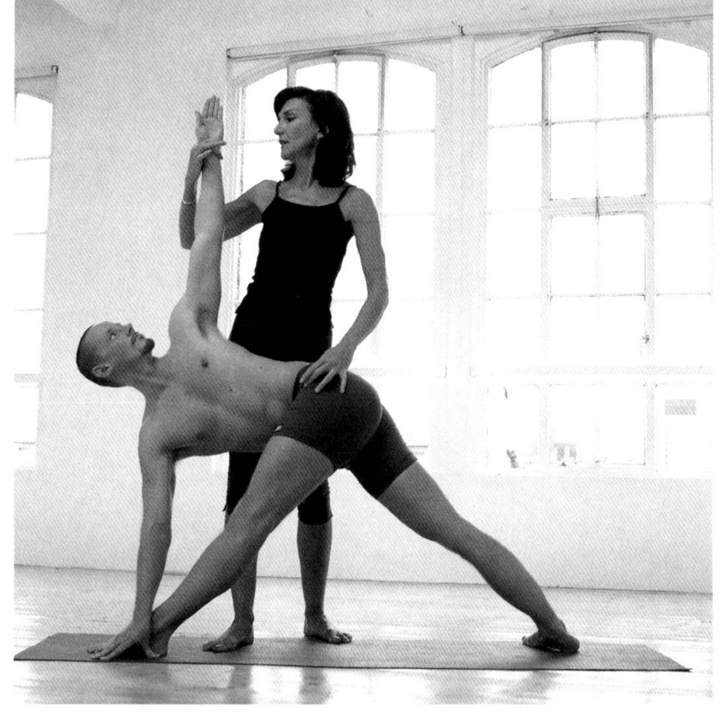

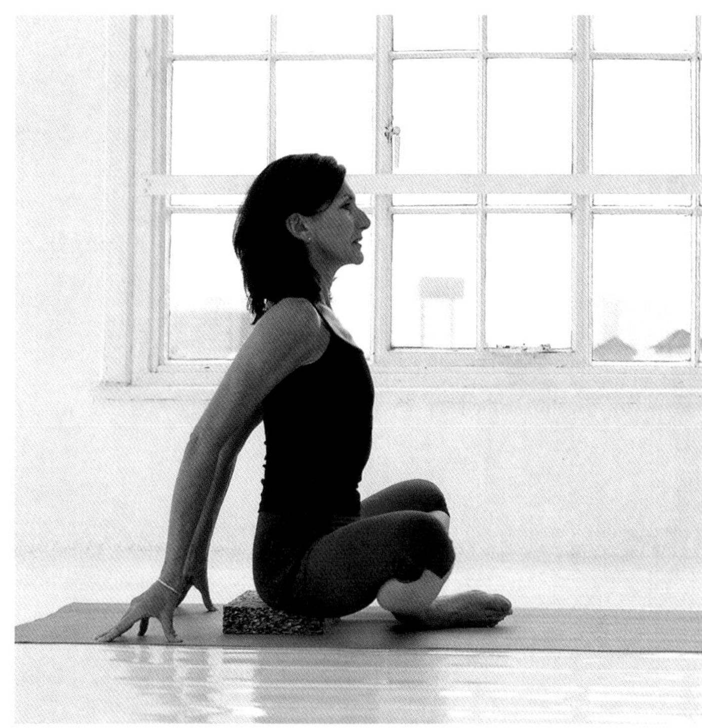

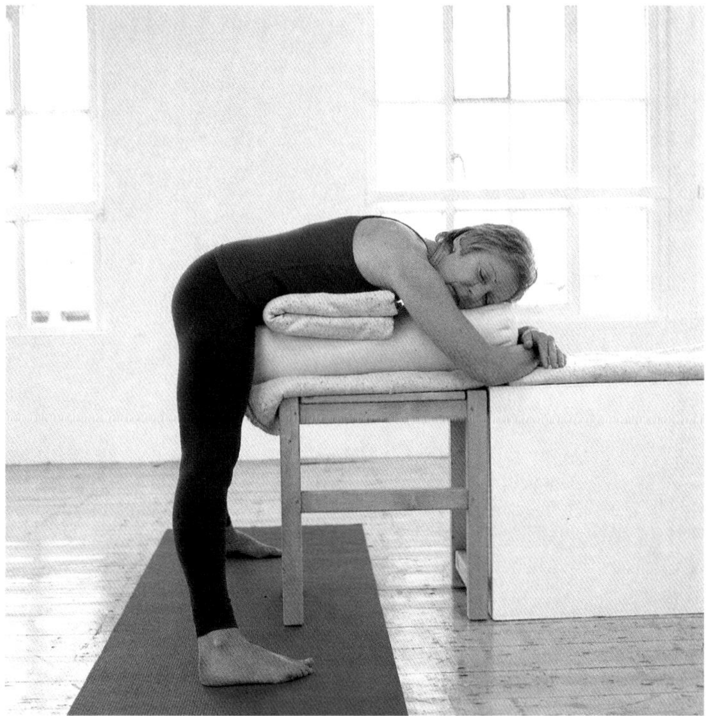

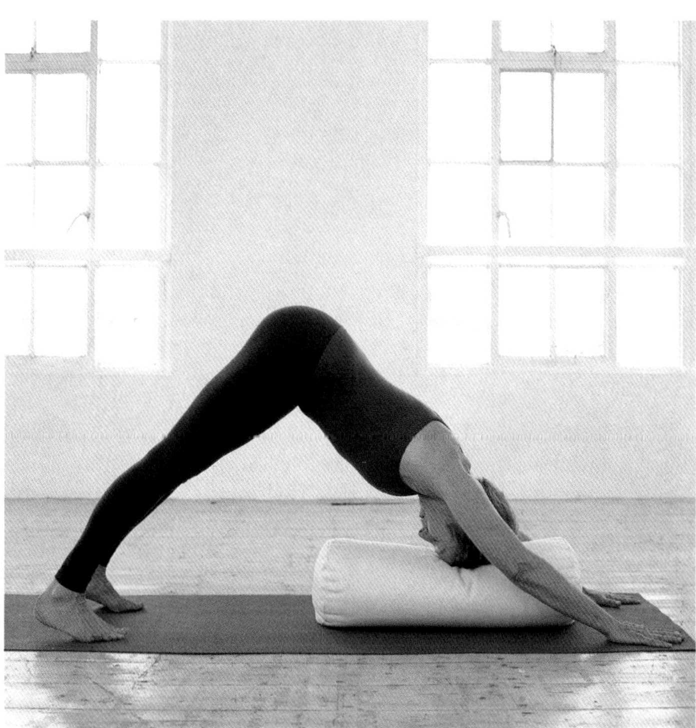

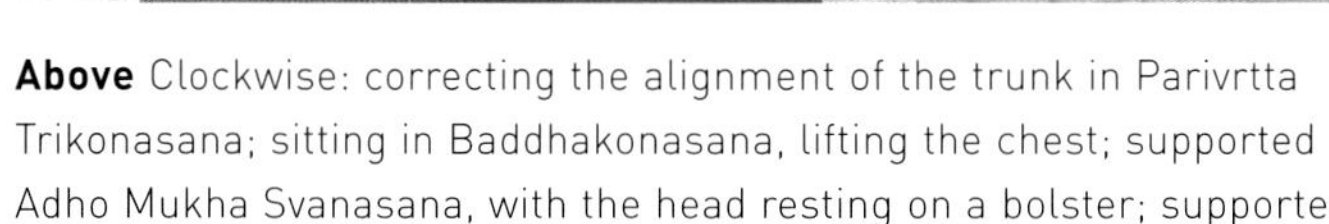

Above Clockwise: correcting the alignment of the trunk in Parivrtta Trikonasana; sitting in Baddhakonasana, lifting the chest; supported Adho Mukha Svanasana, with the head resting on a bolster; supported Prasarita Padottanasana – a quiet, passive posture that allows the brain to stay calm. These are all potentially theraputic postures when used in conjuction with an appropriate routine.

Mental Fatigue and Exhaustion

Stress and physical exertion contribute to fatigue and exhaustion, and if this is not checked it can develop into chronic fatigue syndrome. The pace of daily life has an impact on the body and the emotions.

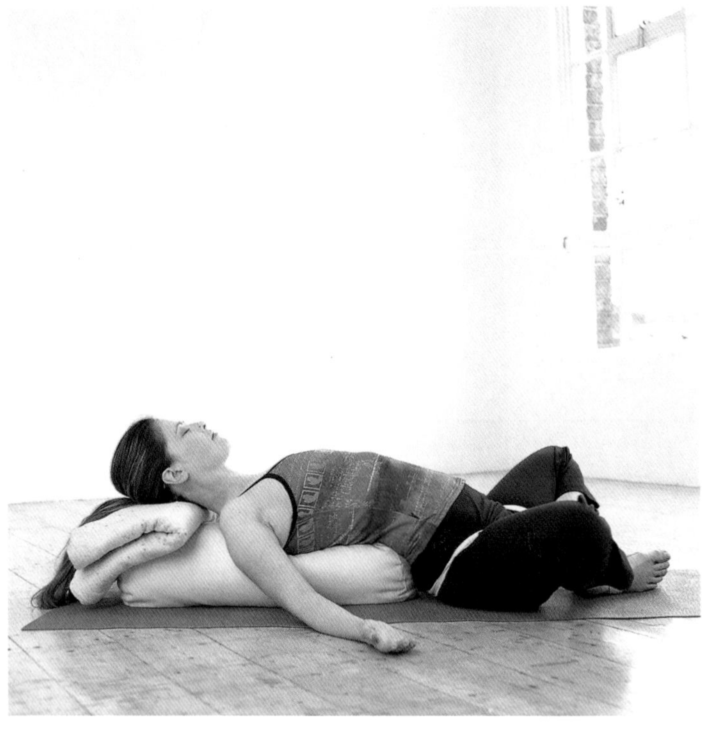

1 **Supta Baddhakonasana** using a bolster and folded blanket to support the head and neck and a strap to keep the feet close to the body.

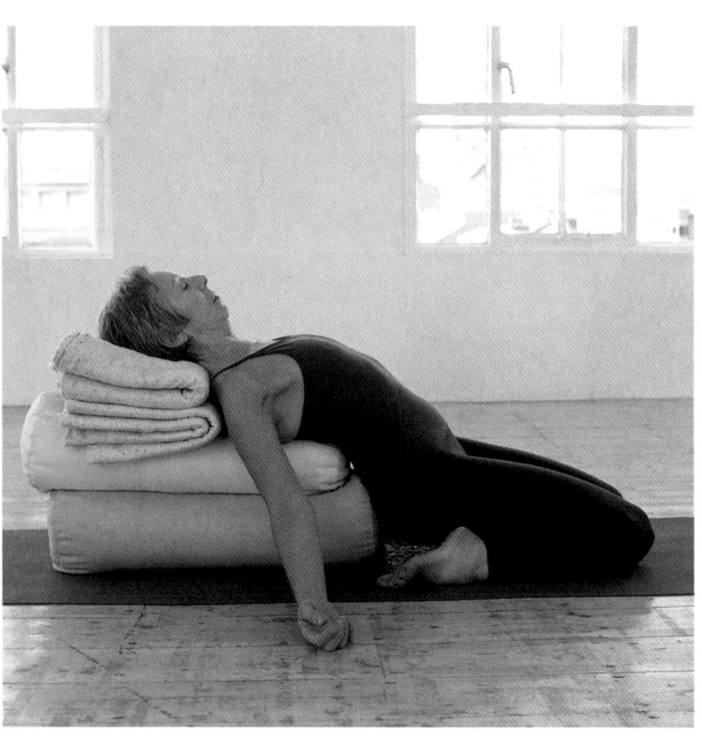

2 **Supta Virasana** with as much support as is needed placed under the spine, neck and head to allow the back and knees to release. Keep the chest open and up and the shoulders relaxed and back.

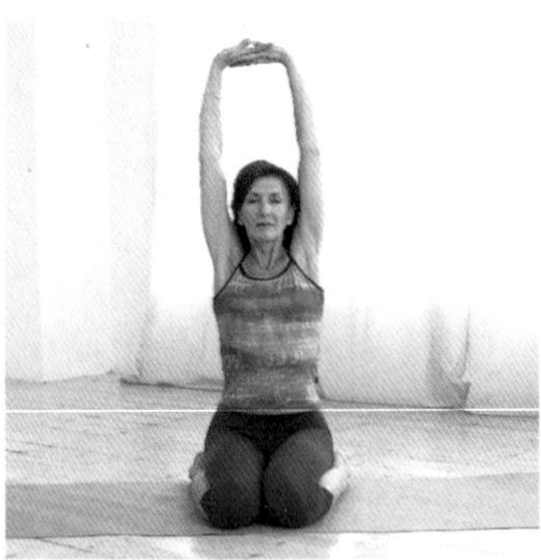

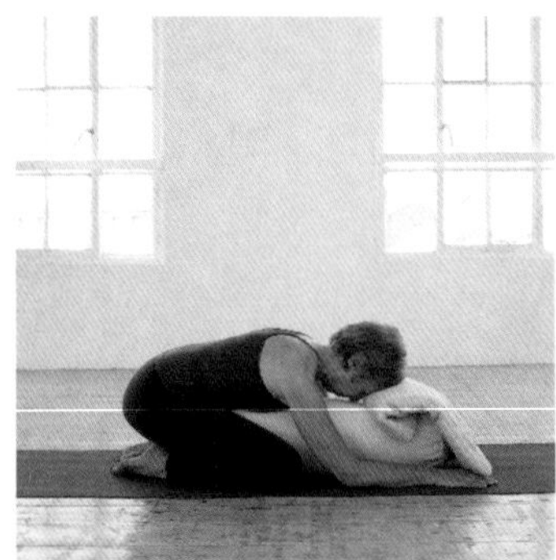

3 **Virasana with Parvatasana** extending the palms towards the ceiling.
4 **Adho Mukha Virasana** with the head and trunk supported on a bolster and/or blanket.

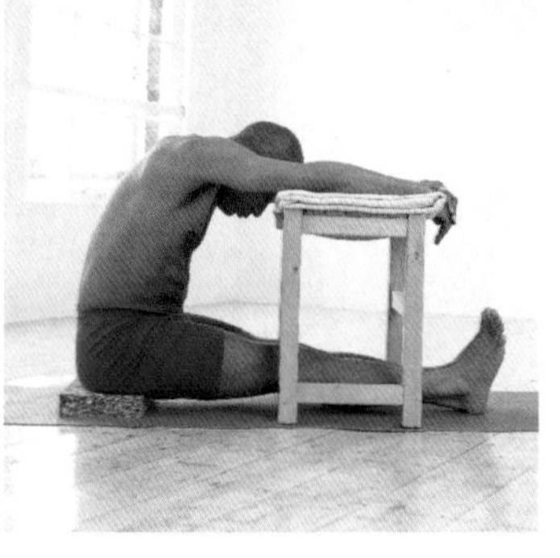

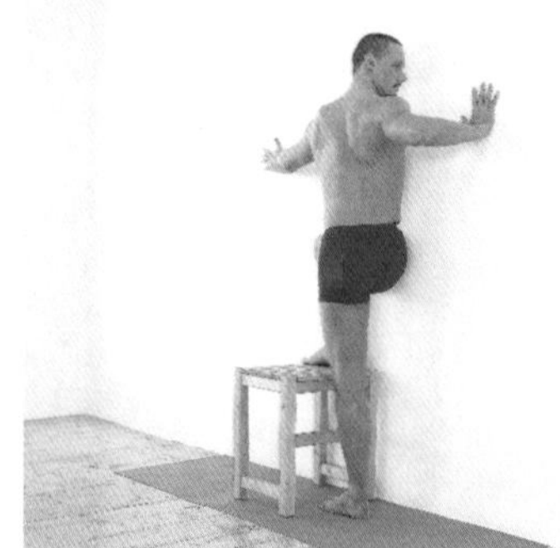

5 **Pascimottanasana** with the forehead supported on a stool so as not to strain the back.
6 **Standing Maricyasana** using the wall and the stool for support.

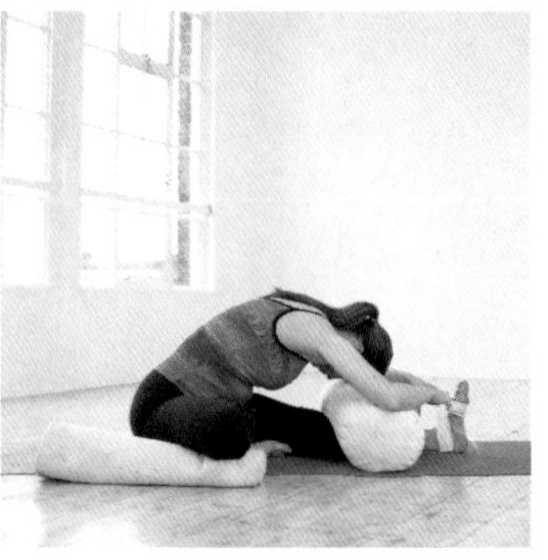

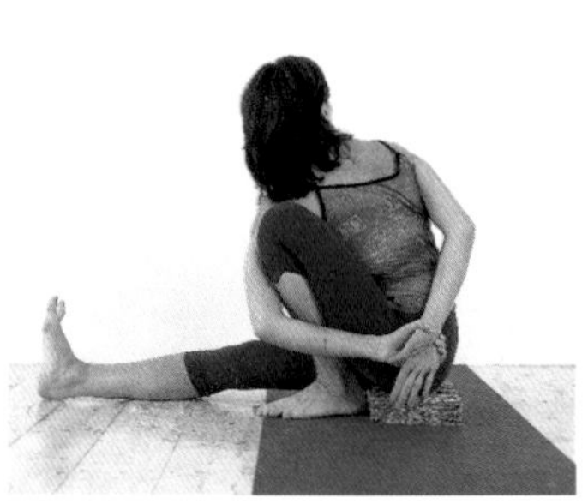

7 **Janusirsasana** with the head, elbows and knee supported on bolsters, and using a strap.
8 **Maricyasana I** sitting on a support to aid the lift of the spine, and turning the chest.

Focus

• In yoga, strong emotions are linked to hormonal imbalances, which leave one vulnerable to infections and illness. This sequence works on stimulating and nourishing the internal organs and the nervous system to pacify and calm the nerves, body and mind.

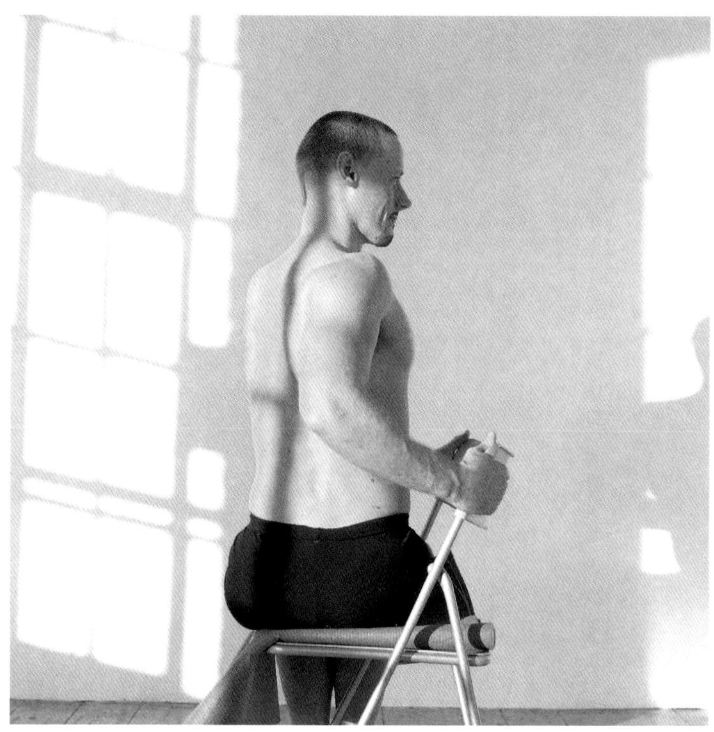

9 **Bharadvajasana (chair)** using the chair to increase the turn. Keep the feet on the floor, parallel to one another, to stabilize the hips. Turn from the waist, moving a little more with each exhalation.

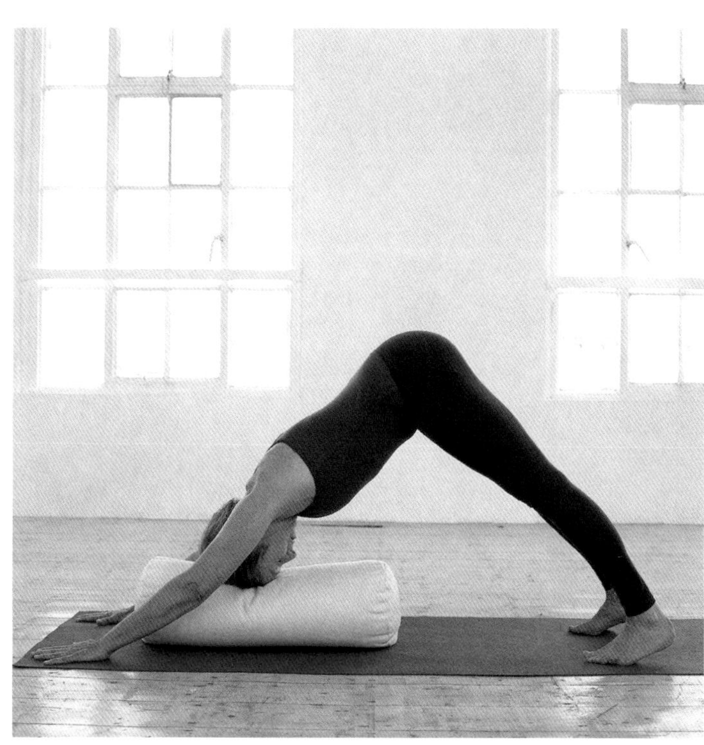

11 **Adho Mukha Svanasana** with the head supported on a bolster to calm the brain.

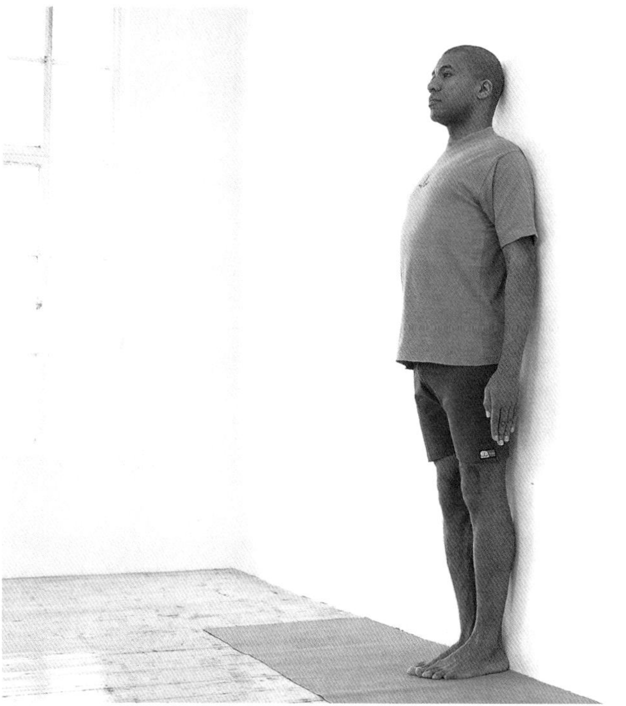

10 **Tadasana** standing against a wall. Use the wall to aid balance, keeping the feet parallel and together and the heels against the wall. Lift the chest, keeping the face and eyes soft.

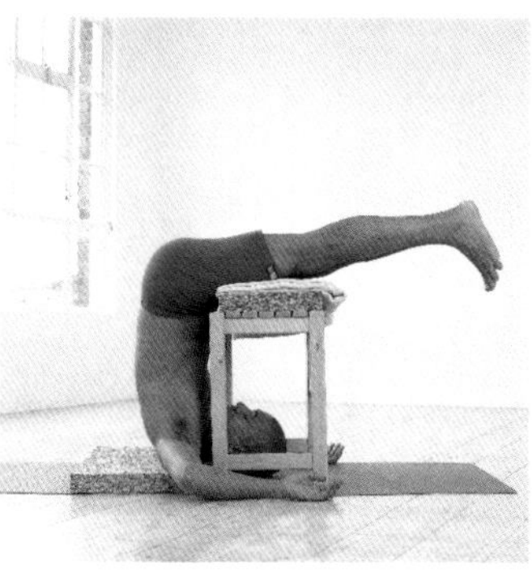

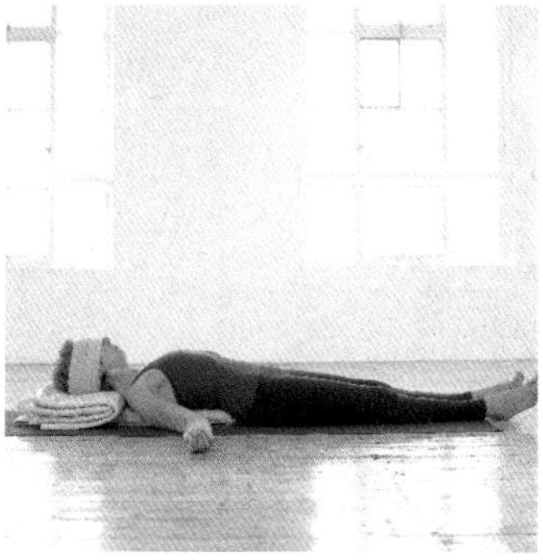

12 **Ardha Halasana** with the legs supported on foam blocks on a stool, and the brain quiet.

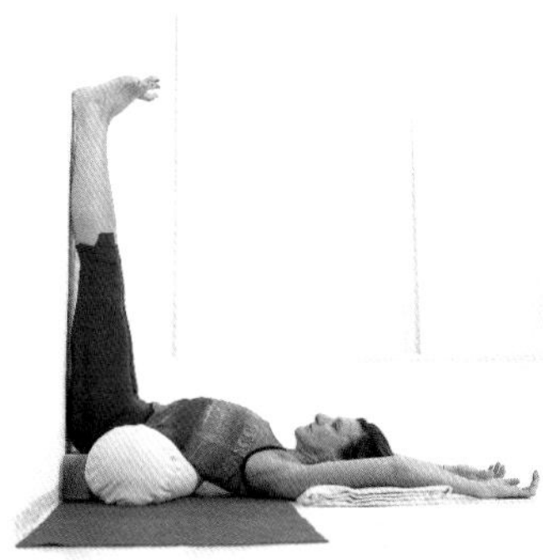

13 **Viparita Karani** using a wooden block and a bolster to support the lower back and hips.

14 **Savasana** with the head and neck supported on a folded blanket, and bandaged eyes.

Headaches / Migraine

This condition is associated with an intense throbbing pain in the head, and in the case of migraine, it may be accompanied with nausea and vomiting. The pain may be a result of tension in the neck muscles and scalp after a stressful event, or due to fatigue and lack of rest.

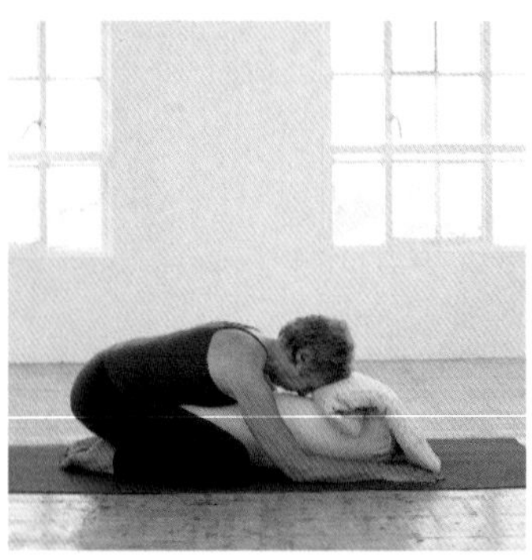

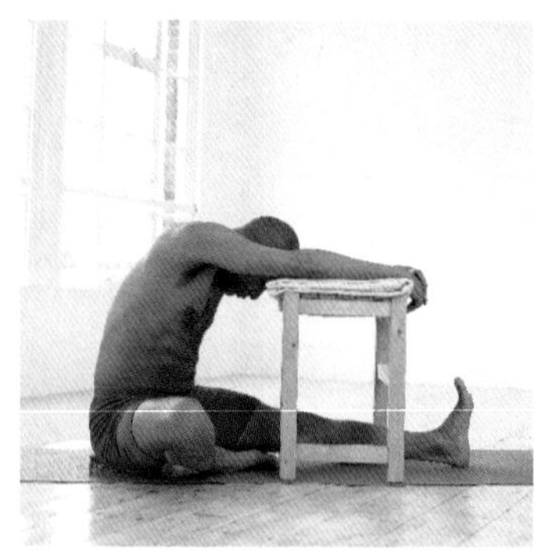

1 **Adho Mukha Virasana** with the head and trunk supported on a bolster and blanket.
2 **Janusirsasnana** with the forehead and arms supported on a stool.

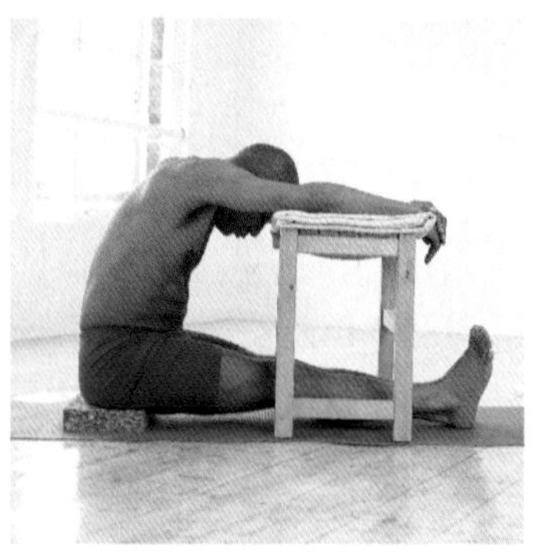

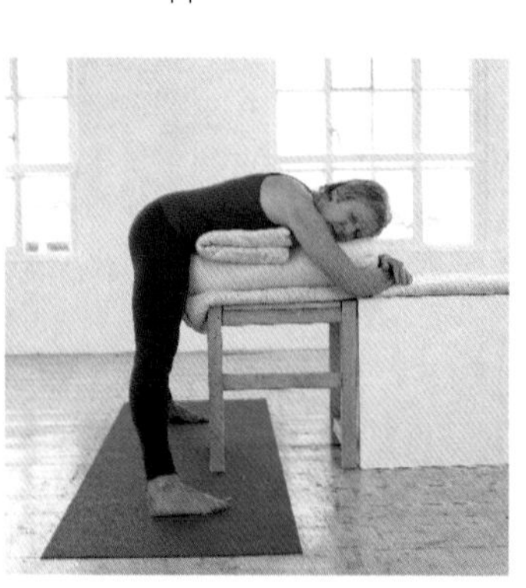

3 **Pascimottanasana** with the forehead and arms supported on a stool.
4 **Prasarita Padottanasana** with the head, trunk and arms supported on a stool and blankets.

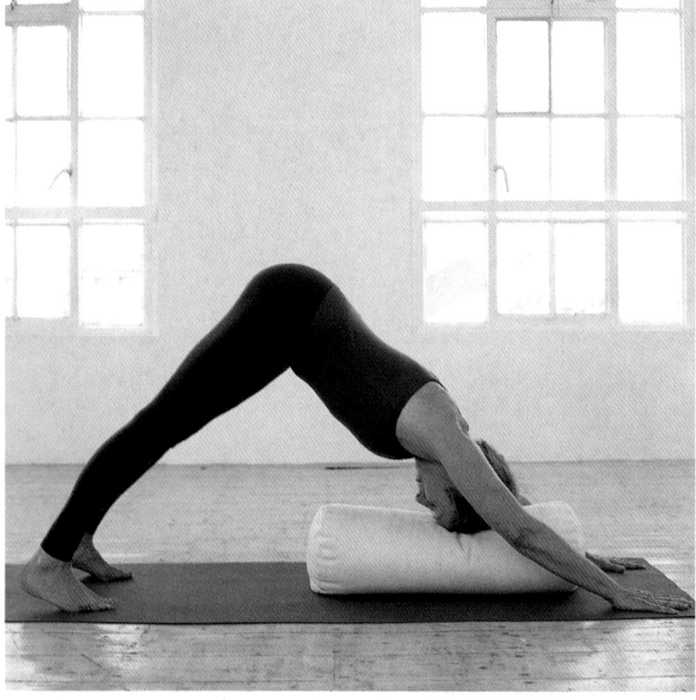

5 **Adho Mukha Svanasana** with the head supported on a bolster, or a pile of blankets, in order to keep the brain calm.

6 **Uttanasana I** with the head and forearms supported on a stool softened with a blanket. This posture, with the head lowered, allows blood to go to the area, helping to relieve any discomfort.

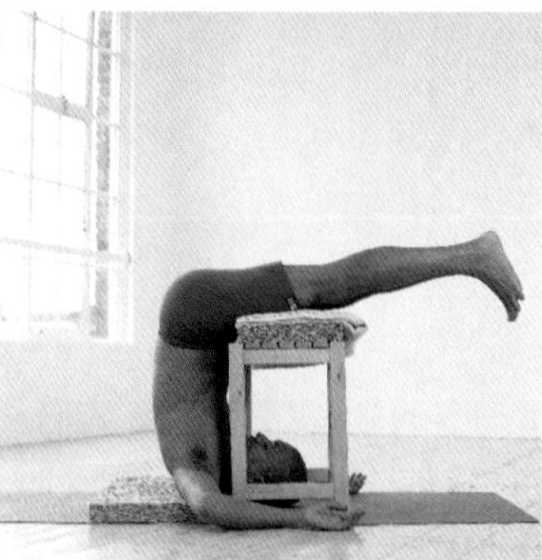

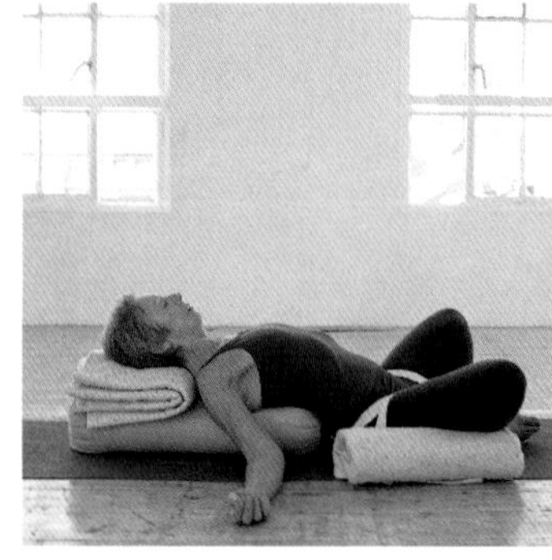

7 **Ardha Halasana** with the legs supported on a stool, the height adjusted with foam blocks.
8 **Supta Baddhakonasana** with a strap around legs, bolster under spine, and head supported.

Focus

- These postures for relieving headaches and migraines increase blood flow to the brain and restore the stability of the nervous system. While doing the postures, be aware of lengthening the muscles of the neck and try to keep the brain as quiet as possible.

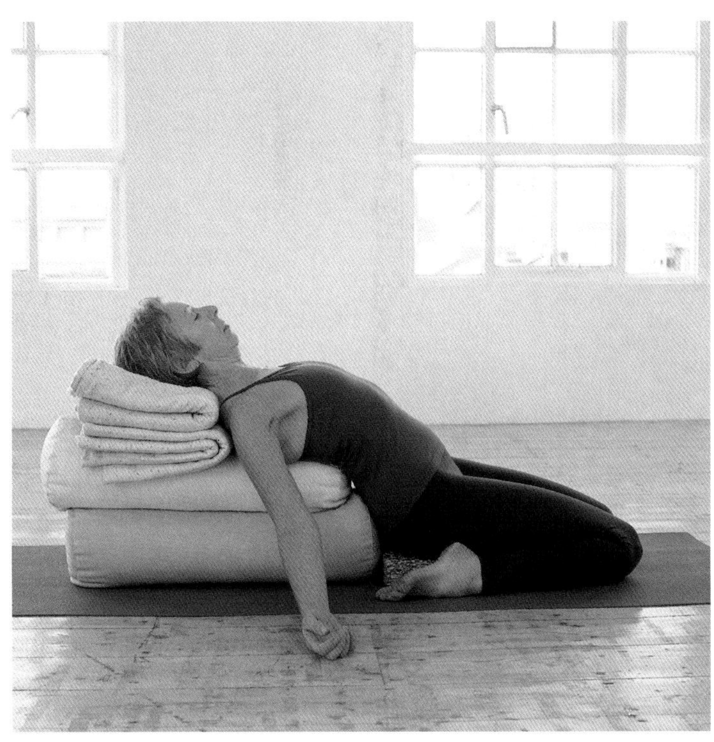

9 **Supta Virasana** with the spine, neck and head supported on two bolsters and two folded blankets.

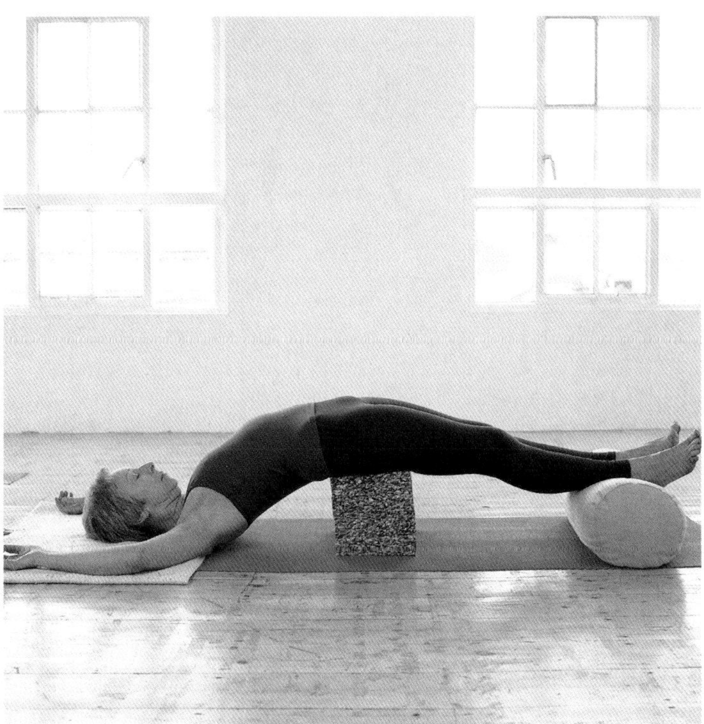

10 **Setu Bandha Sarvangasana** using foam blocks to support the sacrum and a bolster to support the feet, arms extended over the head, palms facing upwards.

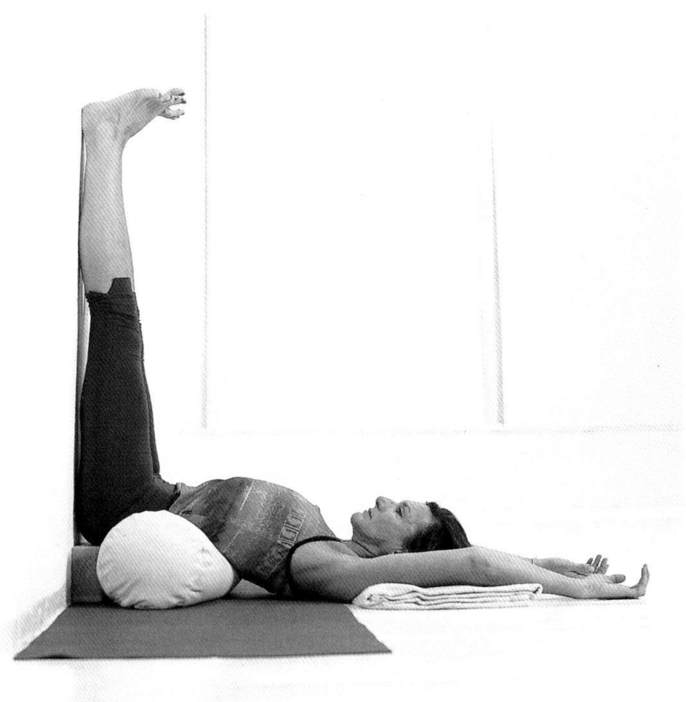

11 **Viparita Karani** with the backs of the legs against the wall and the body lying over a bolster and wooden block. Use a blanket for comfort under the head, arms extended over the head, palms facing upwards.

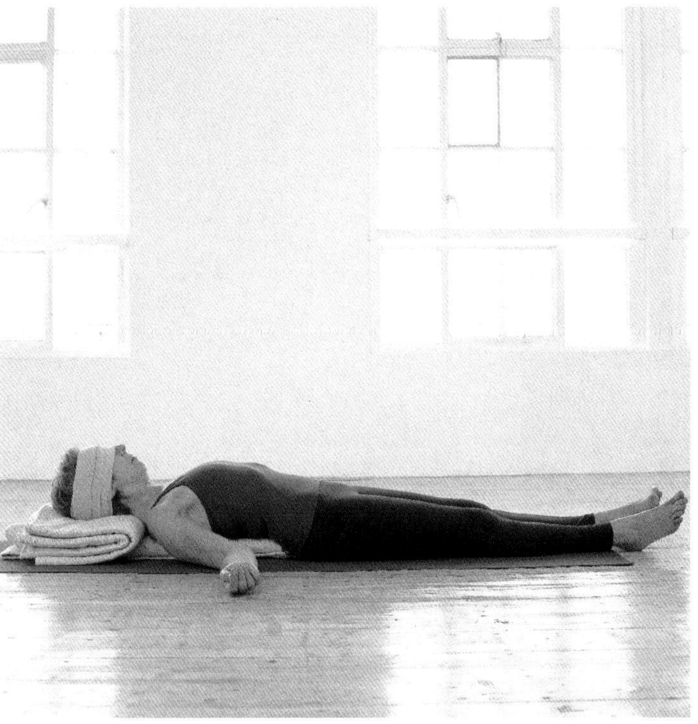

12 **Savasana** with the neck and head supported on a folded blanket. A bandage firmly tied around the head and/or eyes is very soothing and calming, especially when experiencing headaches.

Stress / Anxiety

These postures work on tense muscles and encourage blood to circulate. This stabilizes the heart rate and blood pressure. Shallow, fast breathing becomes deeper, slower and more rhythmical, which results in a higher intake of oxygen, and this helps to remove stress.

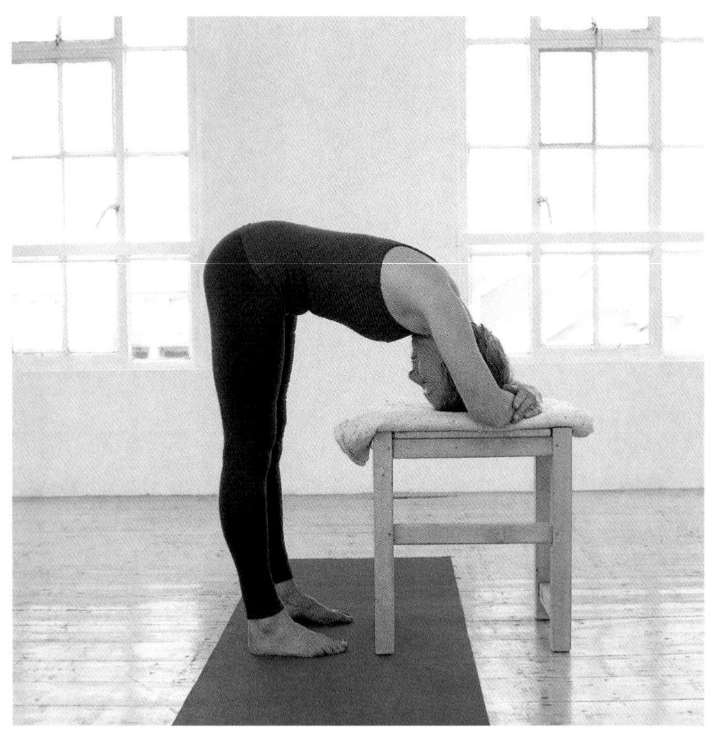

1 **Uttanasana I** with the head supported on a blanket and stool. When one part of the body is strained and tense, circulation to that body part is decreased – increasing it again will help to calm the mind and body.

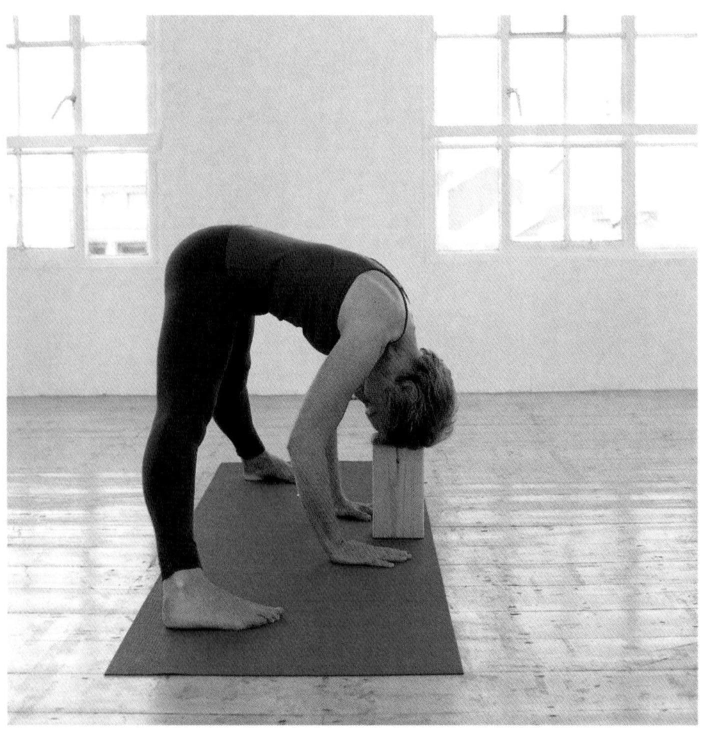

2 **Prasarita Padottanasana** with the head supported on a wooden block. If the hands don't reach the floor, use foam blocks under the palms to raise the floor level. It may be necessary to use more blocks under the head as well.

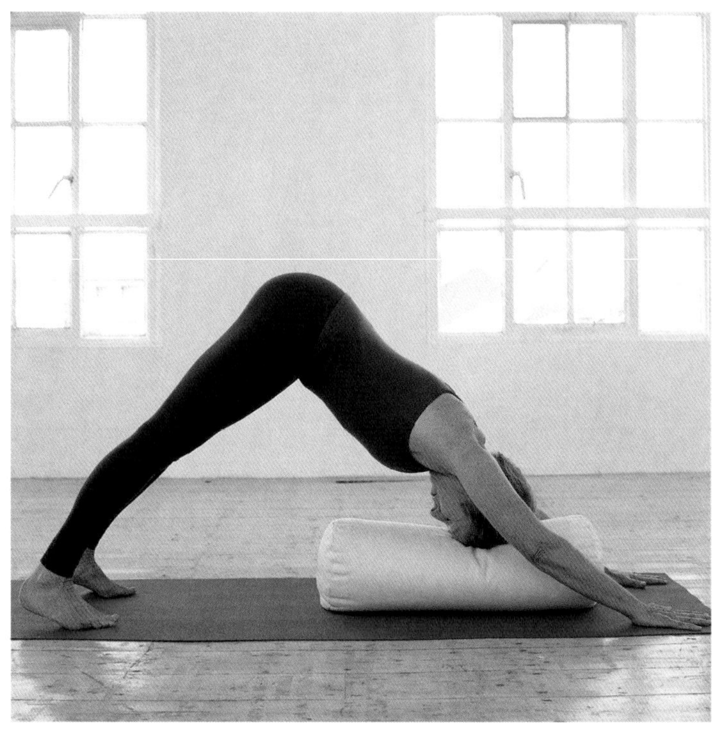

3 **Adho Mukha Svanasana** with the head supported on a bolster to keep the mind quiet.

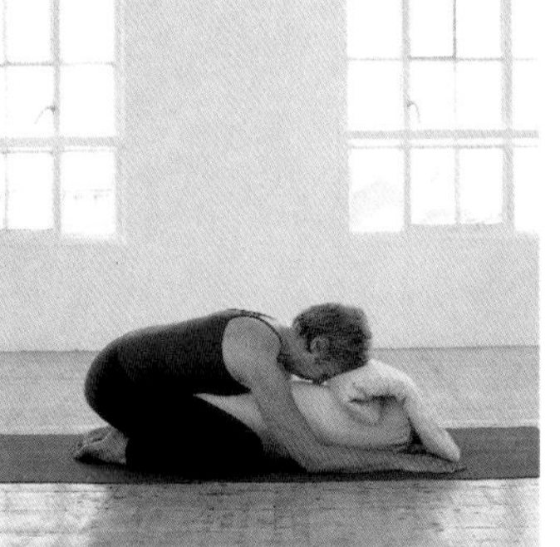

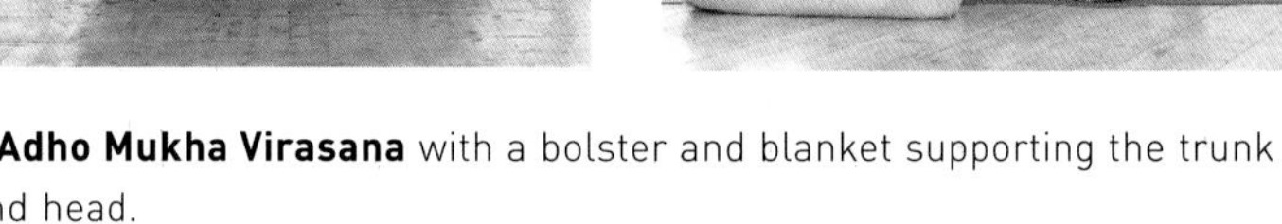

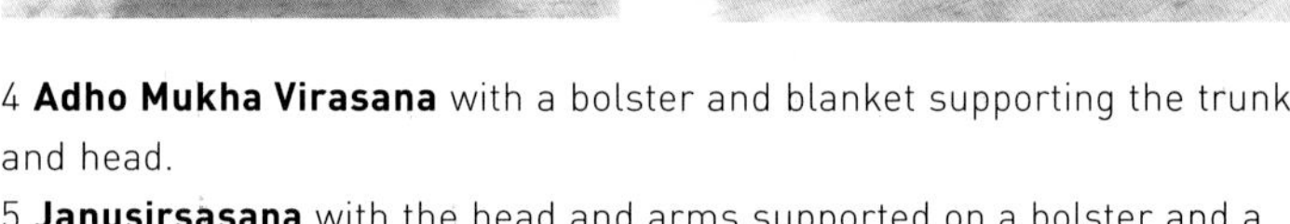

4 **Adho Mukha Virasana** with a bolster and blanket supporting the trunk and head.

5 **Janusirsasana** with the head and arms supported on a bolster and a strap around the foot. If necessary, you may also use a bolster to support the bent knee.

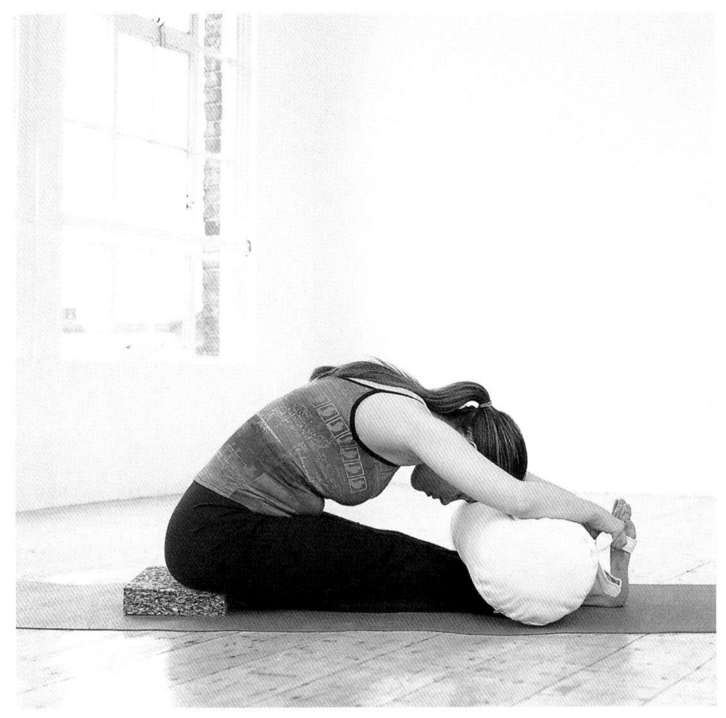

6 **Pascimottanasana** with the head and forearms supported on a bolster and using a strap around the foot. Keep the eyes closed and the mind still and quiet.

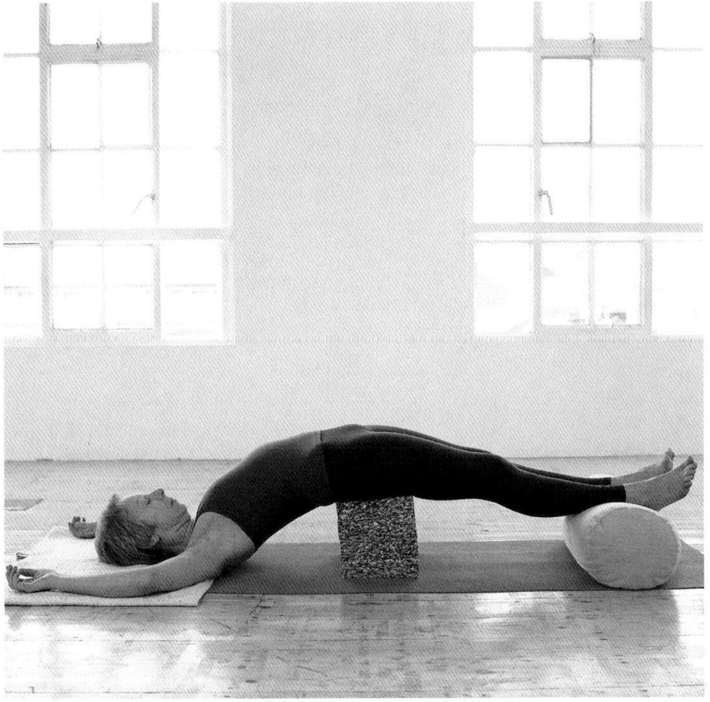

7 **Setu Bandha Sarvangasana** with four foam blocks under the sacrum, feet resting on a bolster and head and shoulders supported on a folded blanket – arms over head, palms facing the ceiling.

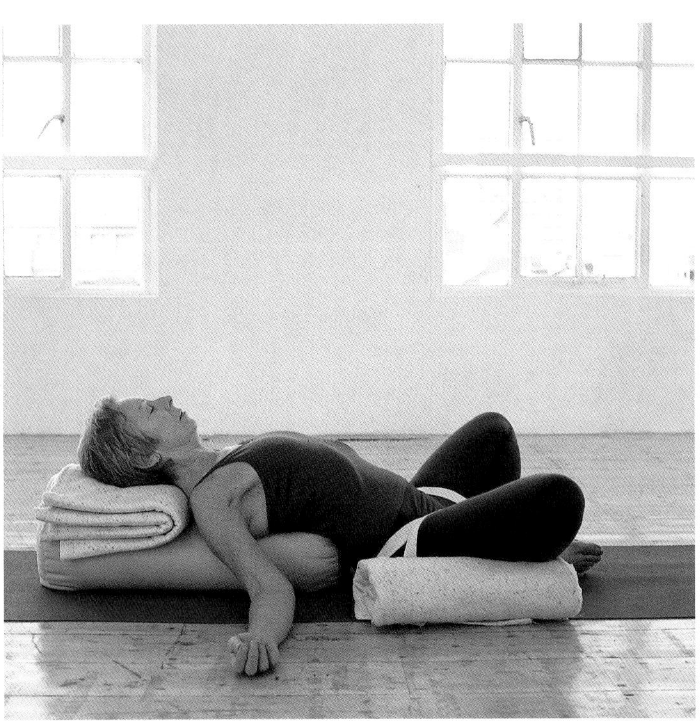

8 **Supta Baddhakonasana** with bolsters and blankets supporting the spine and head, and a strap around the legs and feet. The thighs are supported with rolled-up blankets.

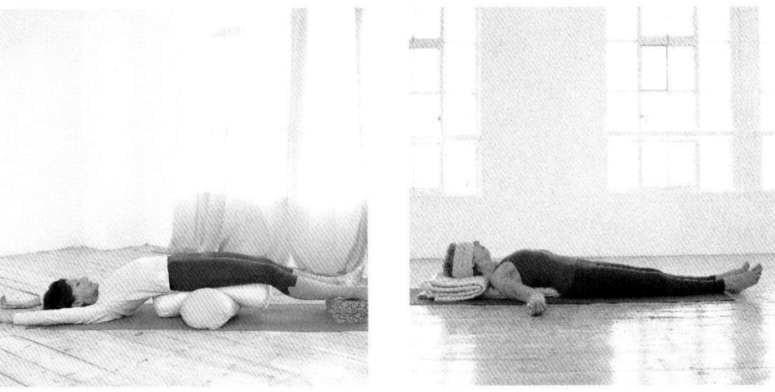

9 **Cross Bolsters** with the feet resting on blocks. This gentle arch opens the chest.

10 **Savasana** with a folded blanket supporting the head and neck, and with the eyes covered.

Focus

- Postures here are done with a support under the head. This allows the brain to become quiet and calm. Breathe normally throughout and focus the mind on the breath. Keep the face, mouth and throat relaxed.
- In order to deal with stress and anxiety, both the mind and body must be treated. Tension associated with stress is stored mainly in the muscles, diaphragm and nervous system and if these areas are relaxed, stress is reduced.

Insomnia

The physiological symptoms of insomnia – raised or lowered blood pressure and exhaustion – can be dealt with by doing these postures with the face, mouth, throat and stomach soft and relaxed, in order to keep the mind and brain quiet.

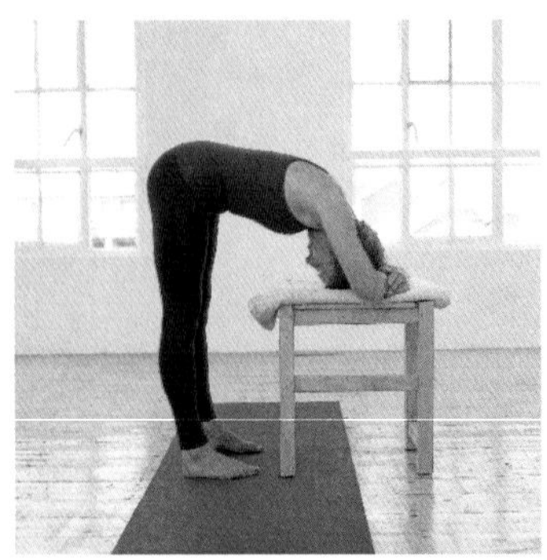

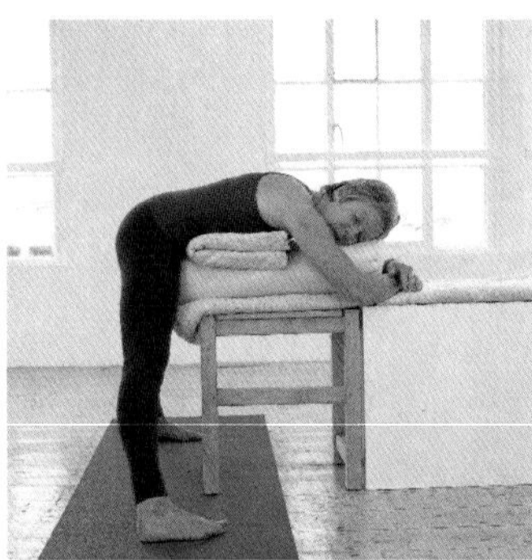

1 **Uttanasana I** with the head and arms supported on a stool.
2 **Prasarita Padottanasana** with trunk, arms and head supported.

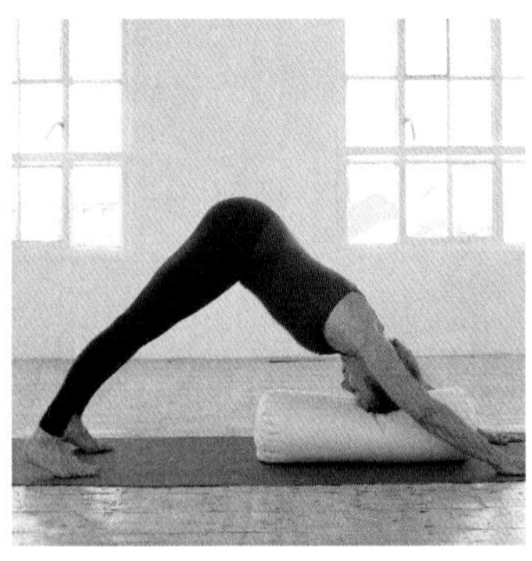

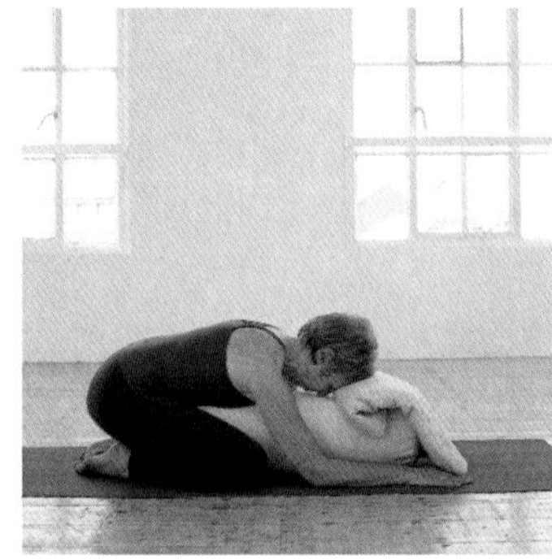

3 **Adho Mukha Svanasana** with the head supported on a bolster.
4 **Adho Mukha Virasana** with the forehead and trunk supported.

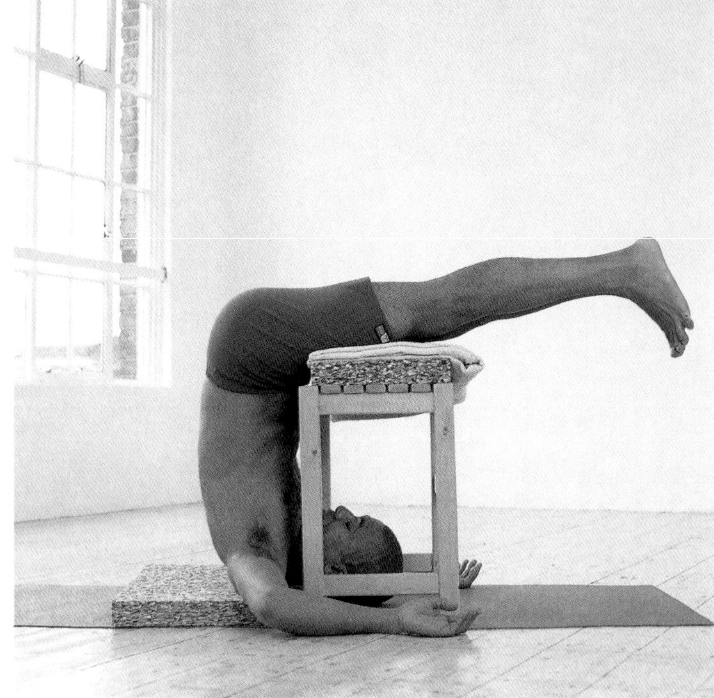

9 **Ardha Halasana** with a stool and foam blocks for support.

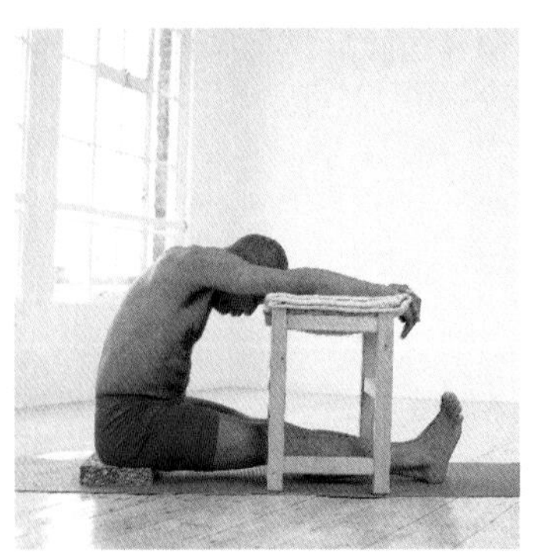

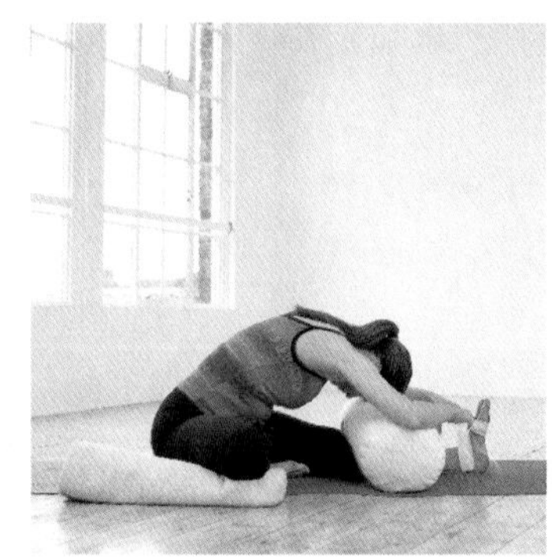

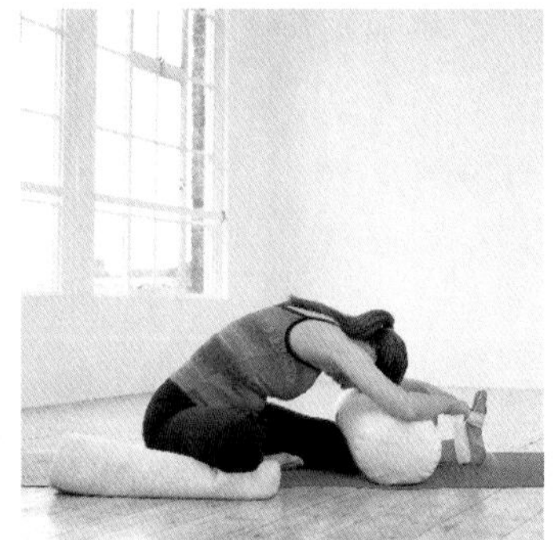

5 **Pascimottanasana** with the forehead and arms supported.
6 **Janusirsasana** with the forehead and arms supported, using a strap.

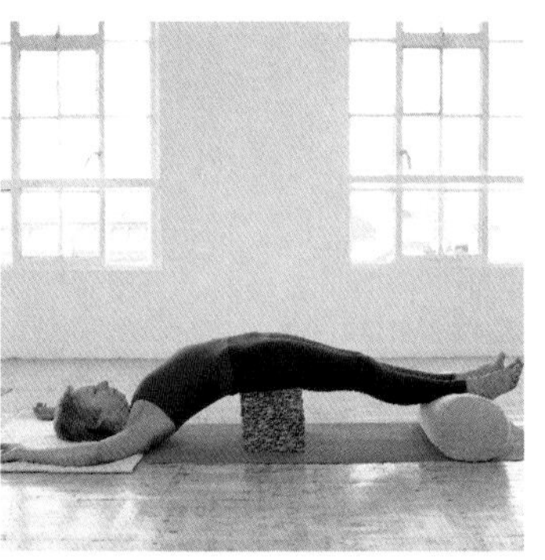

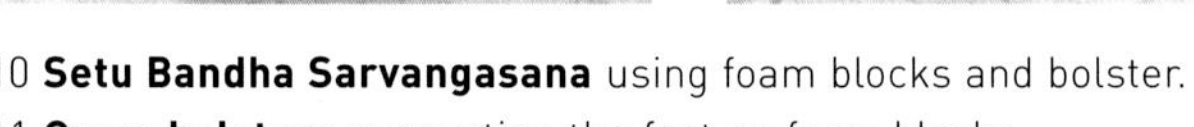

10 **Setu Bandha Sarvangasana** using foam blocks and bolster.
11 **Cross bolsters** supporting the feet on foam blocks.

7 **Supta Baddhakonasana** using a strap and bolster support.
8 **Chair Sarvangasana** shoulder stand using a chair and bolster.

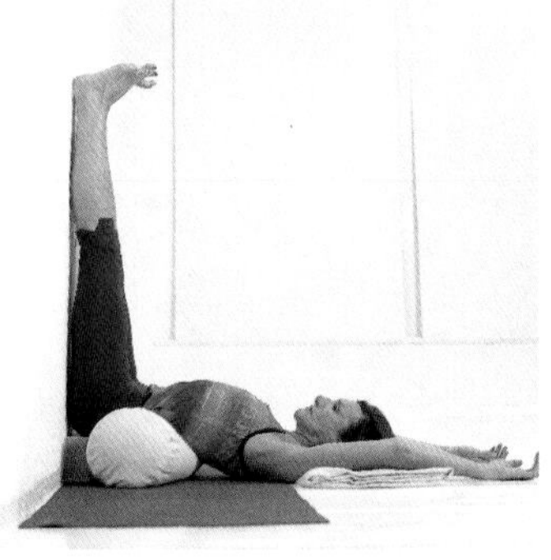

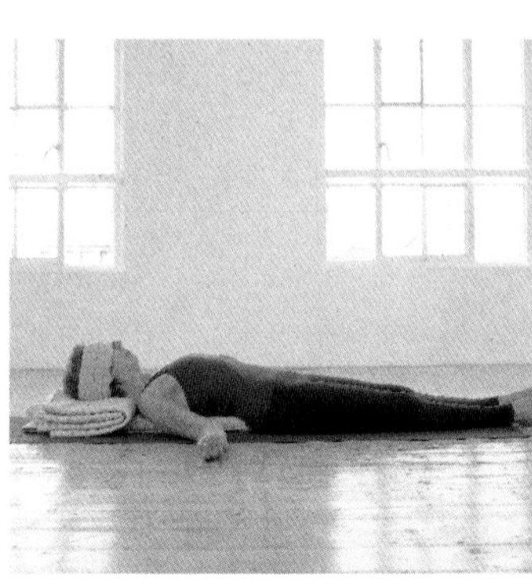

12 **Viparita Karani** legs against wall, support under lower back.
13 **Savasana** head and neck supported, eyes bandaged.

Depression

Whilst performing the postures, there needs to be a balance between the mind, body, emotions, and soul. Since the head is supported in these postures, the mind becomes calm and the heart is energised, bringing about courage and a healthy mental state.

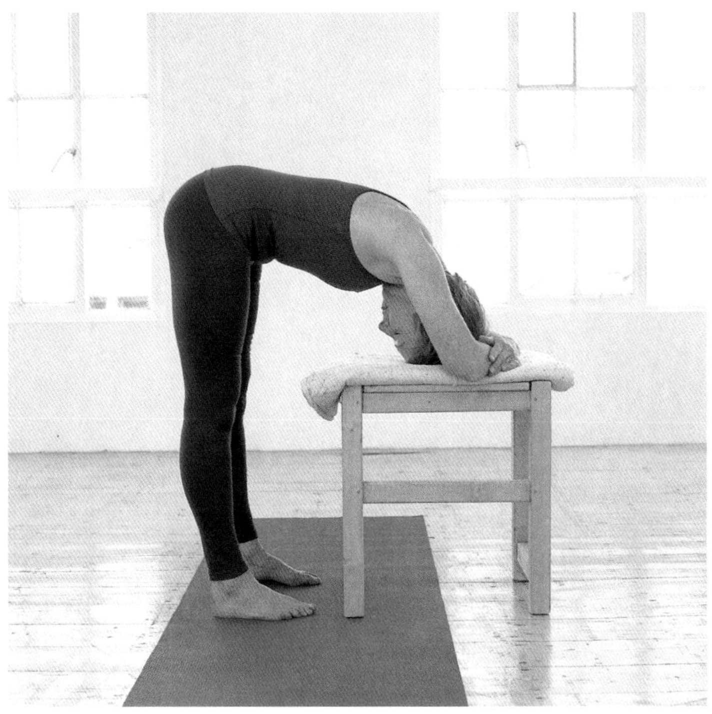

1 **Uttanasana I** with the head and forearms supported on a stool. Since the head is supported in these postures, the mind becomes calm and the heart is energized – this brings about courage and a healthy mental state.

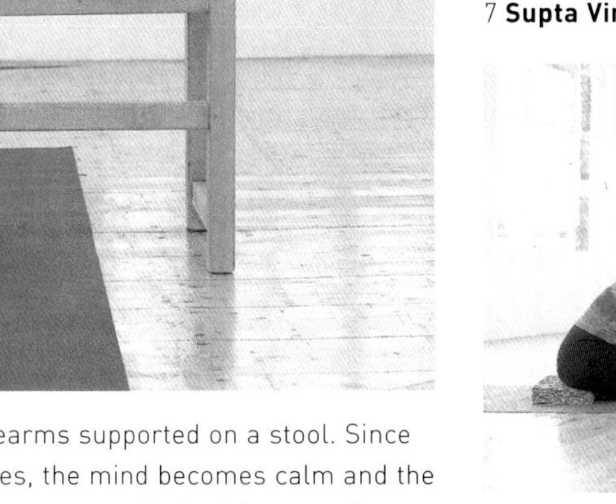

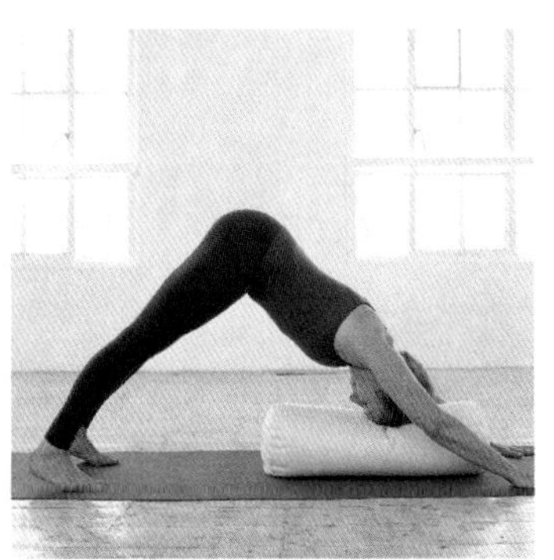

2 **Prasarita Padottanasana** with trunk, head and arms supported.
3 **Adho Mukha Svanasana** with the head supported on a bolster.

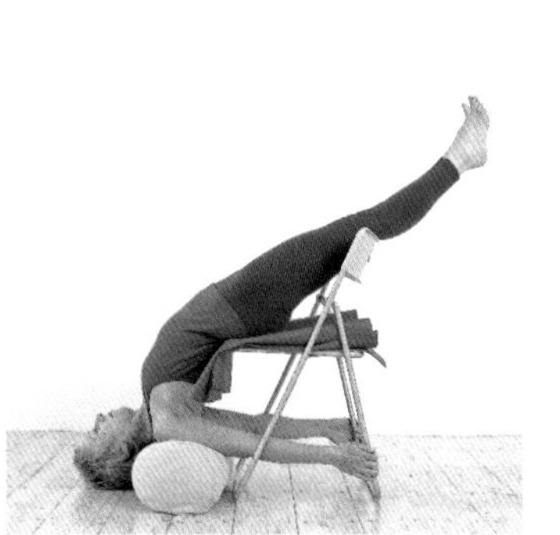

4 **Chair Sarvangasana** using a bolster for the shoulders.
5 **Ustrasana** with a chair and bolsters supporting the spine.

6 **Supta Baddhakonasana** with a strap and supports.
7 **Supta Virasana** with several bolsters for support.

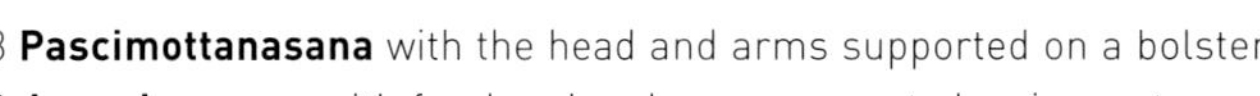

8 **Pascimottanasana** with the head and arms supported on a bolster.
9 **Janusirsasana** with forehead and arms supported, using a strap.

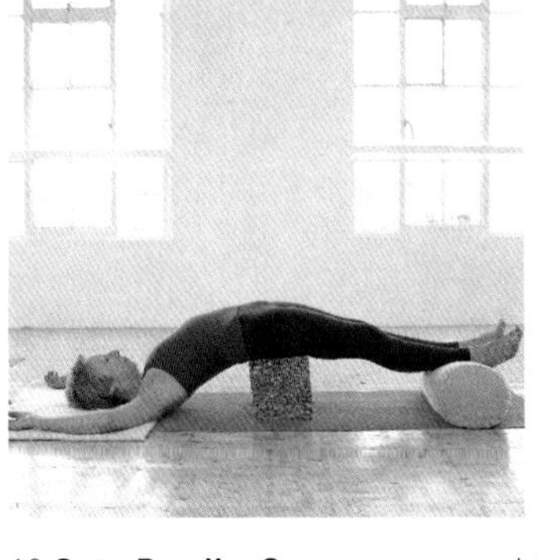

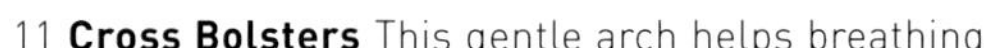

10 **Setu Bandha Sarvangasana** with supports under sacrum/feet.
11 **Cross Bolsters** This gentle arch helps breathing.

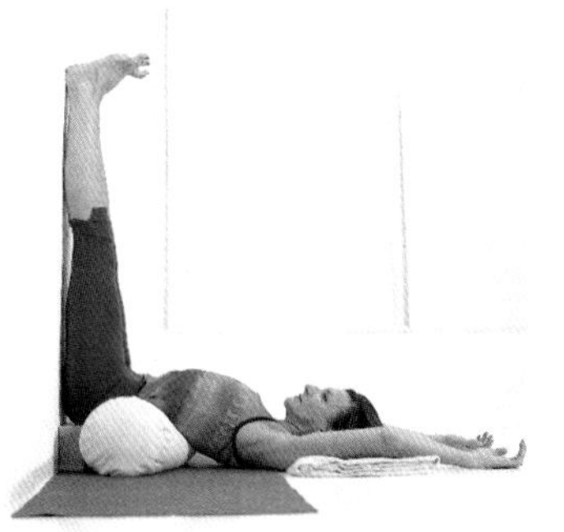

12 **Viparita Karani** with legs up the wall and a bolster for support.
13 **Savasana** using support and with the eyes covered.

Colds

In some of the postures listed below, the head is down, which helps to drain the nasal passages and sinuses. In others, the chest is supported and lifted to facilitate easier breathing.

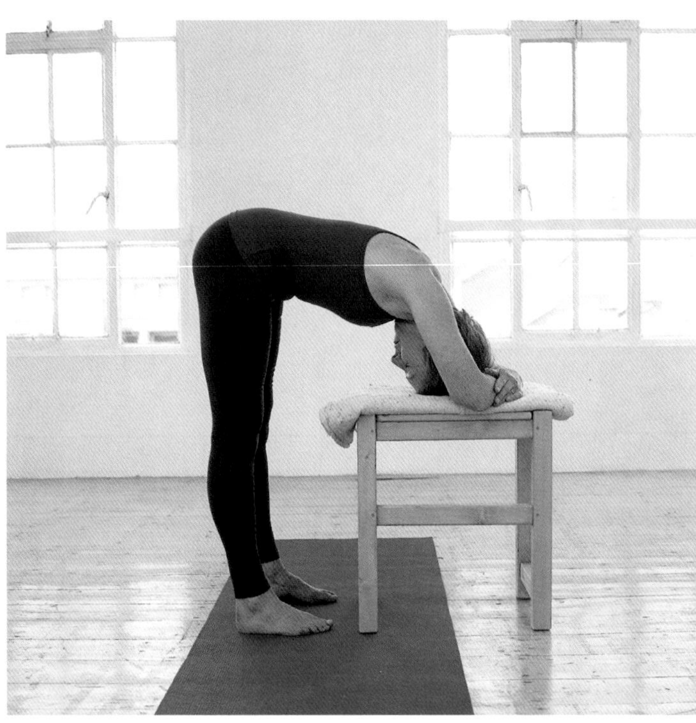

1 **Uttanasana I** with the head and forearms supported on a stool softened with a blanket. Broadening the chest in this posture will facilitate easier breathing.

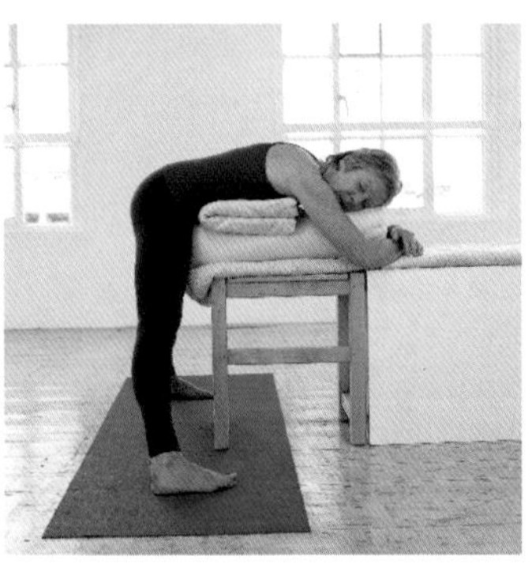

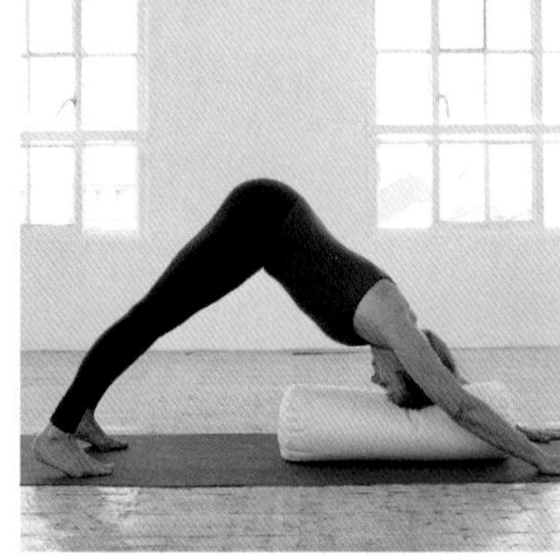

2 **Prasarita Padottanasana** with the arms and trunk supported on a stool, bolster and blankets.
3 **Adho Mukha Svanasana** with the head supported on a bolster.

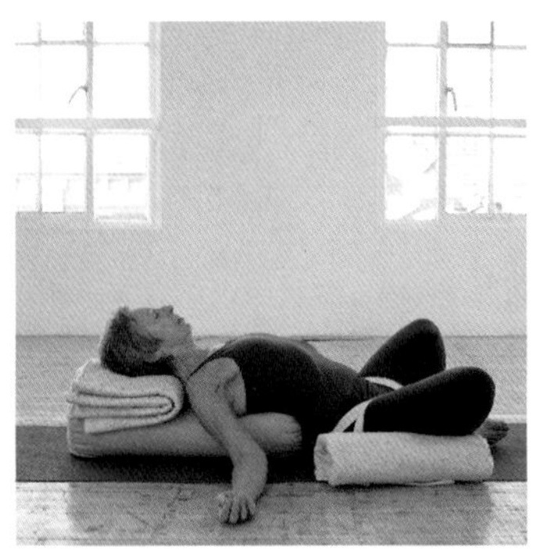

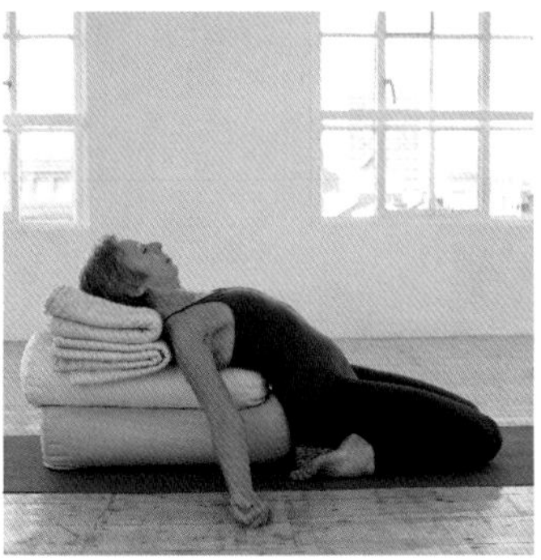

4 **Supta Baddhakonasana** using a strap and bolster support.
5 **Supta Virasana** with bolsters and blankets supporting the spine.

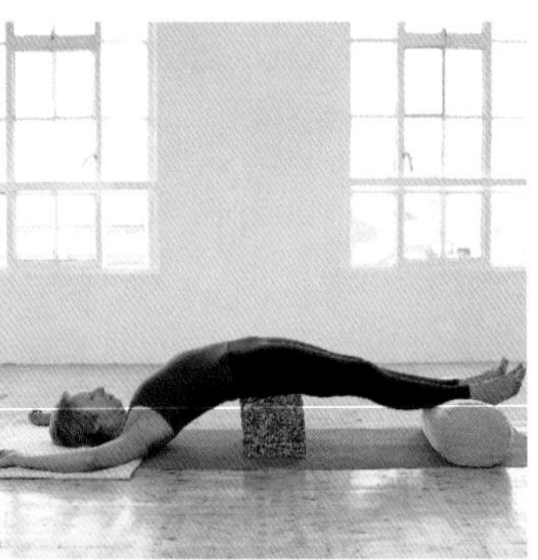

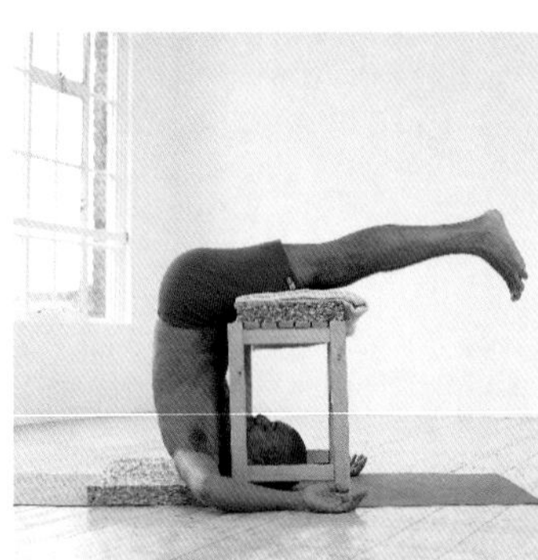

6 **Setu Bandha Sarvangasana** with foam blocks supporting the sacrum.
7 **Ardha Halasana** with thighs supported on a stool and shoulders on a foam block.

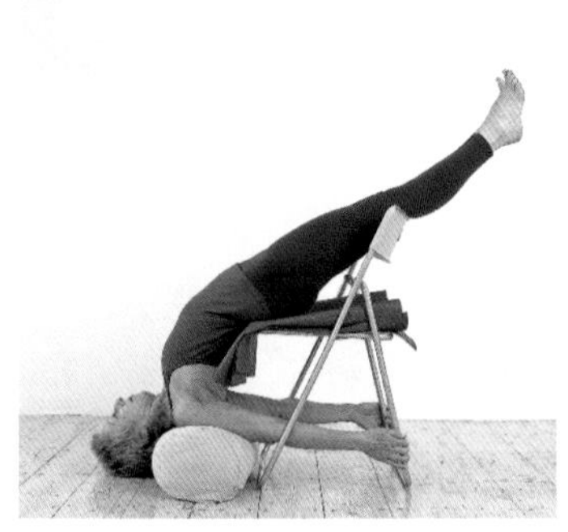

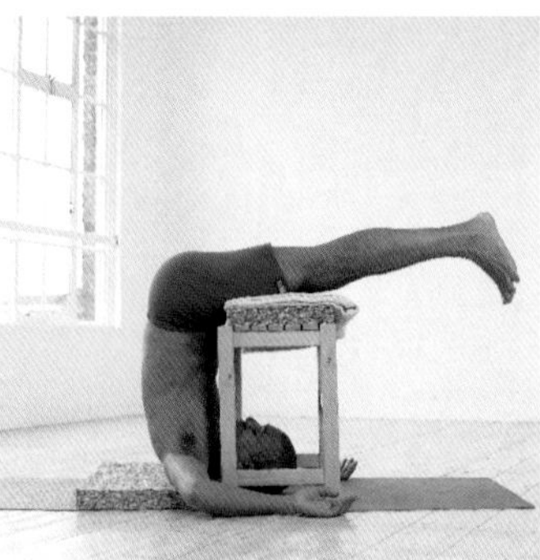

8 **Chair Sarvangasana** with the shoulders and neck supported on a bolster.
9 **Ardha Halasana** with the thighs supported on a stool and the shoulders on a foam block.

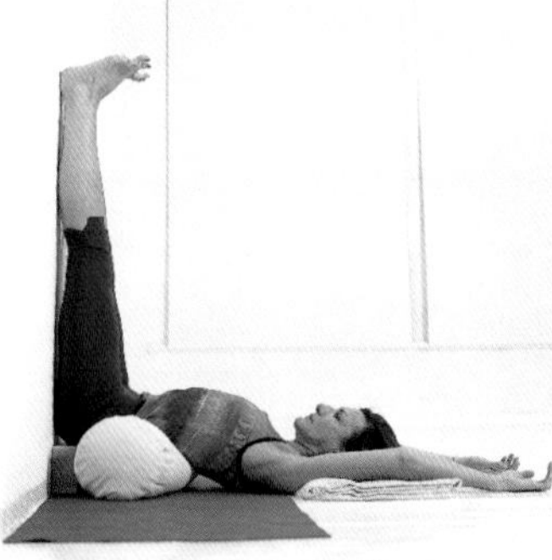

10 **Viparita Karani** with the legs against the wall and the lower back raised with block and bolster.

Focus

- In the sequences for colds and asthma, attention should be paid to opening and broadening the chest while in the postures. Breathing should be normal and the brain passive. Regular practice of these routines will build up the strength of the respiratory system.

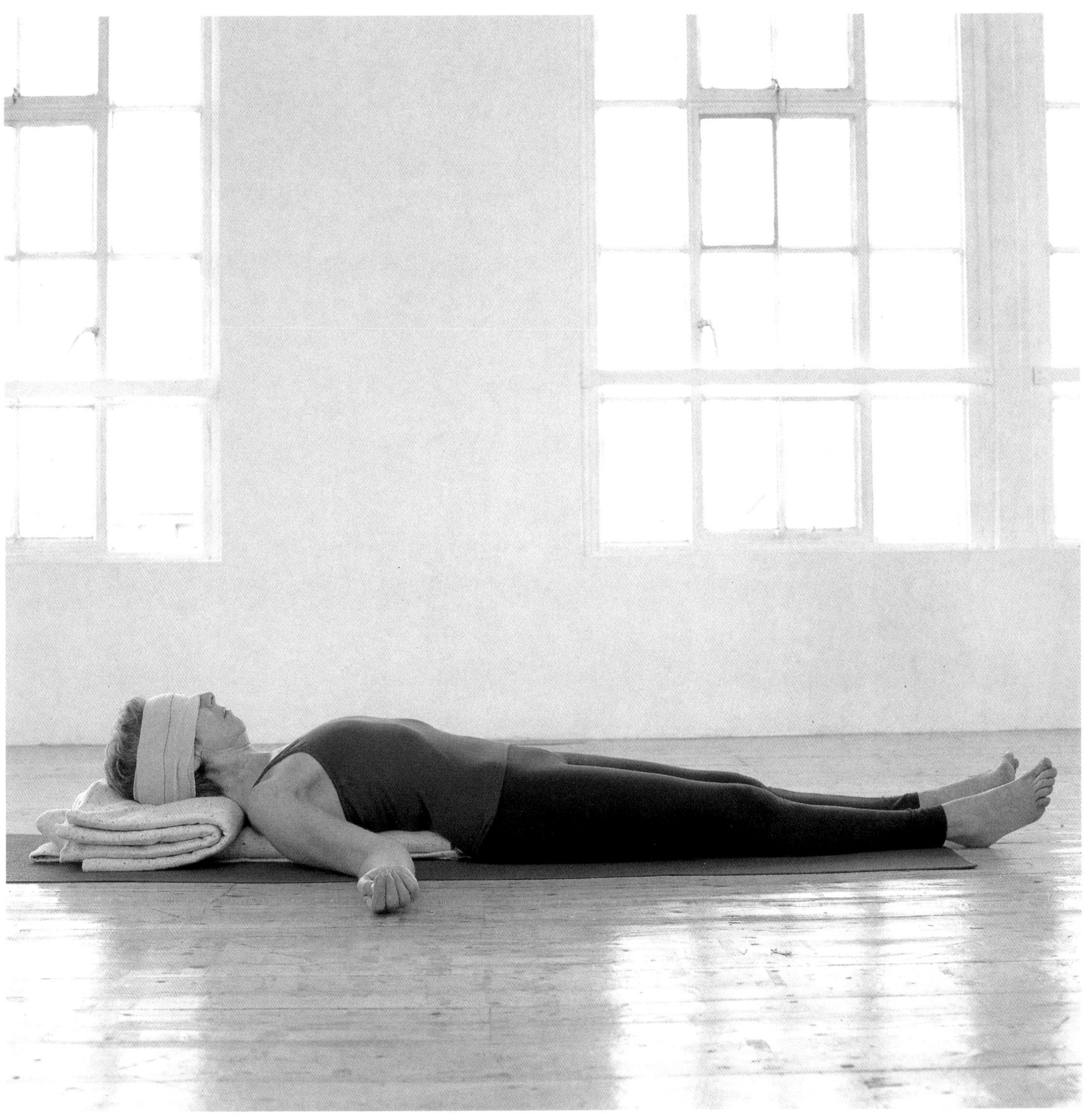

11 **Savasana** with the head supported and eyes covered. Arms out with palms facing upwards. Allow the body to let go completely in this posture. Sink towards the floor. Focus on the breath.

Asthma

These postures facilitate dilation of the air passages in order to make exhalation easier during an attack and help to prevent constriction of these passages, thus reducing the number and intensity of further attacks.

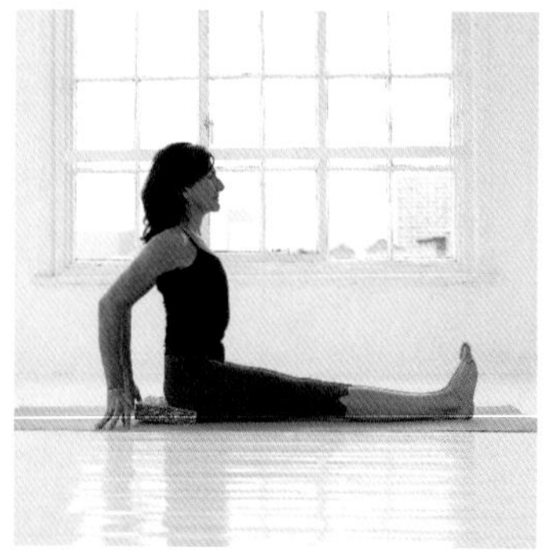

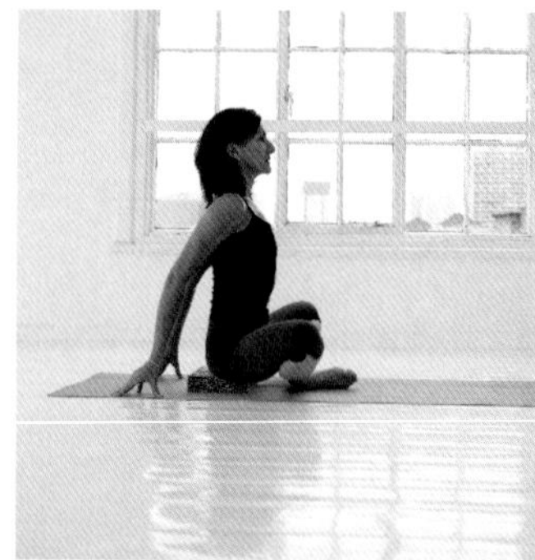

1 **Dandasana** with the inner edges of the feet together and the backs of the legs pressing into the floor.

2 **Baddhakonasana** with the soles of the feet pressed together, sitting up, lifting and opening the chest.

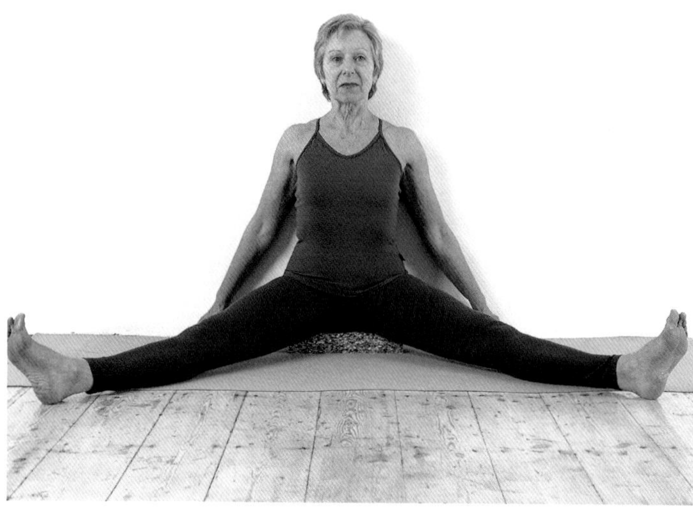

3 **Upavistakonasana** sitting on a foam block for lift, and using the wall to support the back.

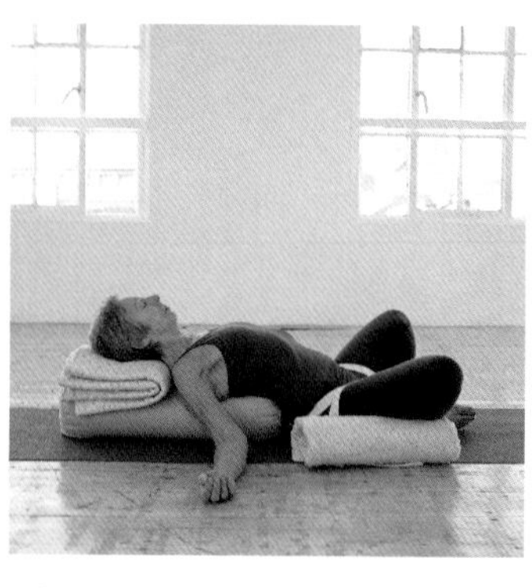

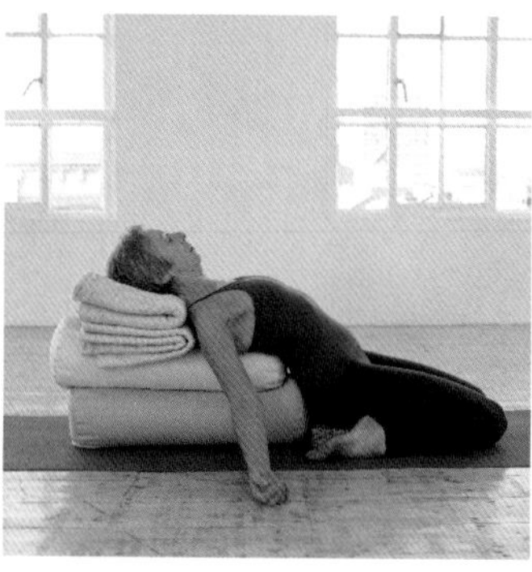

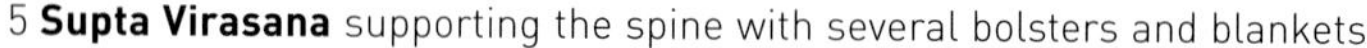

4 **Supta Baddhakonasana** with the head, neck and spine supported by bolsters and blankets.

5 **Supta Virasana** supporting the spine with several bolsters and blankets.

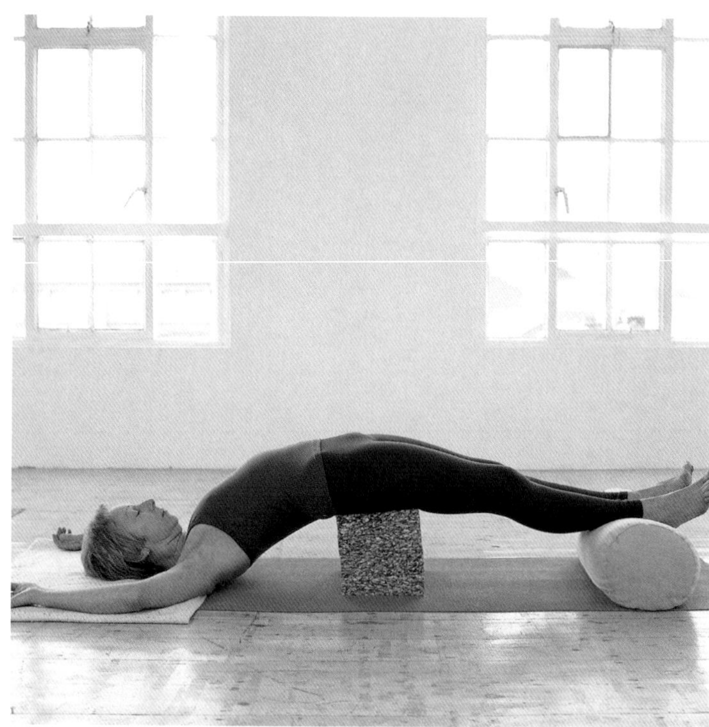

6 **Setu Bandha Sarvangasana** with four foam blocks supporting the sacrum and a bolster to support the feet.

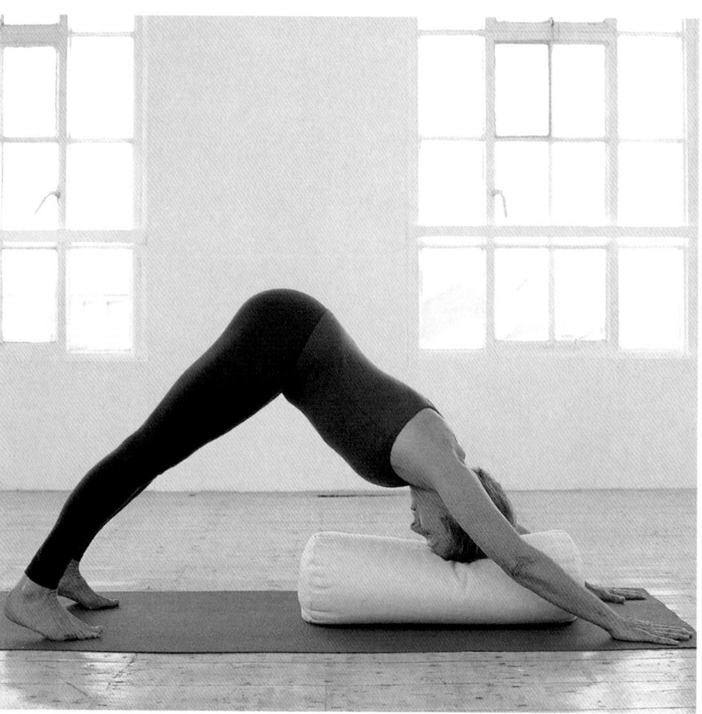

7 **Adho Mukha Svanasana** supporting the head on a bolster.

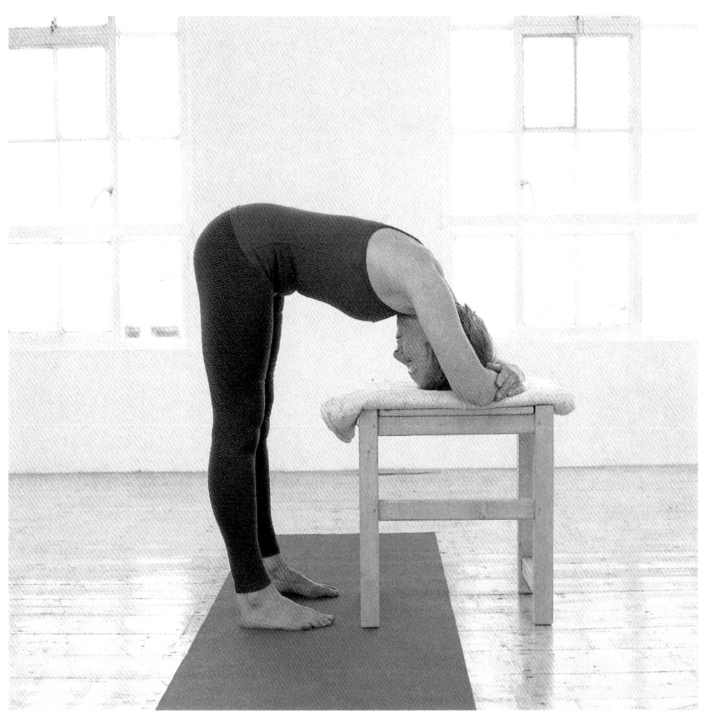

8 **Uttanasana I** with the head and arms supported on a stool softened with a blanket.

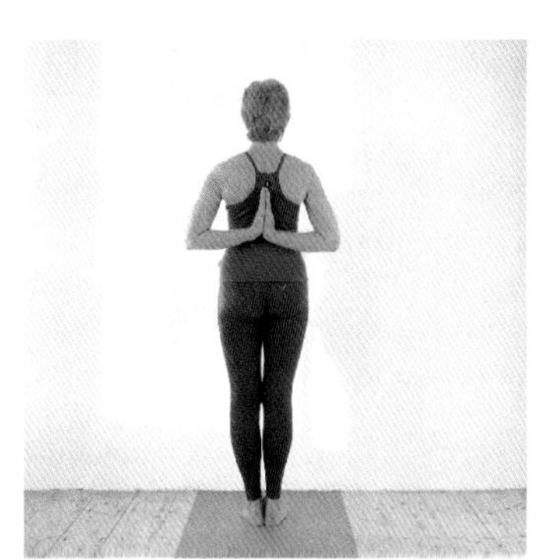

9 **Tadasana** with the hands in Parvatasana, using the wall to support the body.
10 **Tadasana** with the hands in Namaskar, opening the chest.

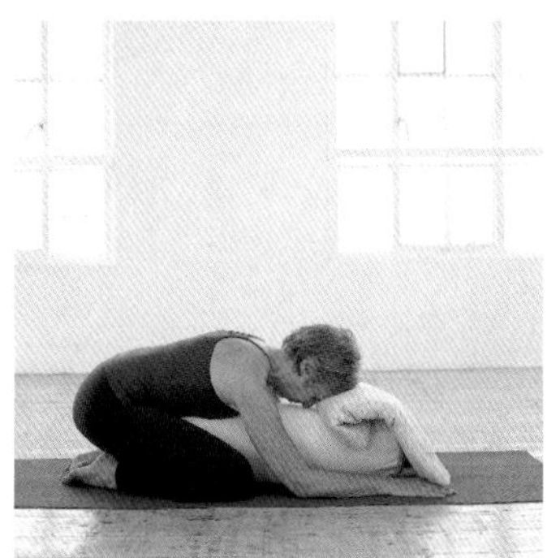

11 **Adho Mukha Virasana** with the trunk and head supported.
12 **Ustrasana** using a support for the spine as it arches back.

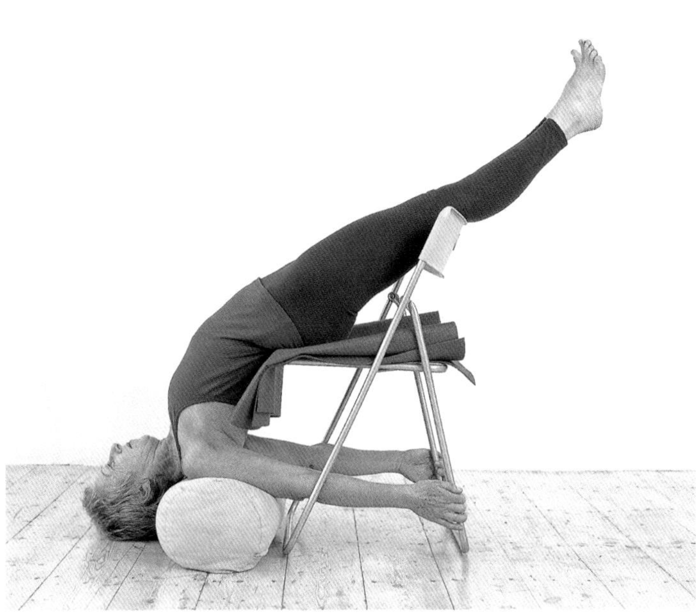

13 **Chair Sarvangasana** using a chair to support the spine and a bolster for the neck and shoulders. Stretch the arms through the chair and pull on the legs to open the chest, keeping the shoulders back.

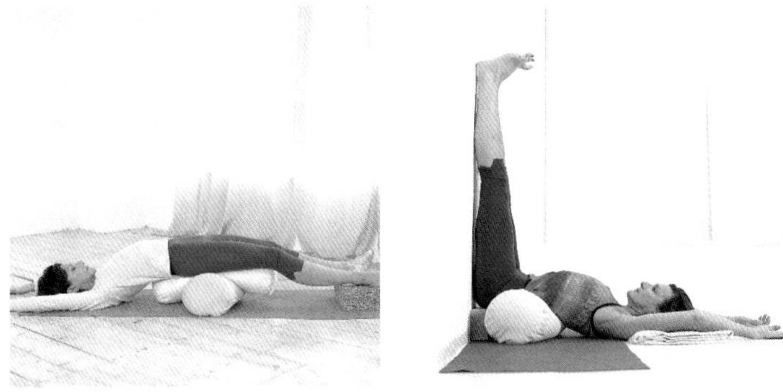

14 **Cross Bolsters** with two bolsters crossing to help lift and broaden the chest.
15 **Viparita Karani** with the legs against the wall and support for the back.

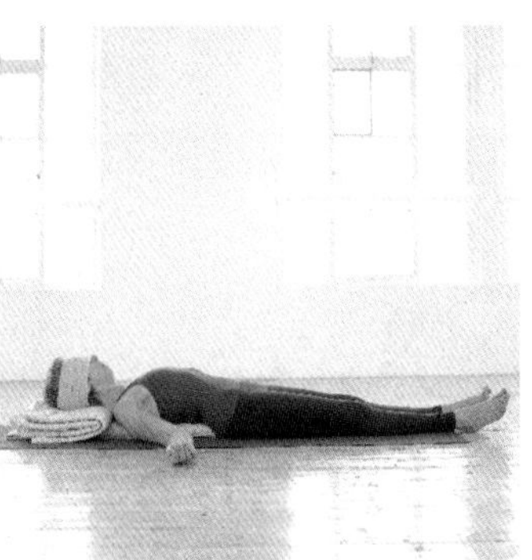

16 **Savasana** using support for the head and with the eyes covered.

Indigestion

Digestion problems occur as a result of the sluggish movement of food through the stomach and the intestines. In these postures there is increased blood flow to the abdominal organs, which improves the functions of the digestive system.

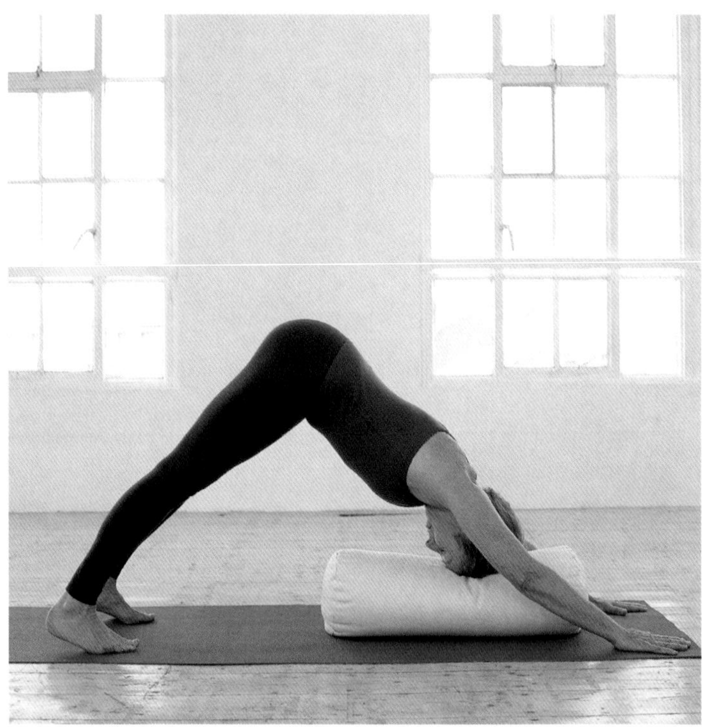

1 **Adho Mukha Svanasana** with the head supported on a bolster. This posture can also be done with the heels resting on a wall for balance.

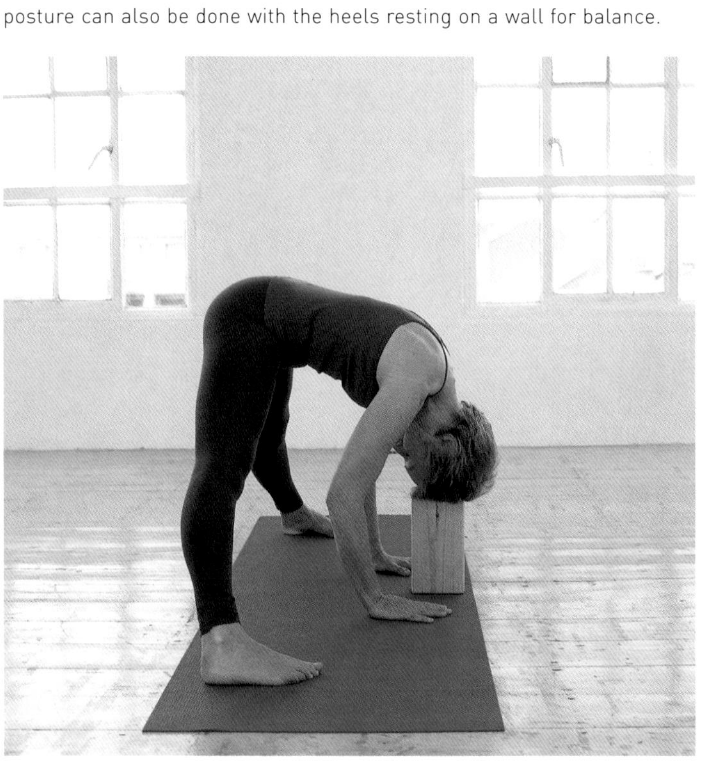

2 **Prasarita Padottanasana** with the legs apart and with the head supported on a wooden block or several foam blocks.

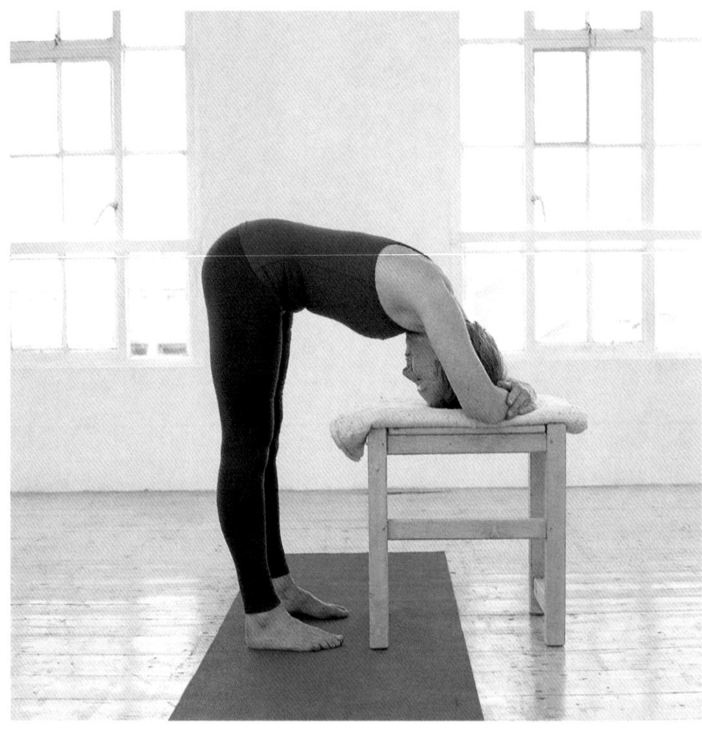

3 **Uttanasana I** with the head and forearms resting on a blanket and stool. If you do not have a Halasana stool, use a chair and blocks.

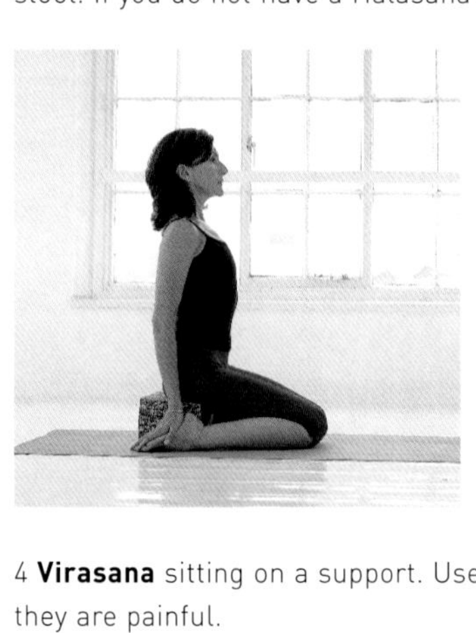

4 **Virasana** sitting on a support. Use a rolled-up blanket under the feet if they are painful.

5 **Virasana (twist)** sitting on a support, turning the trunk, resting the back hand on a block.

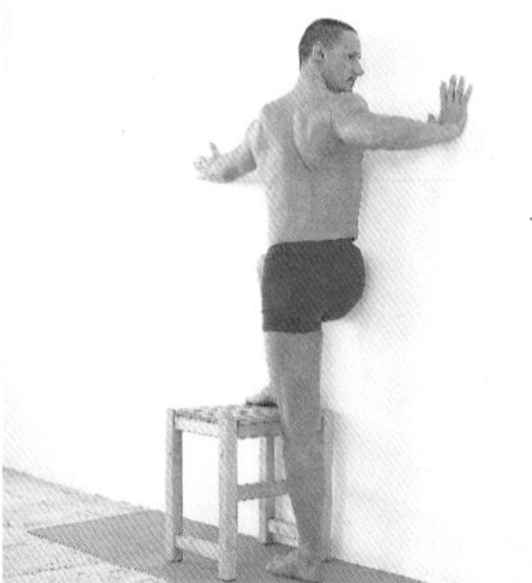

6 **Standing Maricyasana** using the wall and stool as support.

7 **Bharadvajasana (chair)** using the back of the chair to turn.

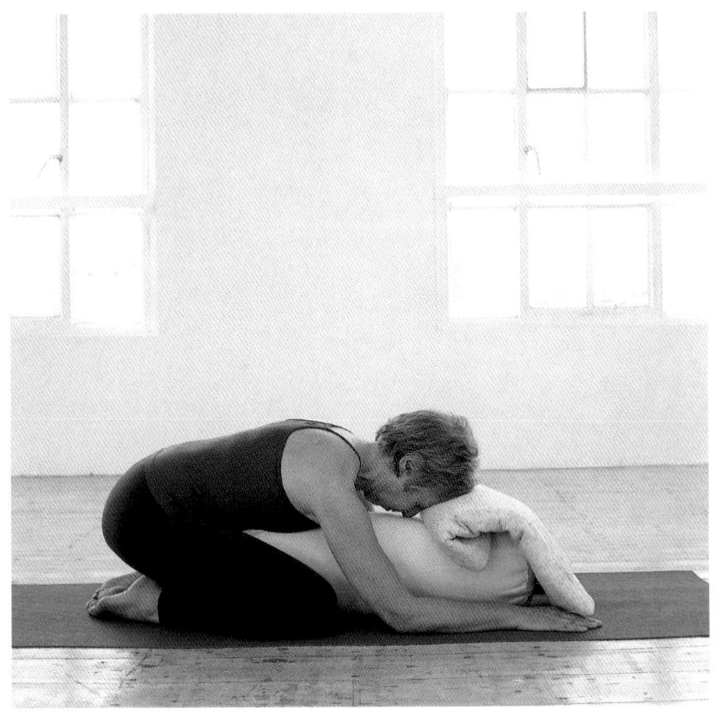

8 **Adho Mukha Virasana** with the head and trunk supported on a bolster and folded blanket.

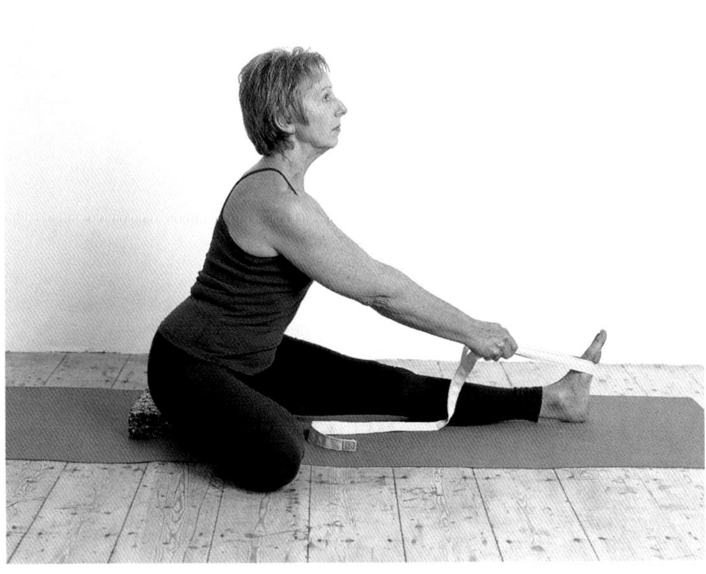

9 **Janusirasana (concave)** using a strap around the foot and keeping the back concave. Hold the strap in a "V" shape, one end in each hand.

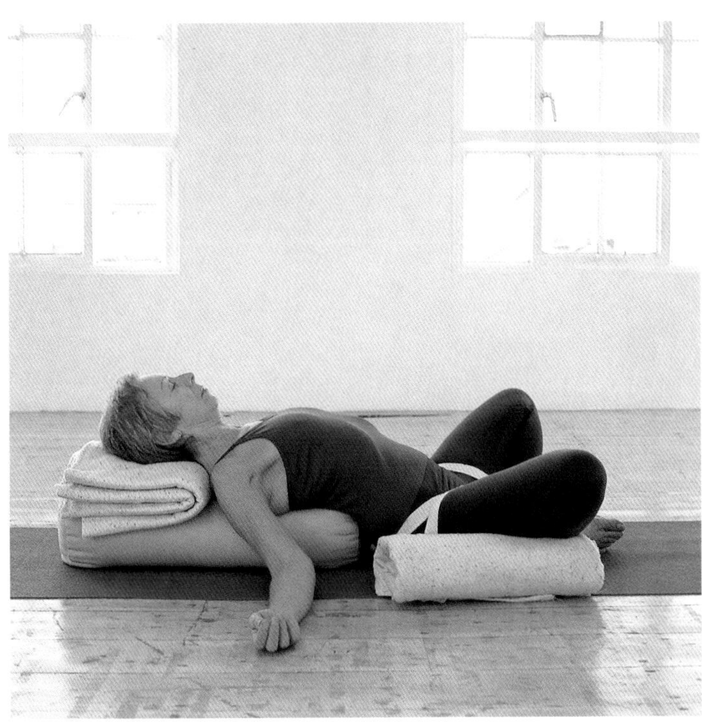

10 **Supta Baddhakonasana** with bolsters and blankets supporting the spine, head and knees, and a strap around the legs and feet.

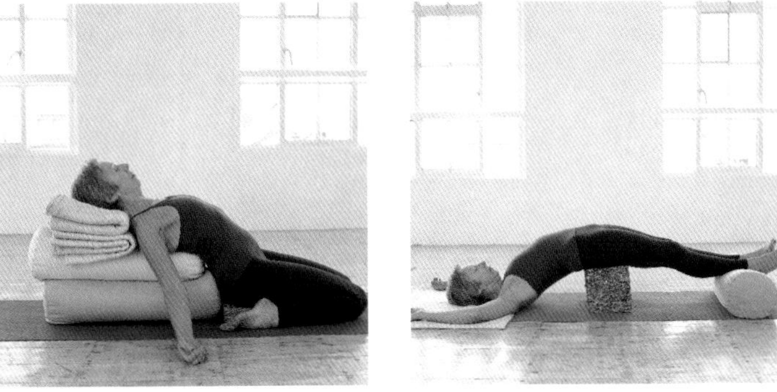

11 **Supta Virasana** using the support of two bolsters and several folded blankets as necessary for comfort.
12 **Setu Bandha Sarvangasana** supported sacrum and raised feet.

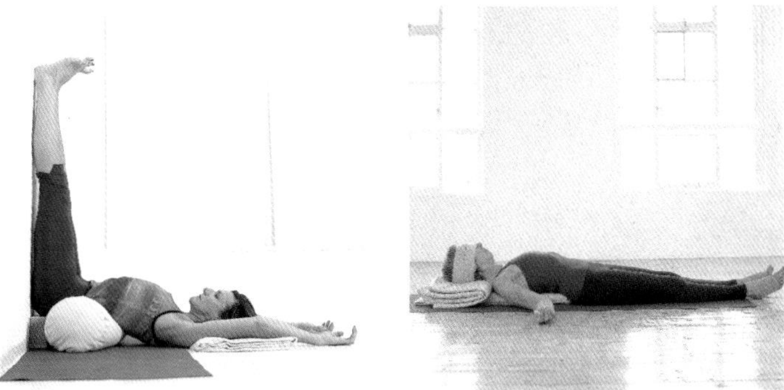

13 **Viparita Karani** with the legs against the wall, bolster and block supporting the lower back.
14 **Savasana** with the head supported by blankets and the eyes covered.

Constipation

In these postures the abdominal organs are compressed and massaged and this improves their digestive, absorptive and excretory functions. In the inverted poses, there is a positive displacement of the abdominal organs, which helps to relieve stress and strain.

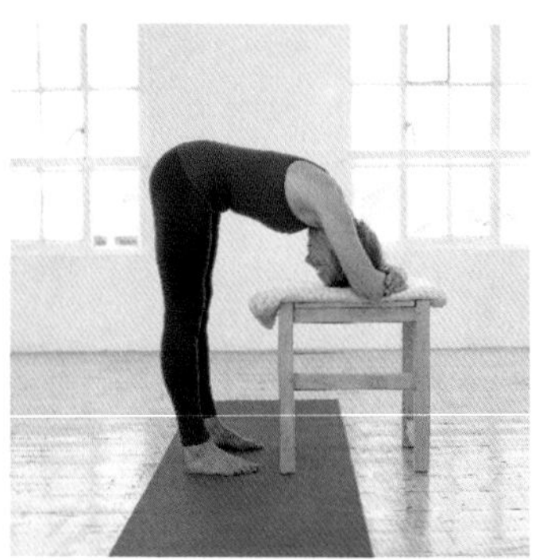
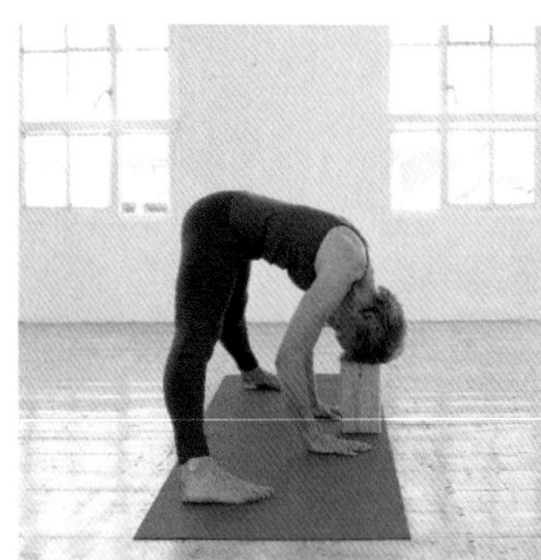
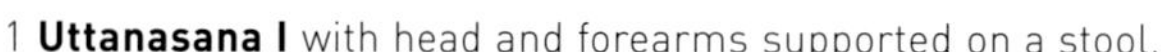

1 **Uttanasana I** with head and forearms supported on a stool.
2 **Prasarita Padottanasana** with the head supported on a wooden block.

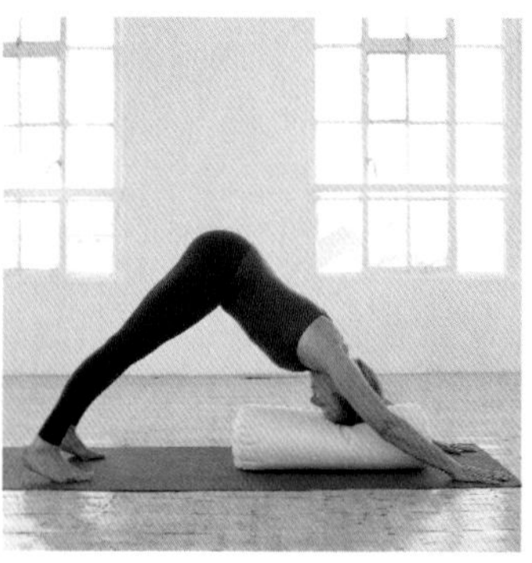
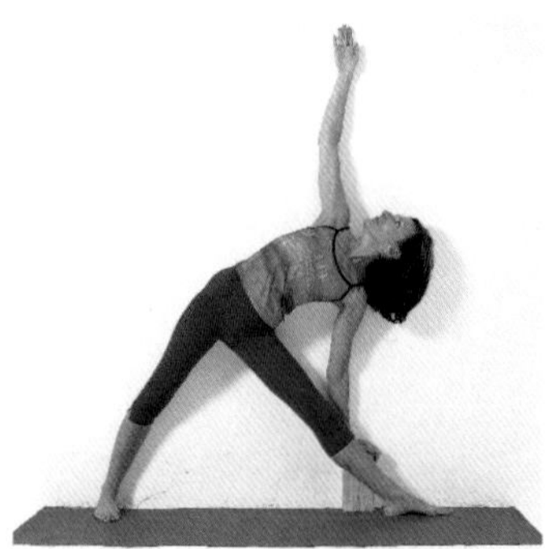

3 **Adho Mukha Svanasana** with a bolster to support the head.
4 **Utthita Trikonasana** against the wall, using a block to support the hand.

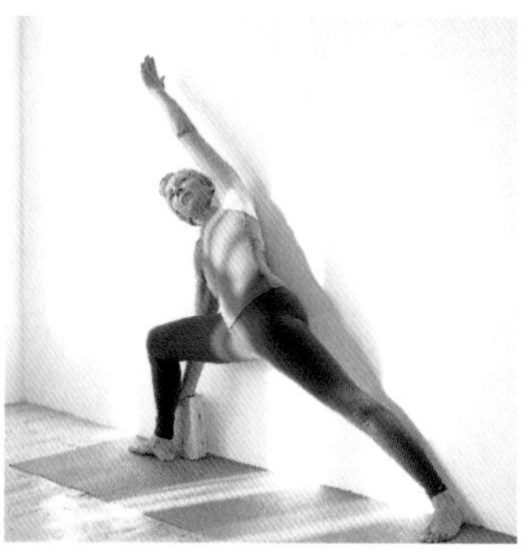
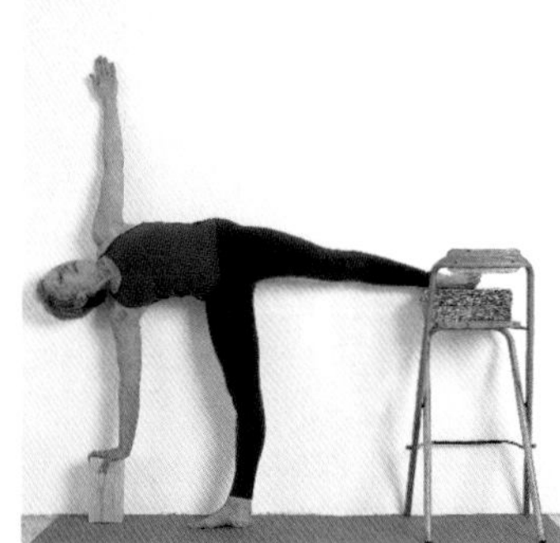

5 **Utthita Parsvakonasana** against the wall, using a wooden block.
6 **Ardha Chandrasana** against a wall supporting the leg with a stool.

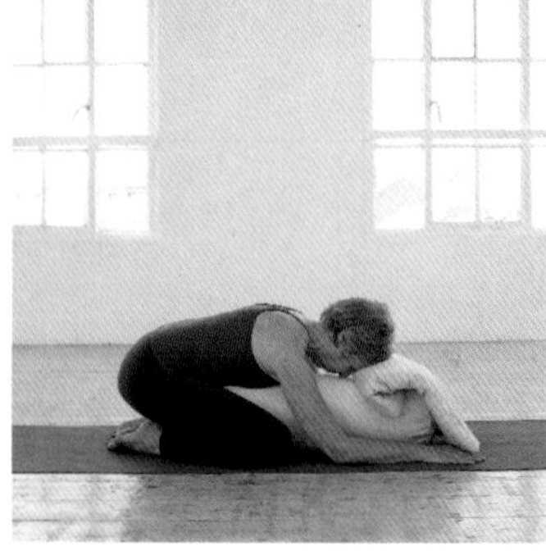
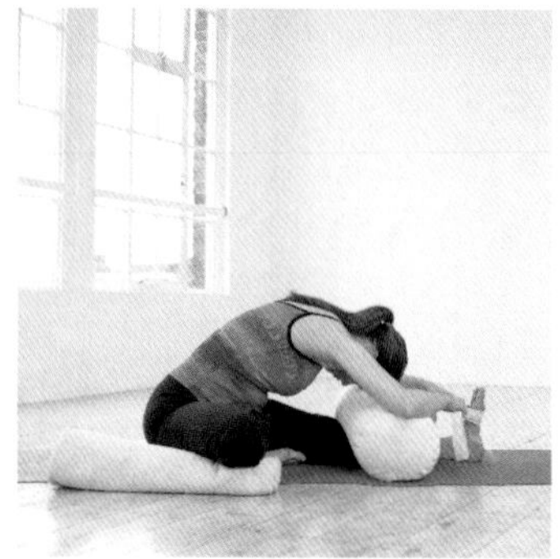

7 **Adho Mukha Virasana** supporting the head with a bolster and blanket.
8 **Janusirsasana** supporting the head and knee with bolsters and strap.

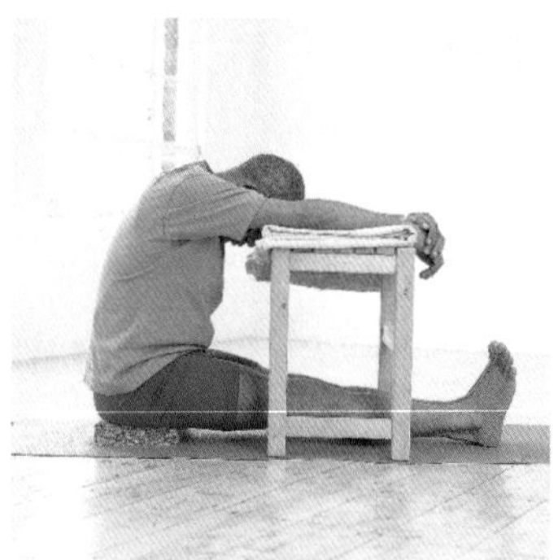
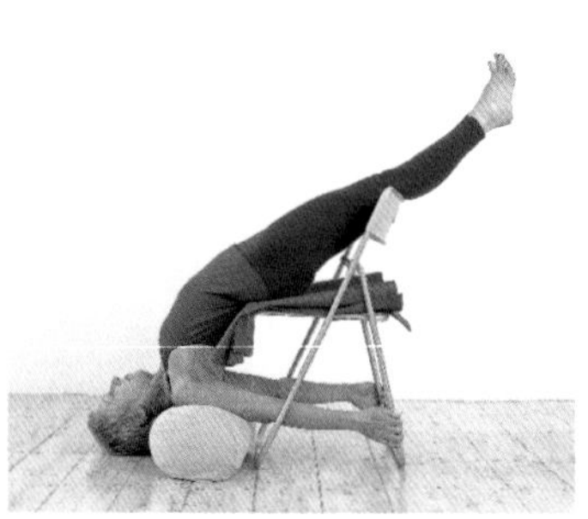

9 **Pascimottanasana** supporting the head on a stool.
10 **Chair Sarvangasana** using a bolster to support the shoulders.

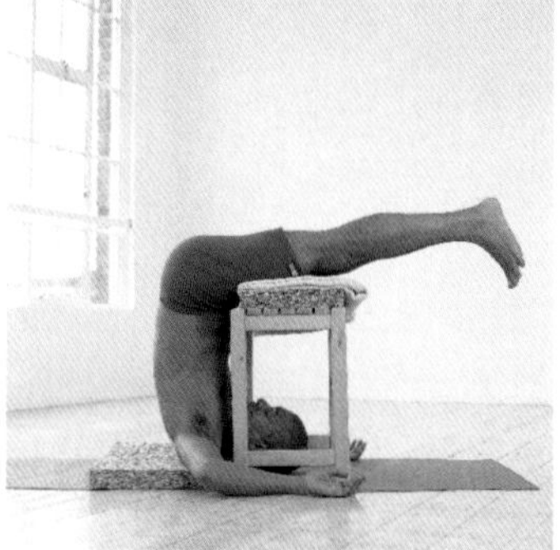
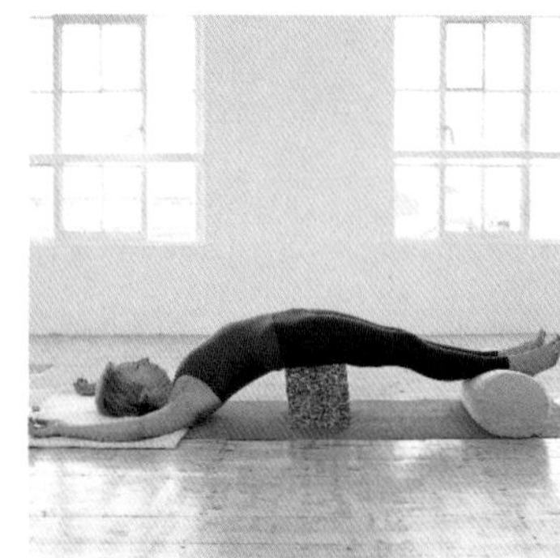

11 **Ardha Halasana** using a stool and blocks to support the thighs and a block for the shoulders.
12 **Setu Bandha Sarvangasana** supporting the sacrum, and feet.

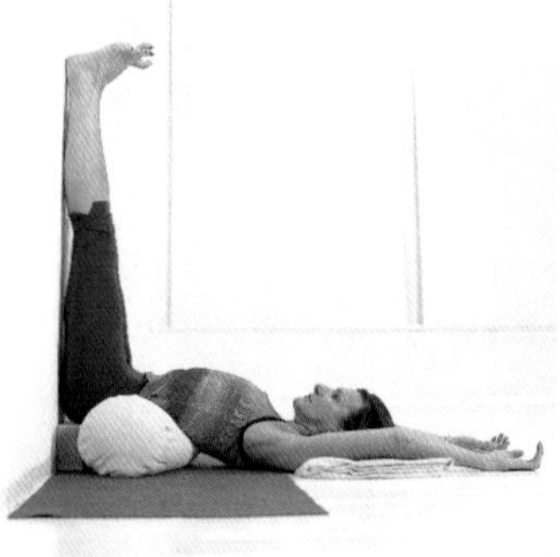
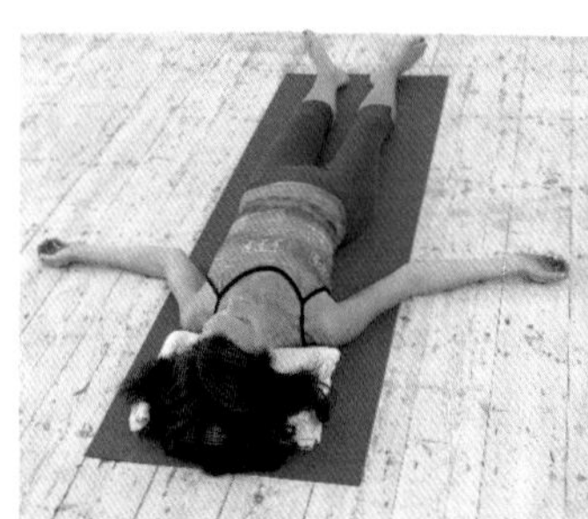

13 **Viparita Karani** with the legs against the wall and a block and bolster to support the lower back.
14 **Savasana** with a blanket supporting the head and neck. Palms are open and up.

Diarrhoea

This condition is often accompanied by abdominal pain or fever. In doing the postures below, the abdomen should remain soft and the brain passive and calm. A combination of restful and stretching potures will aid comfort.

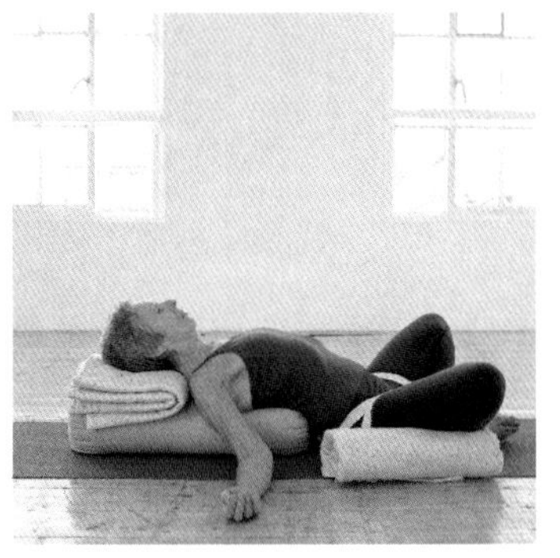

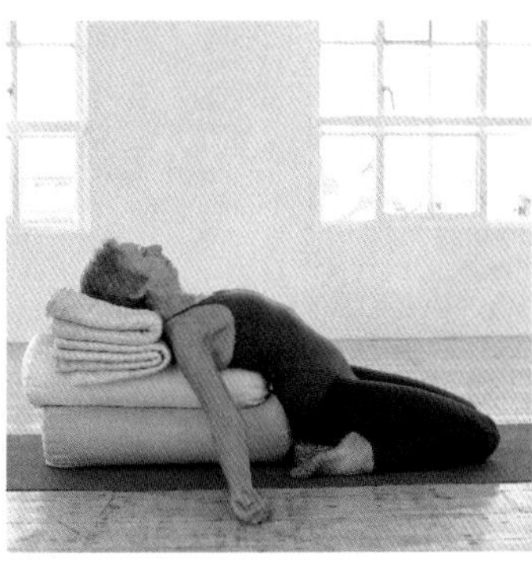

1 **Supta Baddhakonasana** with a strap around the feet and legs, and support for the spine and legs.
2 **Supta Virasana** supporting the back and body on bolsters and blankets.

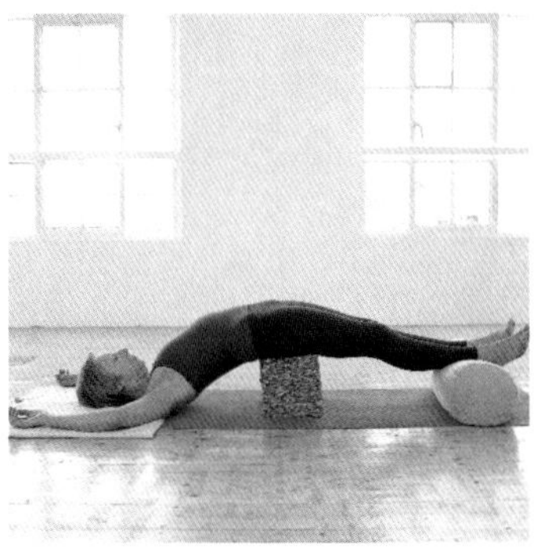

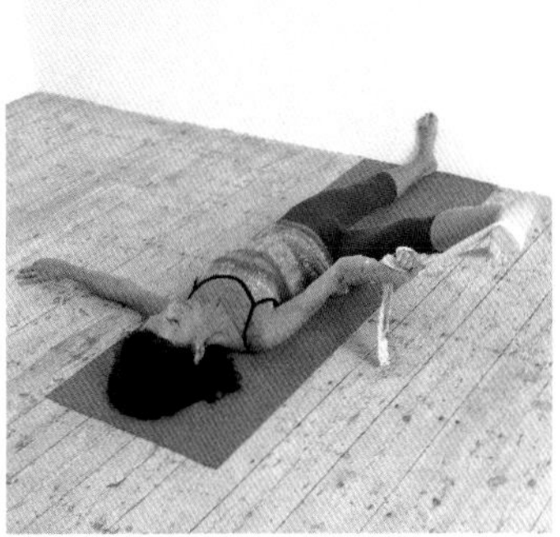

3 **Setu Bandha Sarvangasana** supporting the sacrum with foam blocks.
4 **Supta Padangustasana II** using a strap around the foot, and pressing the other foot to the wall.

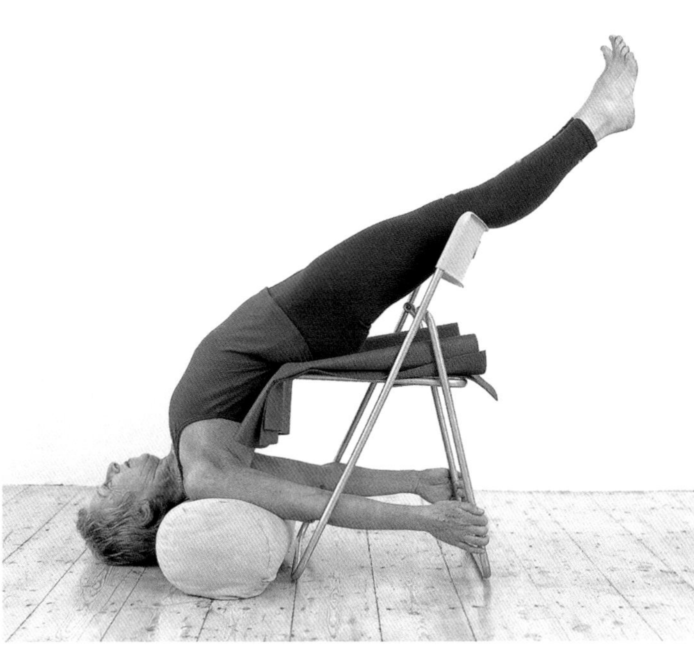

5 **Chair Sarvangasana** using a bolster to support the shoulders and neck. Inversions will help to relieve any stress on the bowels and abdomen.

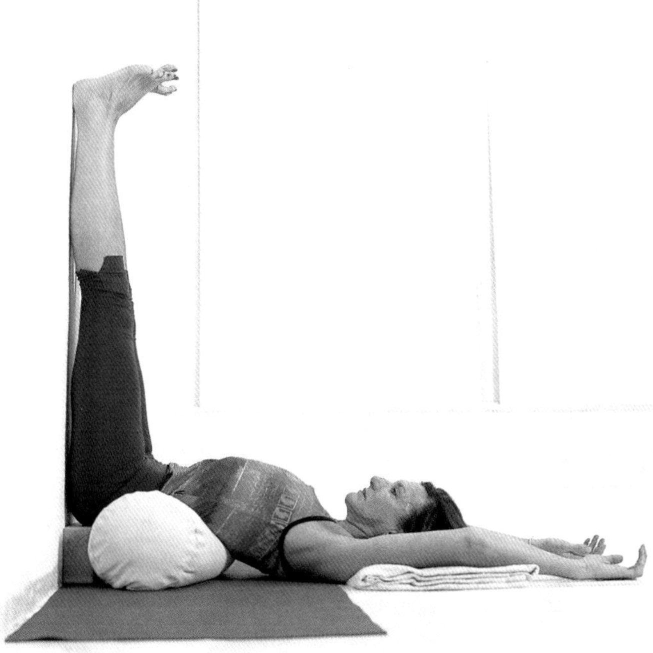

6 **Viparita Karani** with the backs of the legs against the wall and a bolster and wooden block supporting the lower back. Use a folded blanket to support the head and shoulders.

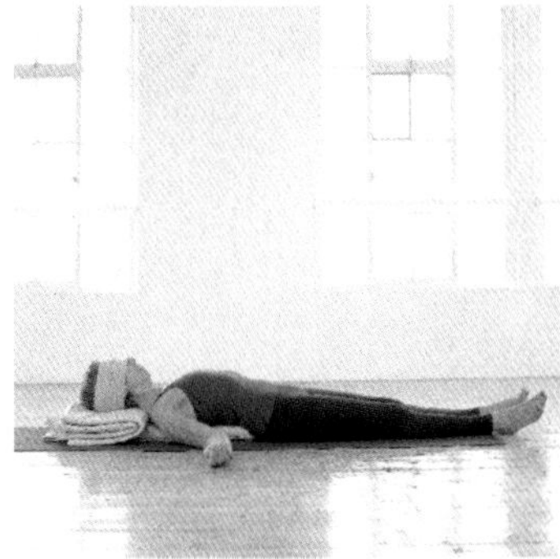

7 **Savasana** with the head and neck on a folded blanket, and the eyes loosely covered. Keep the whole body relaxed, allow the feet to drop and the arms to be loose, with the palms facing the ceiling.

Focus

- These sequences to aid digestion include standing postures that stimulate, as well as twists and forward bends that "squeeze" and massage the abdominal organs. While performing these postures, ensure that the abdomen is not restricted or cramped.

Backache

The following five sequences offer poses that will strengthen bones, stretch muscles and help to free and release the affected areas. Flexibility and mobility improve with sustained practice, and pain and discomfort diminish.

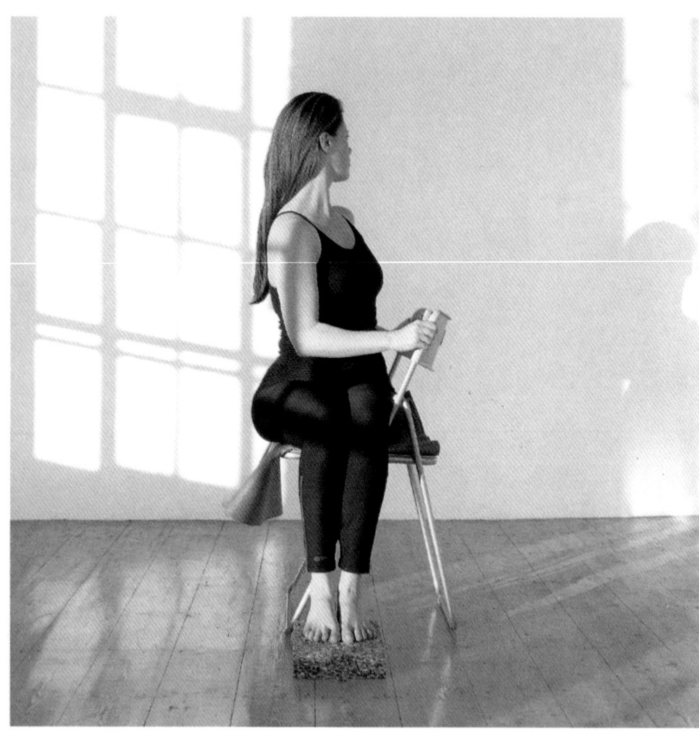

1 **Bharadvajasana (chair)** with hands on chair back to help safely rotate the spine. Try to turn a little more on each exhalation, turning from the waist. Use a block under the feet if they don't touch the floor easily.

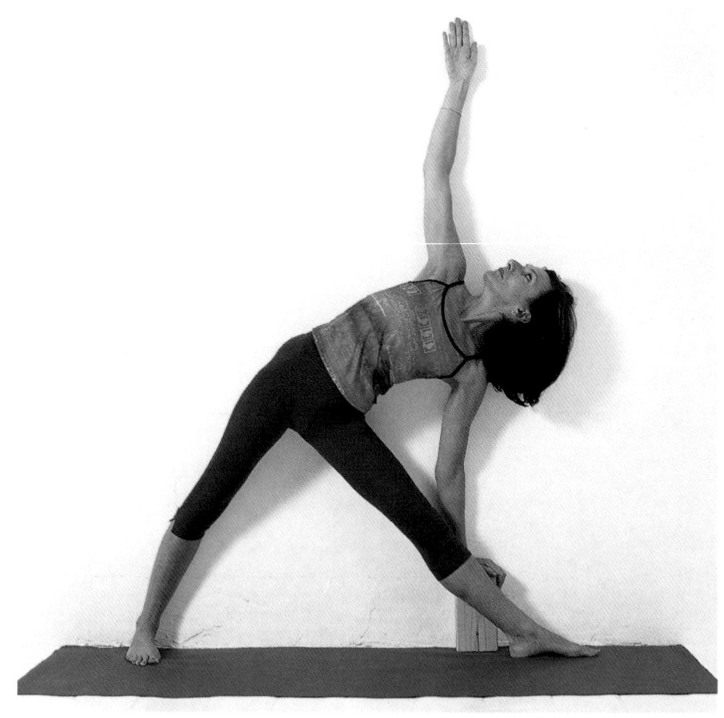

3 **Utthita Trikonasana** against the wall for balance, using a wooden block to support the hand.

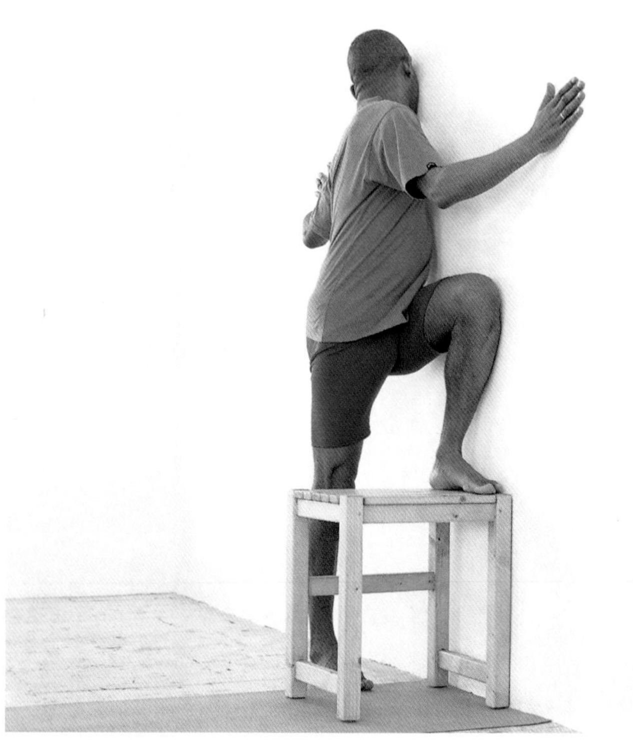

2 **Standing Maricyasana** using a stool to support the foot of the bent leg and the wall to support the hands in order to turn the trunk.

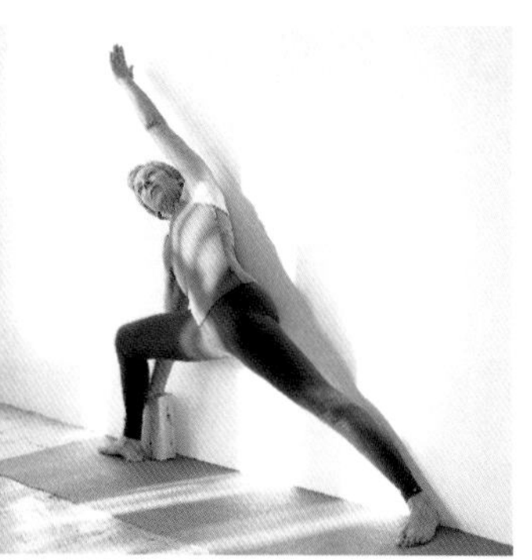

4 **Utthita Parsvakonasana** against the wall, using a wooden block to support the hand.
5 **Ardha Chandrasana** against a wall, using a stool for the foot.

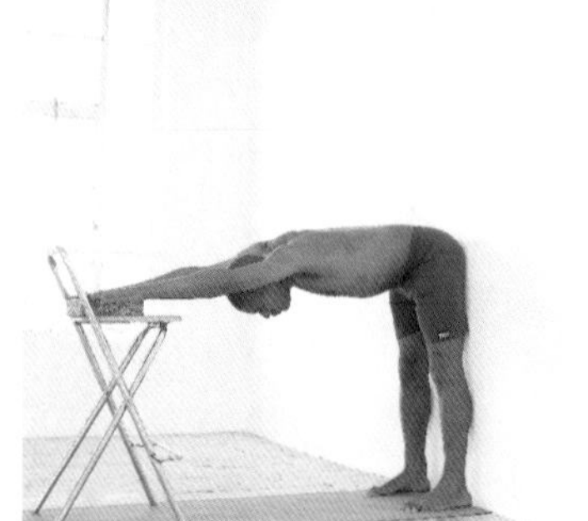

6 **Uttanasana I** against a wall, with the arms supported on a stool.

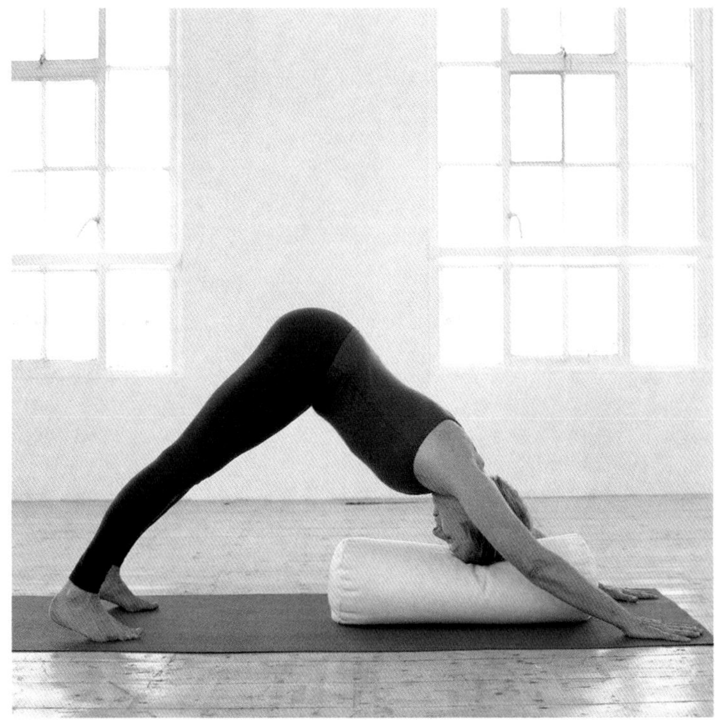

7 **Adho Mukha Svanasana** with the head supported on a bolster.

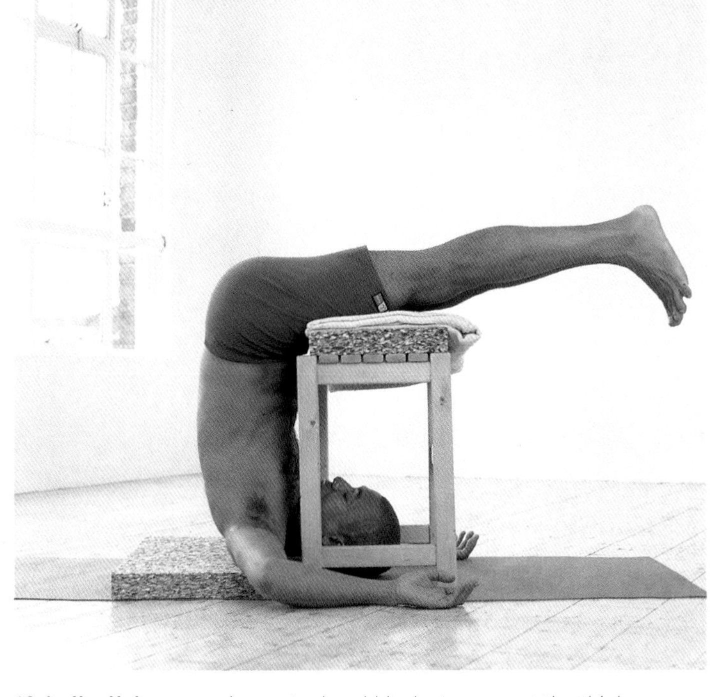

10 **Ardha Halasana** using a stool and blocks to support the thighs.

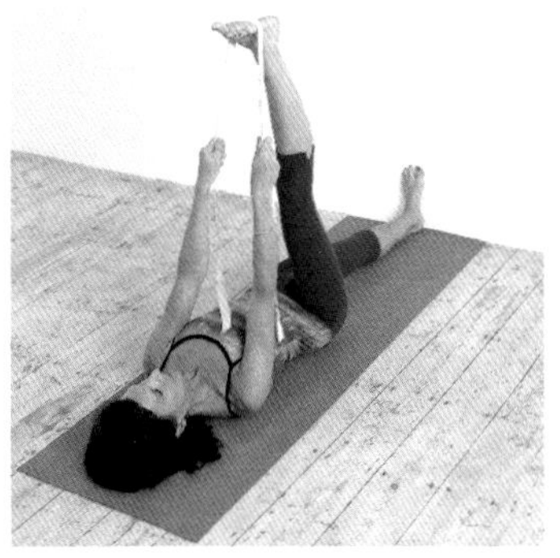

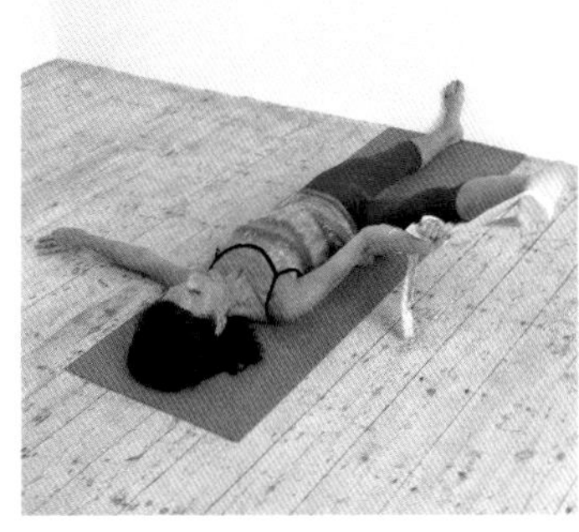

8 **Supta Padangustasana I** with a strap around the foot and other foot against the wall.
9 **Supta Padangustasana II** using a strap around the foot, leg going out to the side.

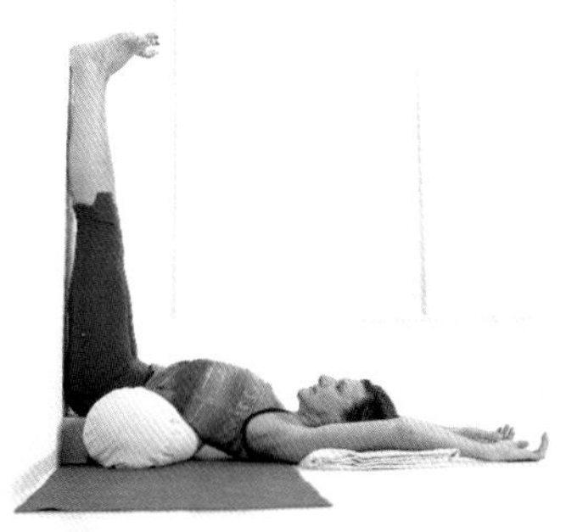

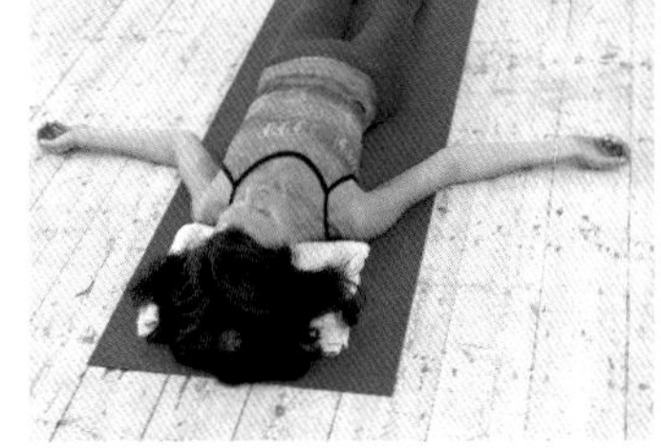

11 **Viparita Karani** with the legs against the wall and a block and bolster to support the lower back.
12 **Savasana** with a blanket supporting the head and neck. Palms are open and up.

Focus

• Back problems are caused by a number of factors – stiffness in lower back muscles, weak abdominal muscles, muscle strain, arthritis, slipped discs or inflammation of muscles and tendons.

• The spine is made up of 32 vertebrae, which work in unison. Weakness and strength is transmitted from one vertebra to another. If one of the vertebra is overworked it weakens itself, and other bones, and the muscles and ligaments begin to take the strain until they too begin to weaken.

• When doing postures for backache, the spine must always be lifted, particularly in the lower back. Never hold the breath – breathe normally in the postures, and keep the neck and facial muscles relaxed.

Sciatica

This condition is due to inflammation and compression of the sciatic nerve. These postures help to strengthen the leg muscles, increase flexibility in the hips and improve circulation in the legs.

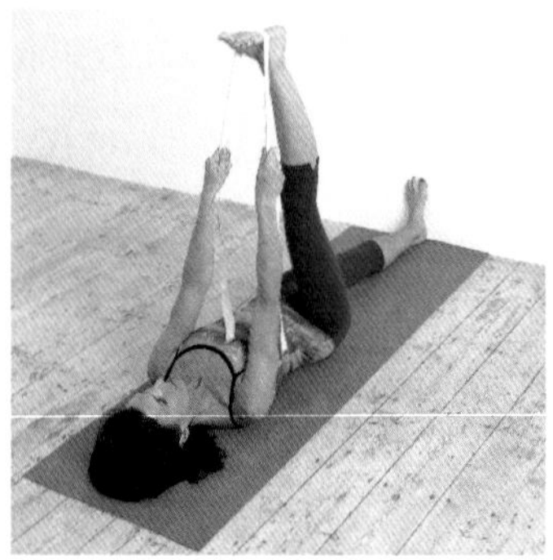

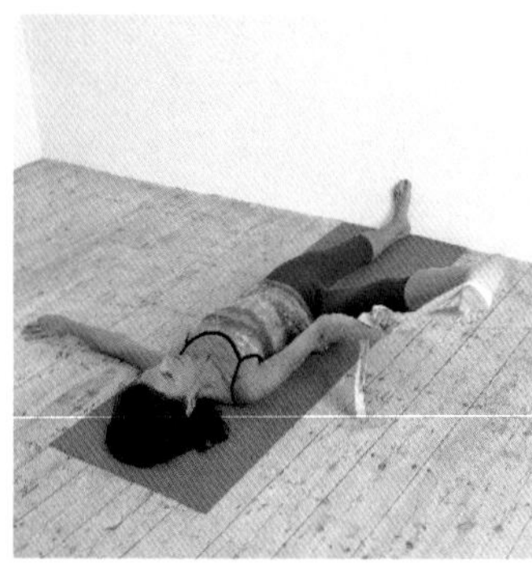

1 **Supta Padangustasana I** with a strap around the foot and the other foot against the wall.
2 **Supta Padangustasana II** using a strap, leg going out to the side.

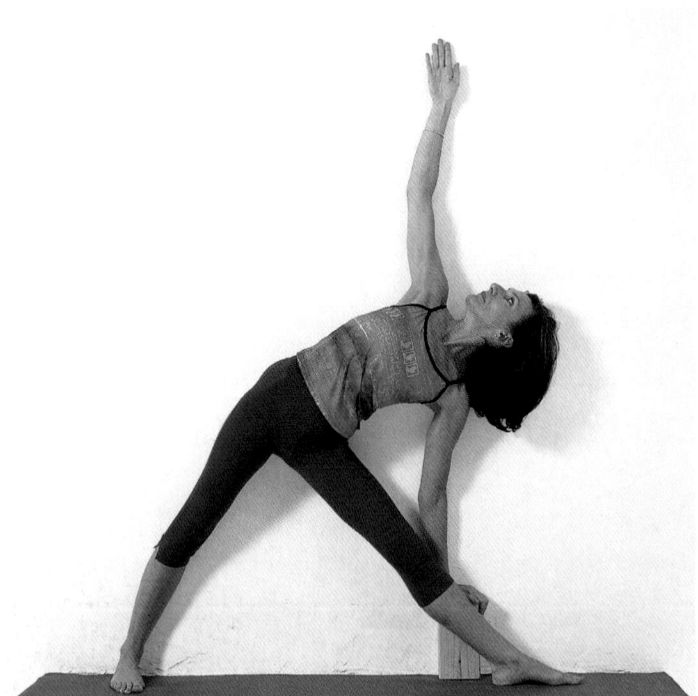

3 **Utthita Trikonasana** against a wall for balance, and using a wooden block to support the hand.

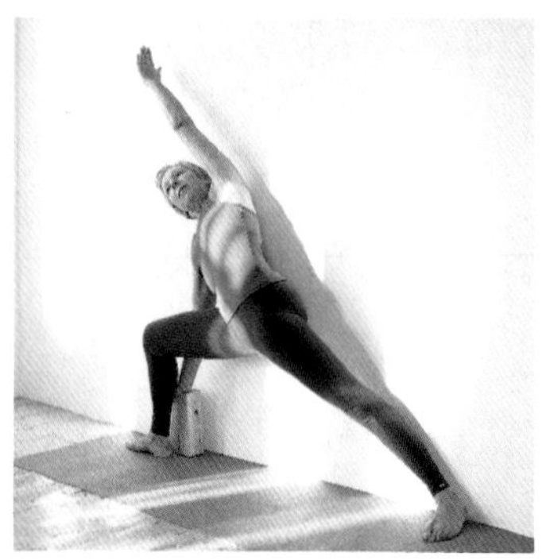

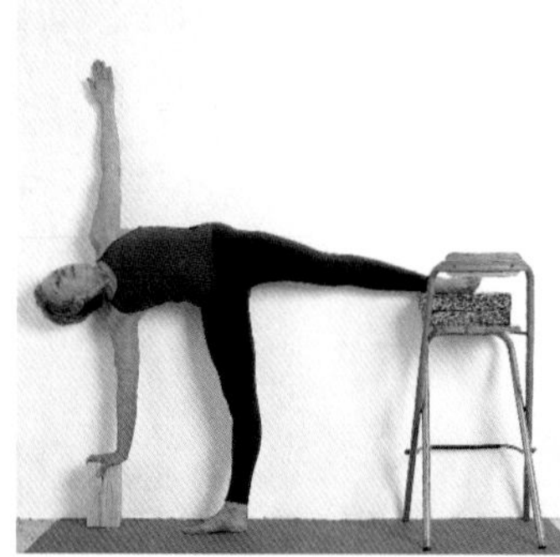

4 **Utthita Parsvakonasana** against a wall, using support for the hand.
5 **Ardha Chandrasana** against a wall, using a foam block on a stool to support the extended leg.

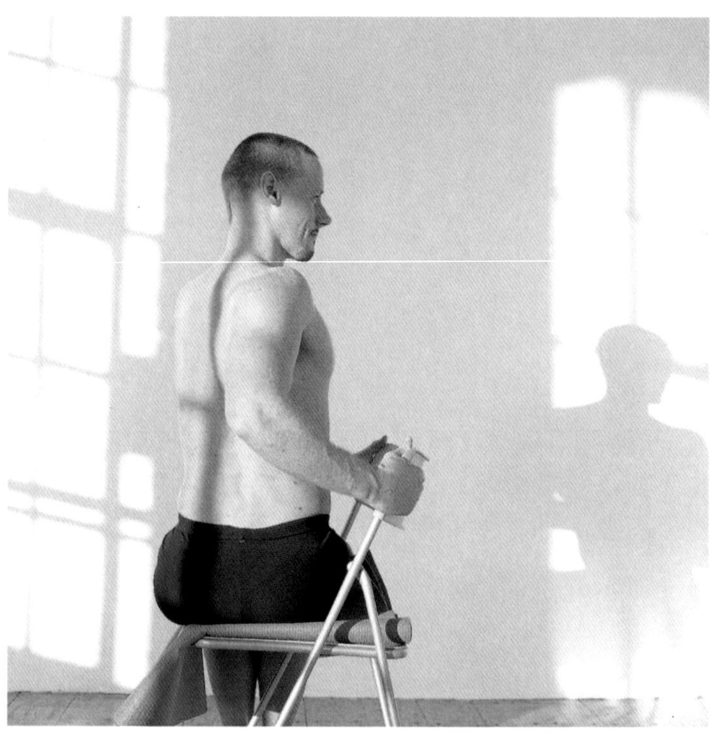

6 **Bharadvajasana (chair)** with the feet parallel on the floor and using the hands to help turn.

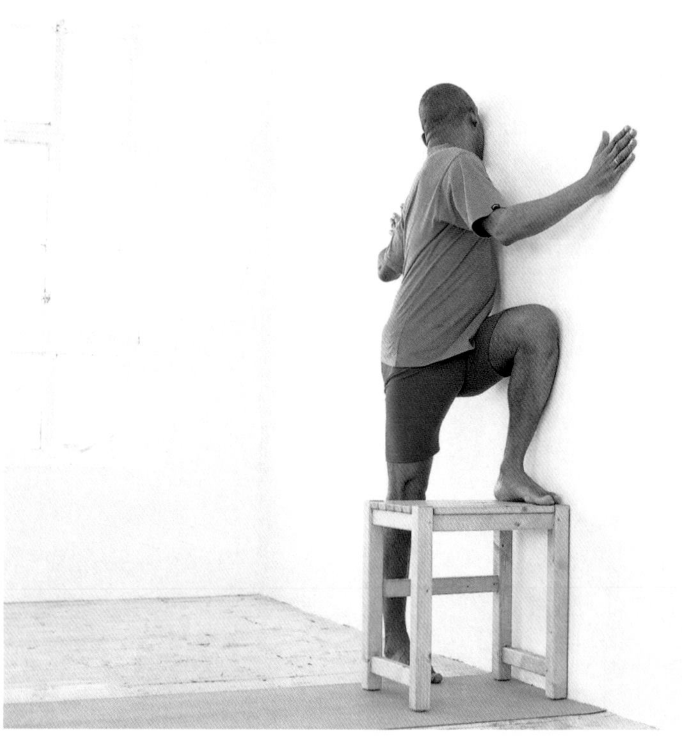

7 **Standing Maricyasana** against a wall, with the foot on a stool. Push the hands into the wall to turn.

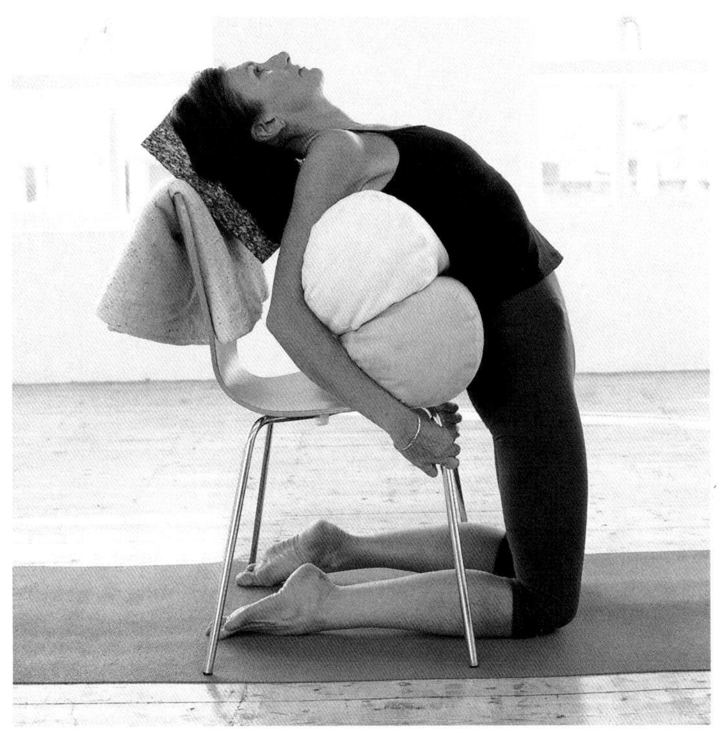

8 **Ustrasana** using a chair and bolsters to support the arch of the spine. Lean back, allowing the head and neck to relax backwards.

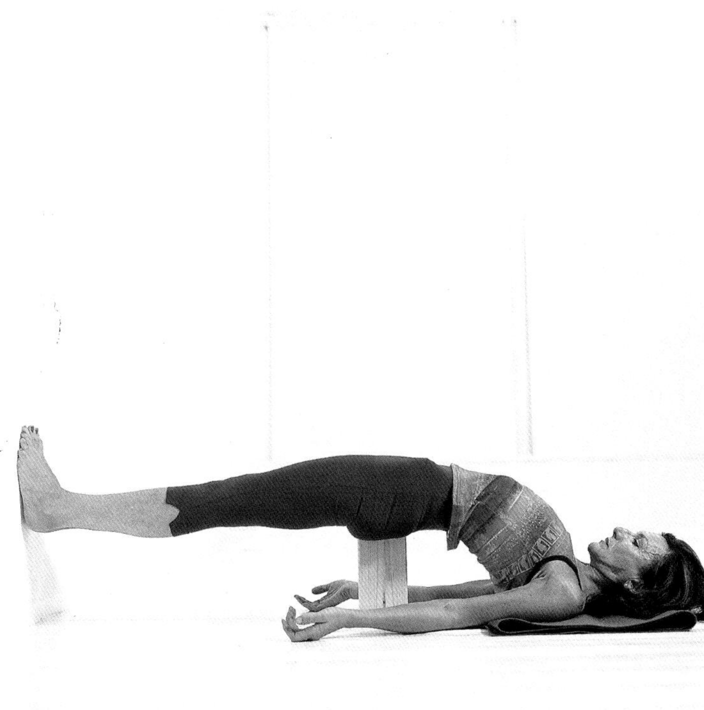

10 **Setu Bandha Sarvangasana** using a wooden block, feet pressing into the wall.

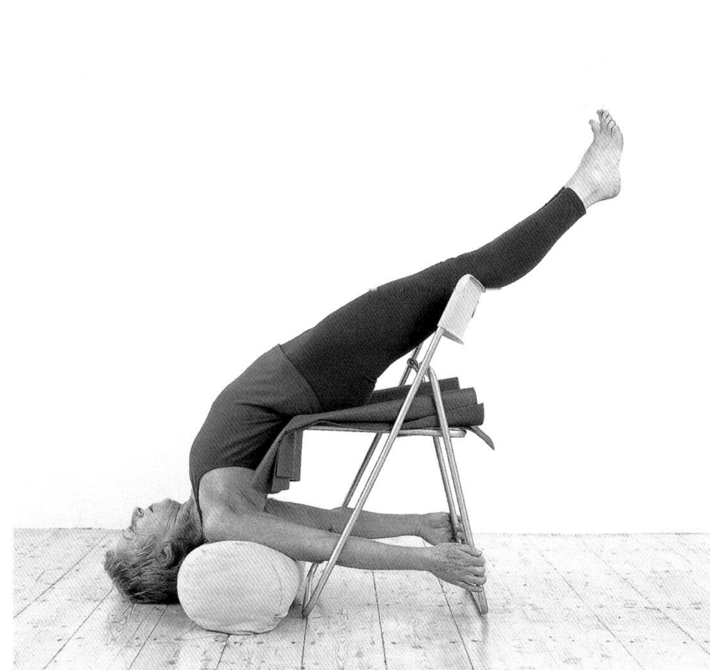

9 **Chair Sarvangasana** using a bolster to support the neck and shoulders.

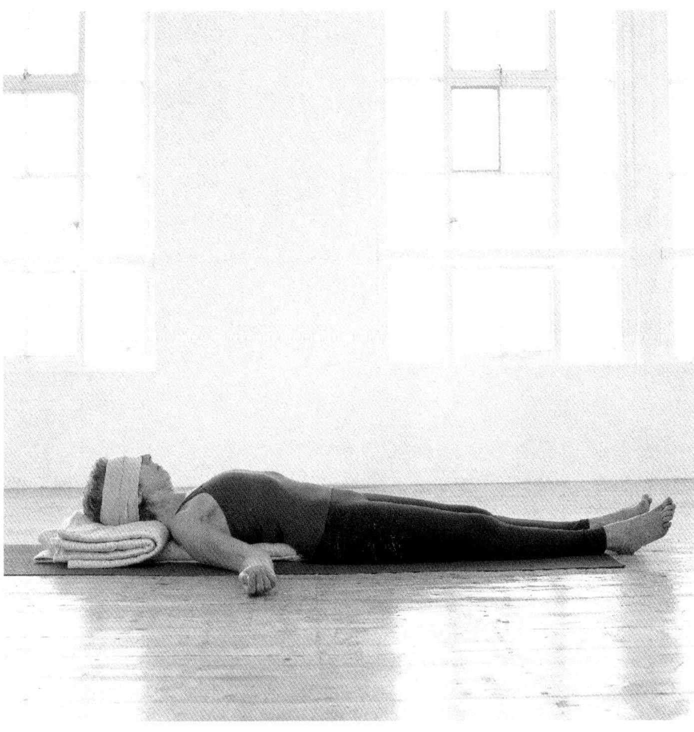

11 **Savasana** relaxing with a blanket supporting the head and neck, and the eyes loosely covered.

Shoulders and Neck

These postures, which tone and stretch the trapezius muscles and release tension in the neck, must be done with attention to rolling and extending the muscles at the back of the neck down the back, and drawing the shoulders away from the ears.

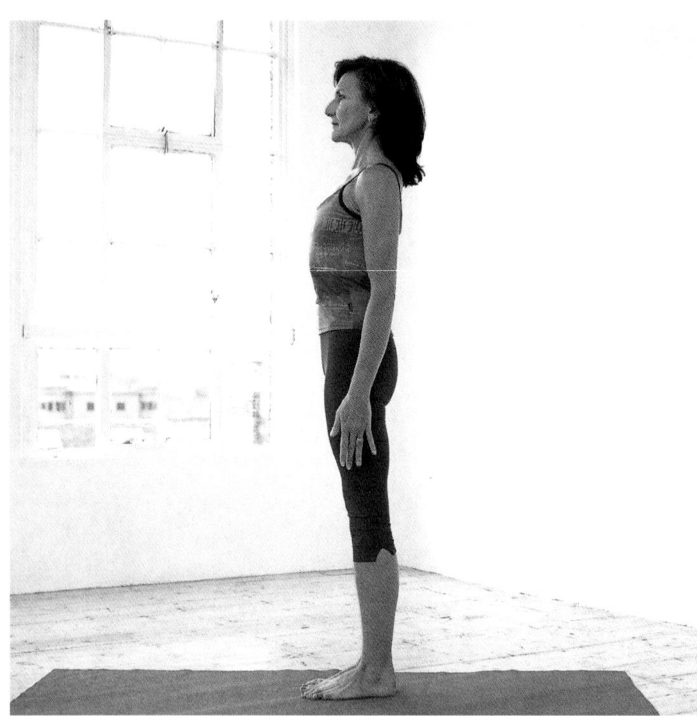

1 **Tadasana** standing up straight and moving the shoulders towards the body. Keep the feet together, tuck in the bottom and sacrum, and keep the legs strong and active.

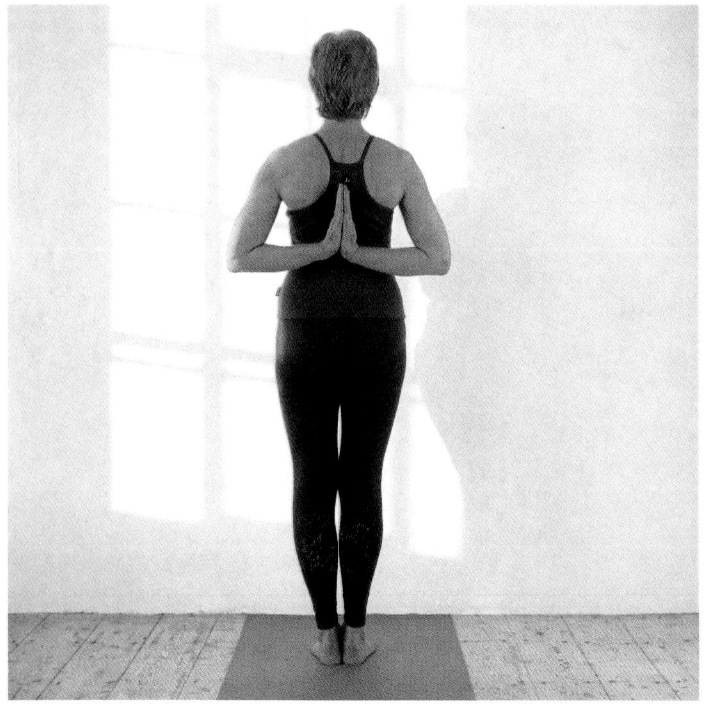

2 **Tadasana with hands in Namaskar** Stand in Tadasana and place the palms of the hands completely together behind the back. Move the shoulders into the body, keeping the hands as high as possible.

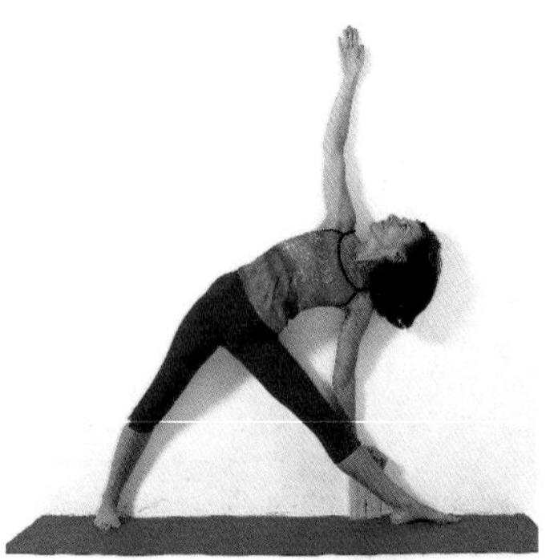

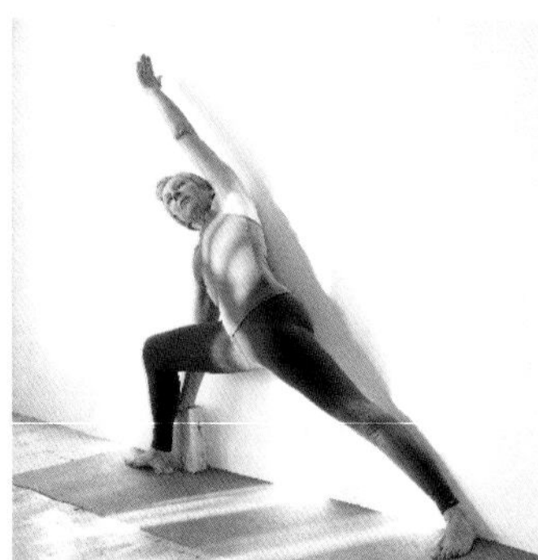

3 **Utthita Trikonasana** against a wall with wooden block.
4 **Utthita Parsvakonasana** against a wall with wooden block.

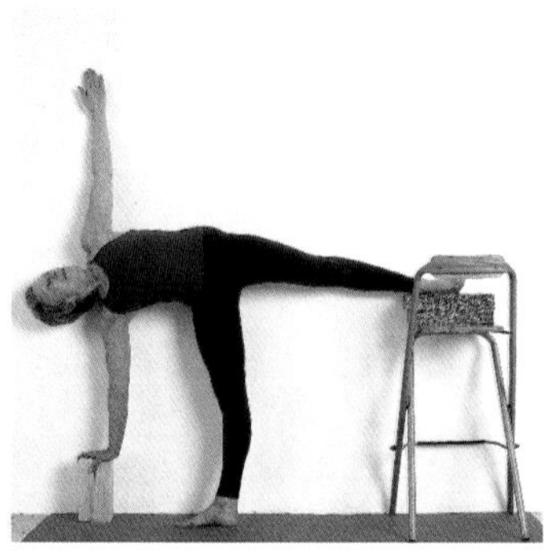

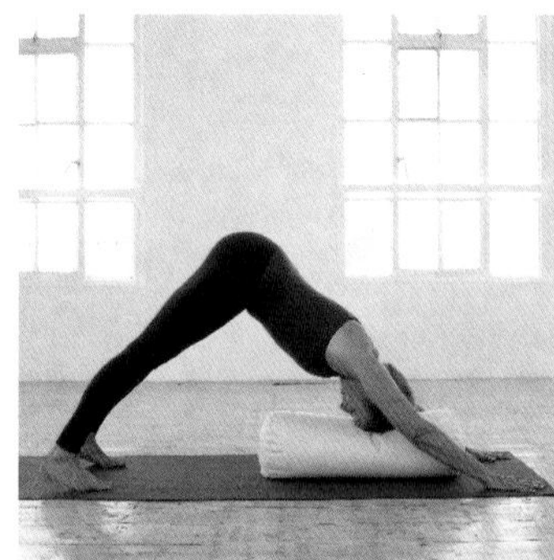

5 **Ardha Chandrasana** against the wall, with the foot supported by foam blocks on a stool.
6 **Adho Mukha Svanasana** with the head supported on a bolster.

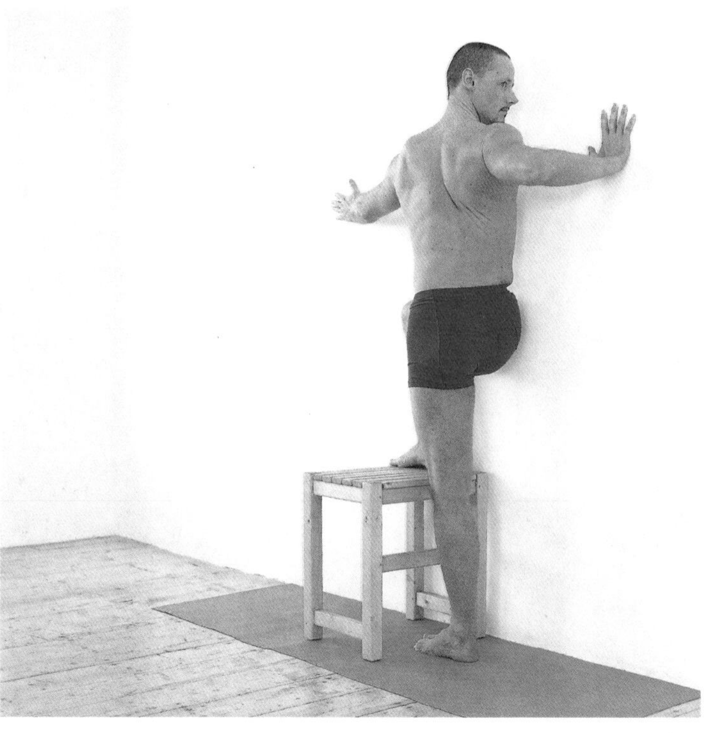

7 **Standing Maricyasana** using the stool, raise one foot up, and use the wall to turn the spine.

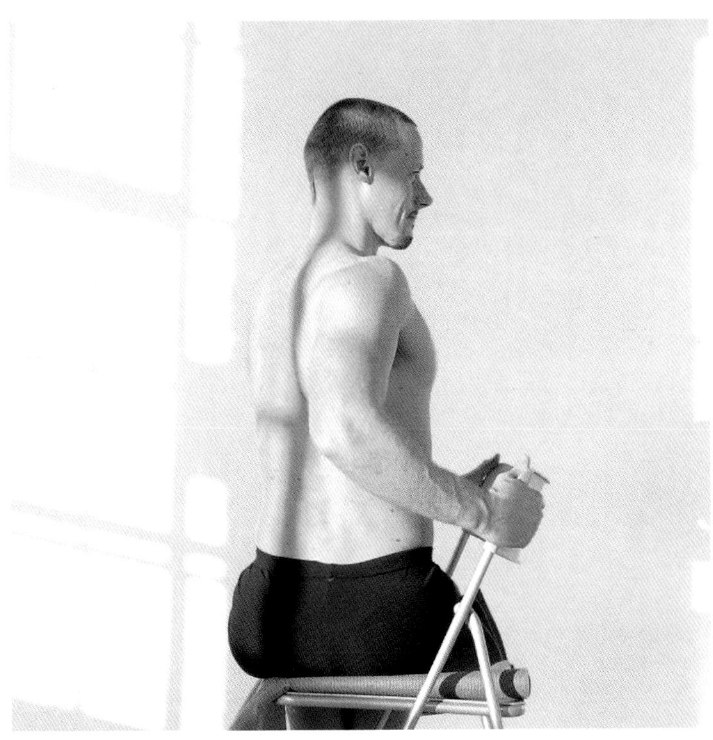

8 **Bharadvajasana (chair)** with hands on the chair back to turn the spine.

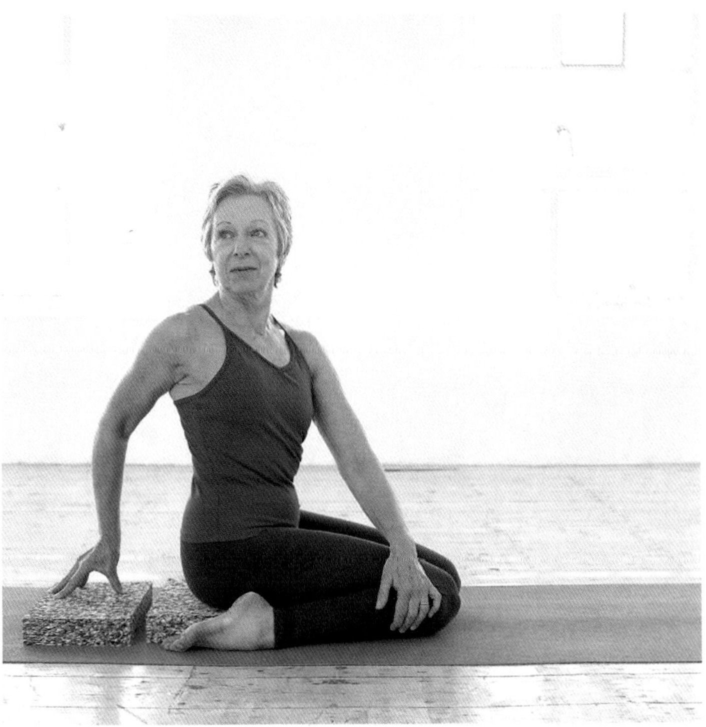

9 **Virasana (twist)** sitting on a support, and using another foam block for the hand if necessary.

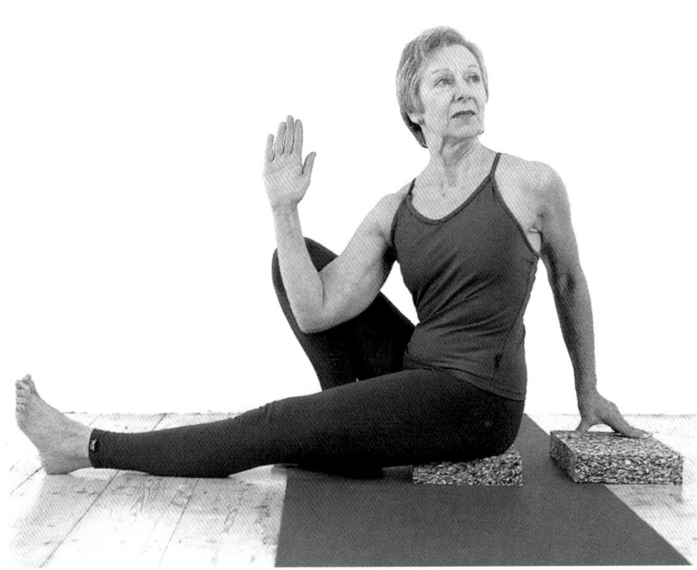

10 **Maricyasana I** sitting on a foam block as a support and using another block to support the back hand. Press into the block to turn the spine.

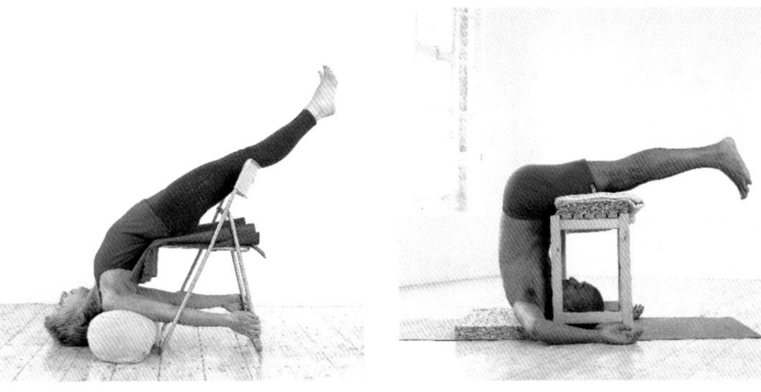

11 **Chair Sarvangasana** holding on to the back legs of the chair.
12 **Ardha Halasana** with the thighs supported on a stool.

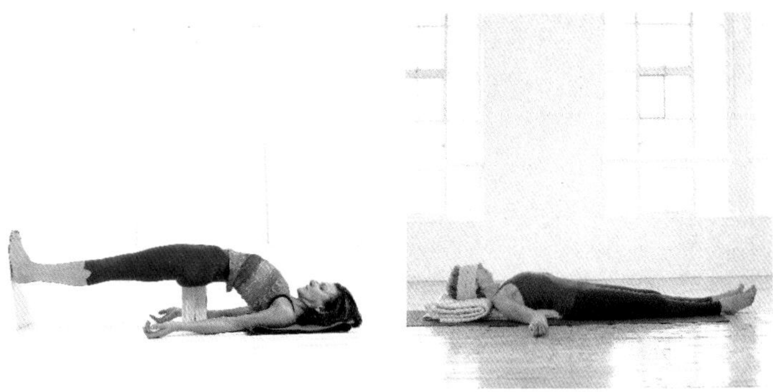

13 **Setu Bandha Sarvangasana** using the wall to raise the legs.
14 **Savasana** with the head and neck supported on a blanket and the eyes covered.

Knees

These postures bring flexibility to the knee joint. Distortions of the knee joint caused by tears in the cartilage or knee injuries will be relieved. When practising, try to create space in the knee joint.

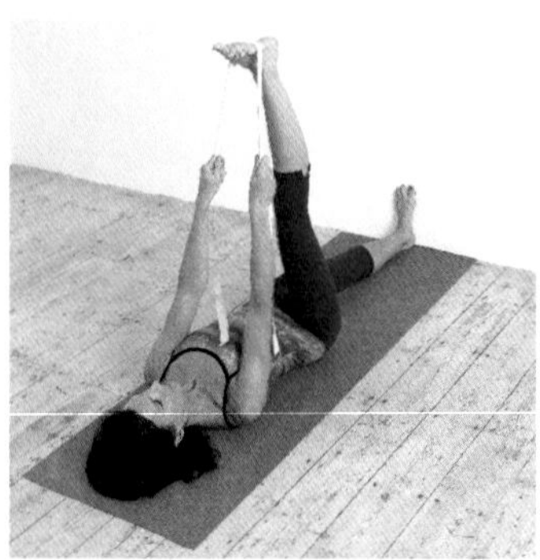

1 **Supta Padangustasana I & II** with a strap around the raised foot

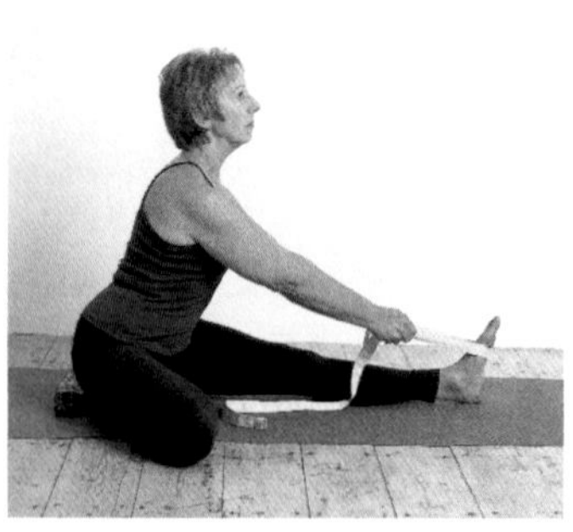

2 **Janusirsasana (concave)** with a strap around the foot.

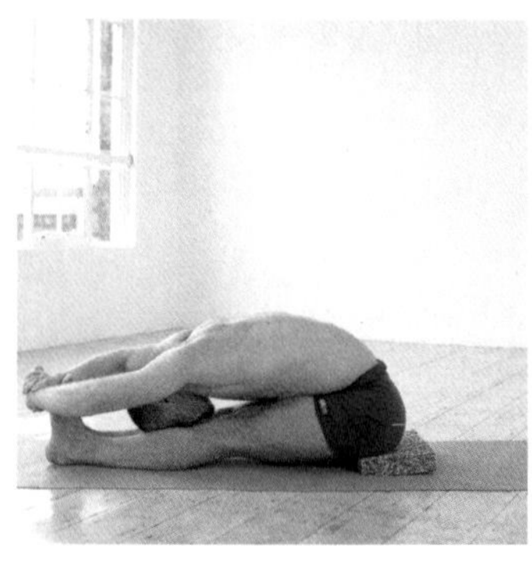

3 **Pascimottanasana** with one hand holding the other wrist.

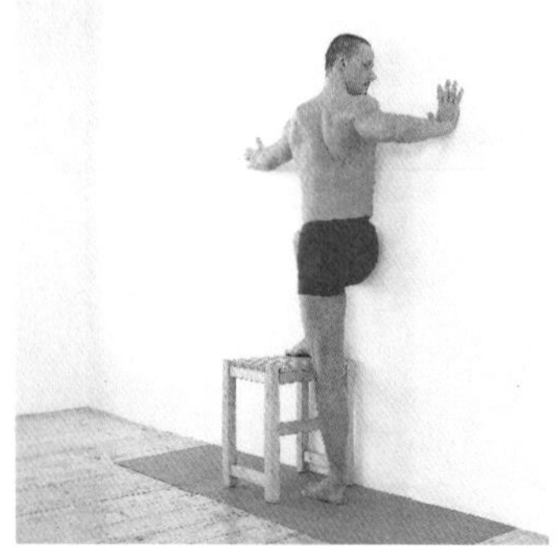

4 **Standing Maricyasana** using a stool and the wall to help twist.

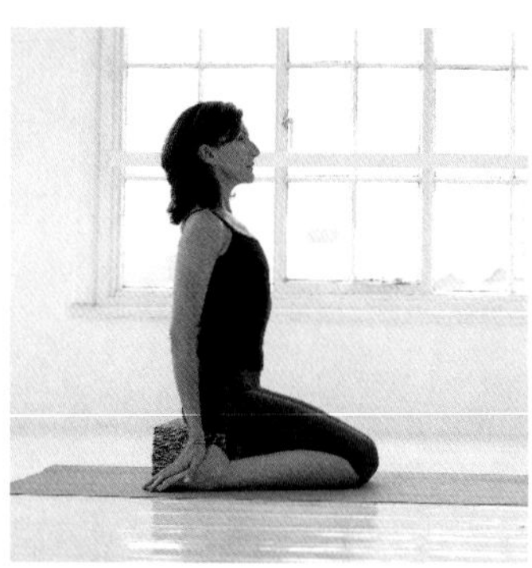

5 **Virasana** using as much support as necessary to relieve the knees.

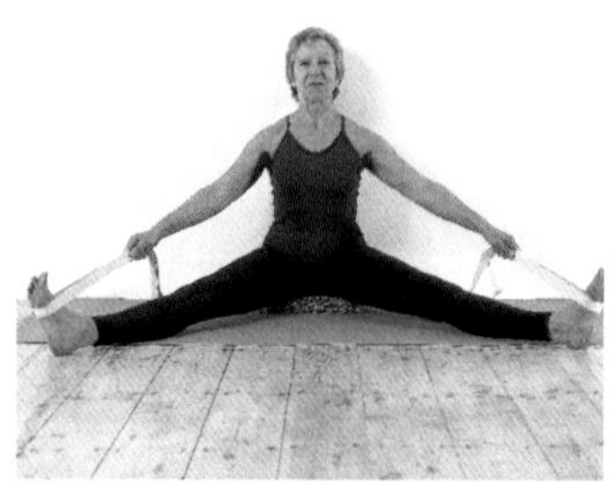

6 **Upavistakonasana** leaning against the wall and with straps.

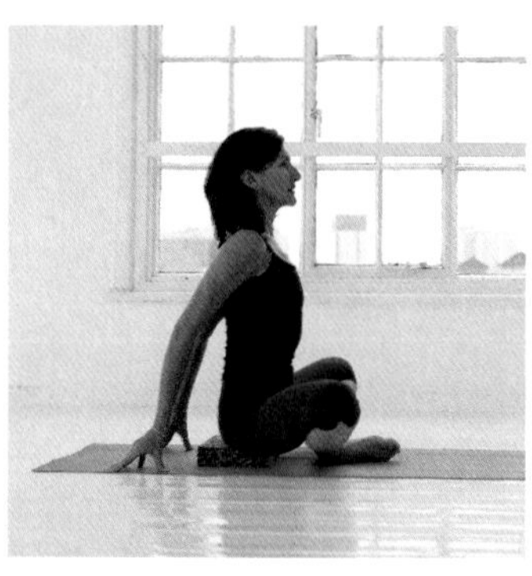

7 **Baddhakonasana** sitting on a support, with the feet together

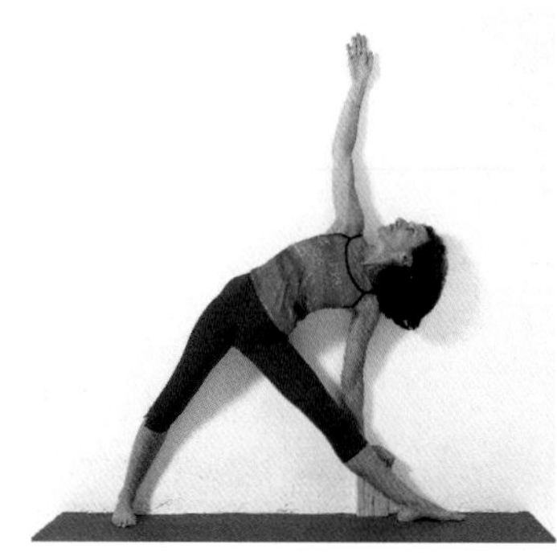

8 **Utthita Trikonasana** against a wall, and using a wooden block.

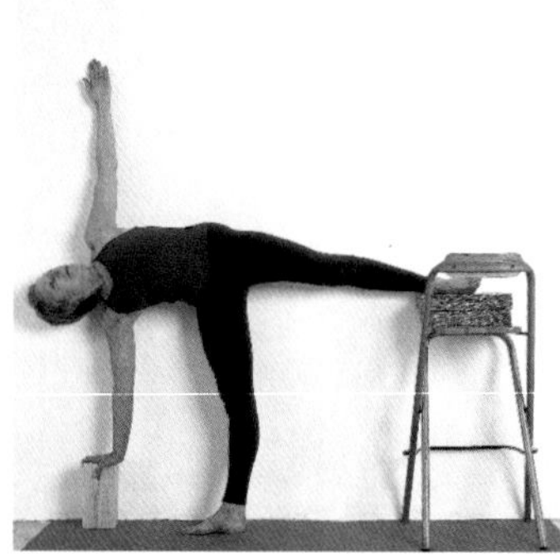

9 **Ardha Chandrasana** against a wall, foot supported by stool.

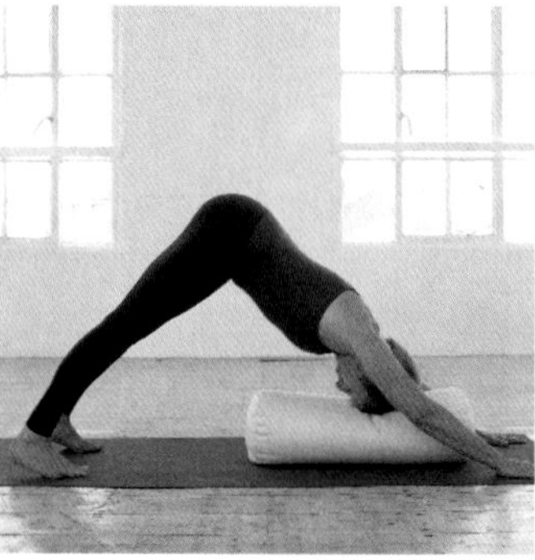

10 **Adho Mukha Svanasana** with the head supported on a bolster.

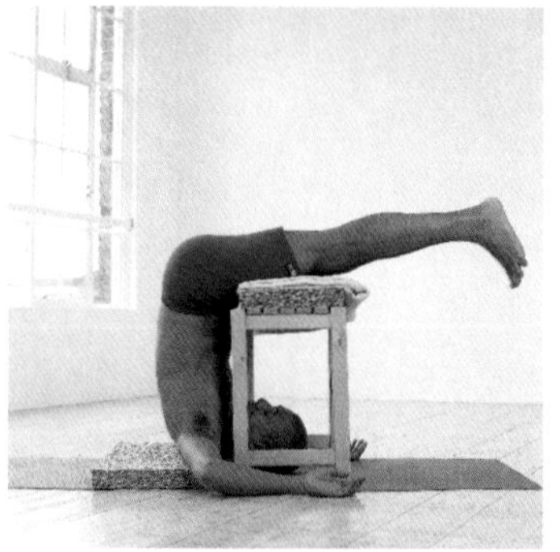

11 **Ardha Halasana** with the thighs supported on a stool.

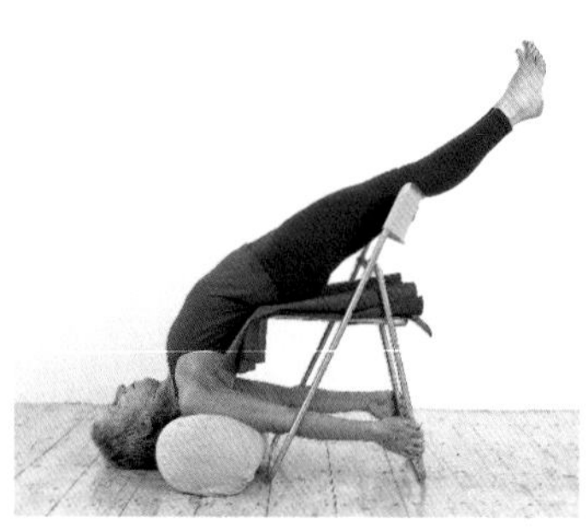

12 **Chair Sarvangasana** supporting the shoulders.

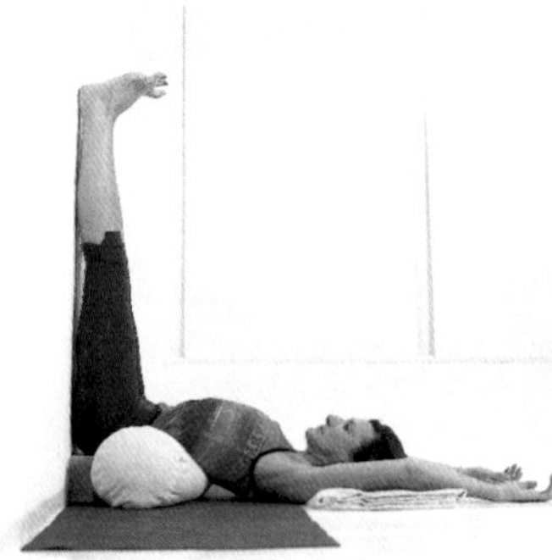

13 **Viparita Karani** with the sacrum on a block and bolster.

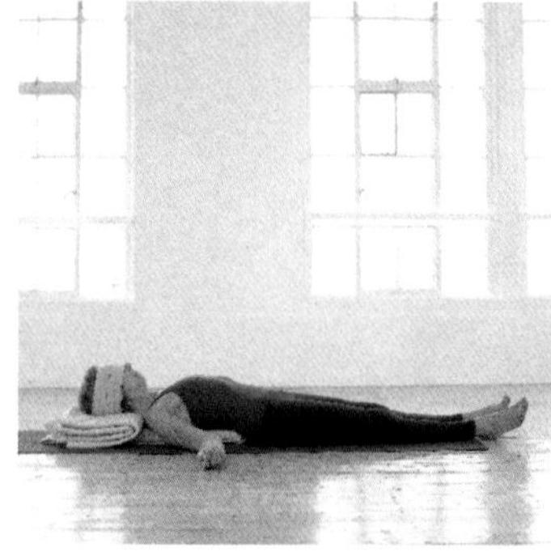

14 **Savasana** relaxing with the head and neck supported.

Focus

- When practising the standing postures, ensure that no sudden jerky movements are made (such as jumping)
- Draw the thigh muscle strongly up towards the top of the leg to create space in the knee joint.

Hips

The hip joint is prone to stiffness as it bears a great deal of body weight. As one gets older, the spinal and hamstring muscles become stiff and the range of movement in the spine and hip joint is reduced.

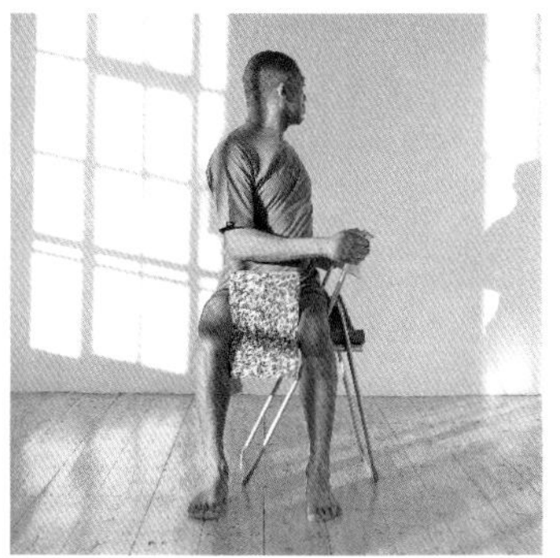
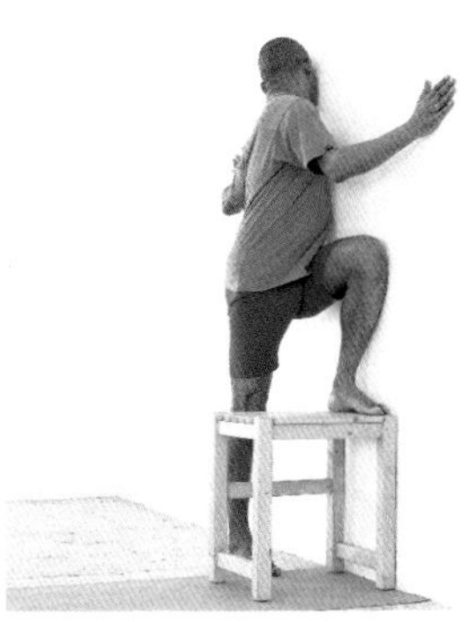

1 **Bharadvajasana (chair)** using a block between the knees.
2 **Standing Maricyasana** using a stool to raise the foot.

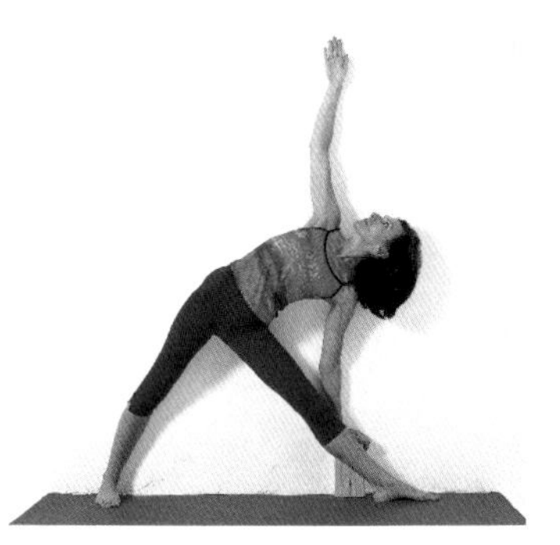
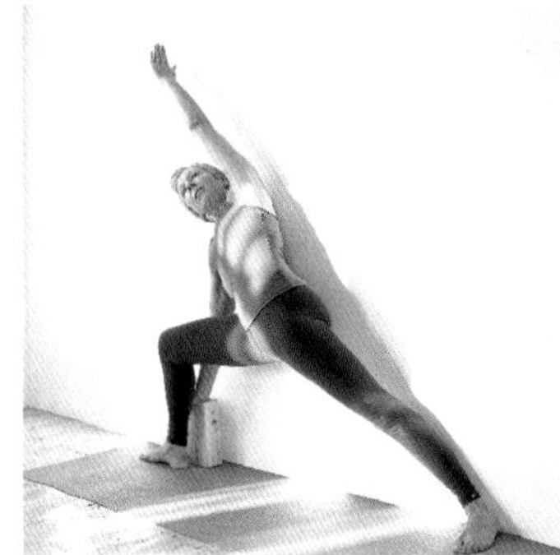

3 **Utthita Trikonasana** against the wall with the hand supported.
4 **Utthita Parsvakonasana** against the wall with wooden block

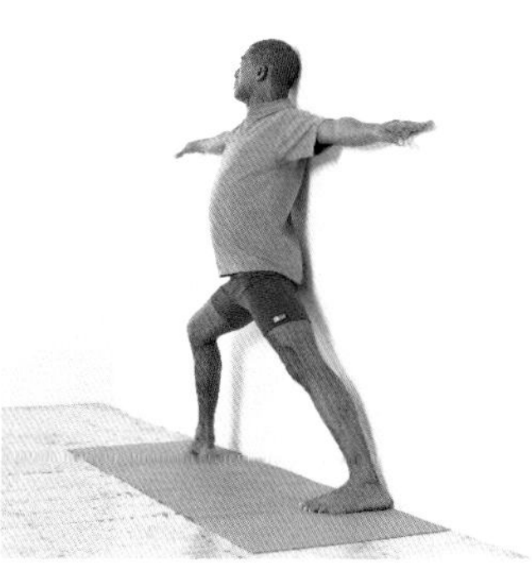
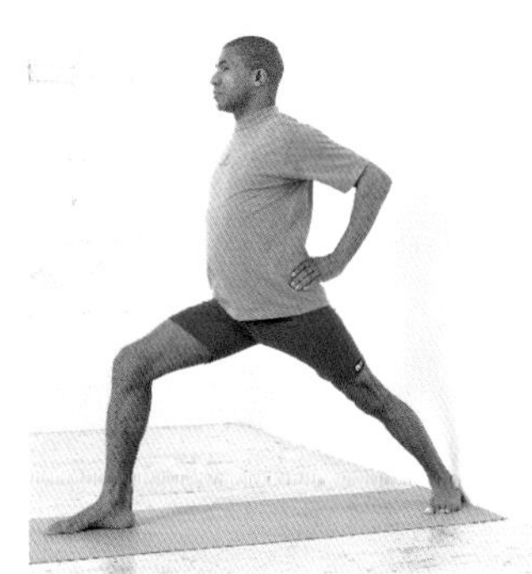

5 **Virabhadrasana II** using the wall for support.
6 **Virabhadrasana I** with hands on hips to protect the back.

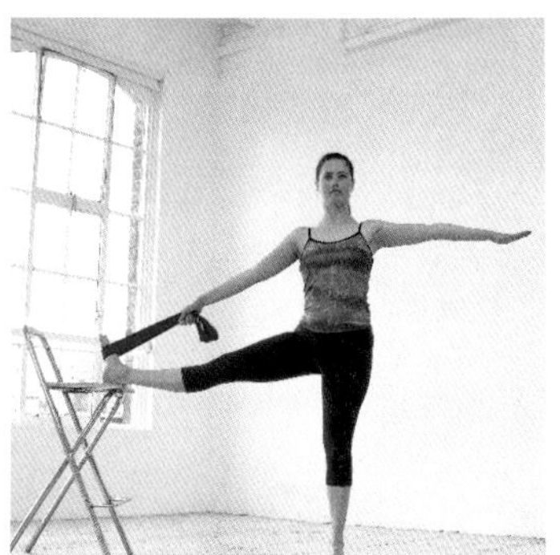
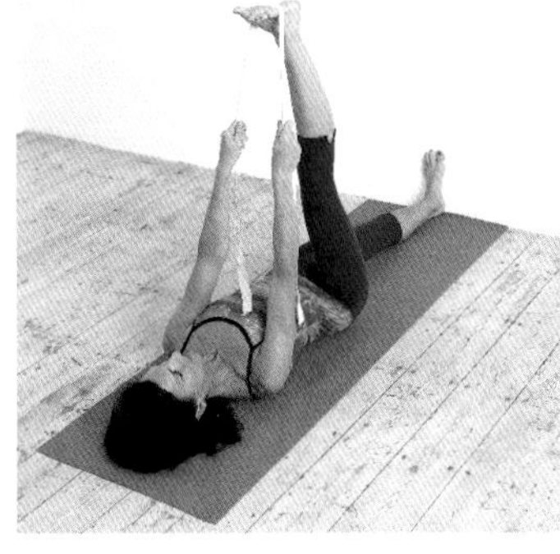

7 **Utthita Hasta Padangusthasana I & II** using the stool for support.
8 **Supta Padangusthasana I & II** using a strap to hold the foot.

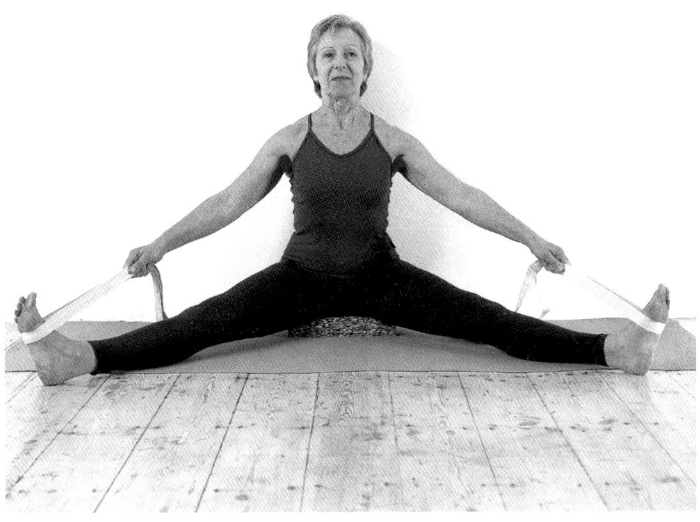

9 **Upavistakonasana** sitting on a foam block against the wall for support, with straps around the feet.

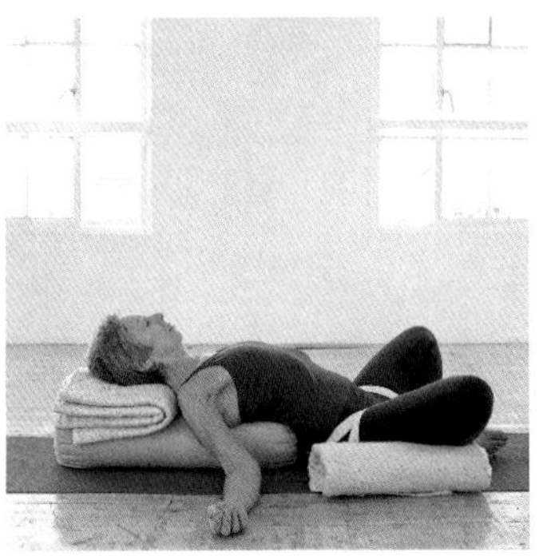
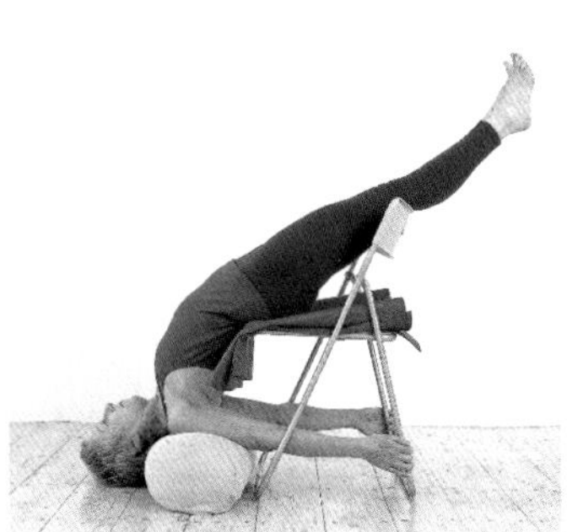

10 **Supta Baddhakonasana** with a bolster and blanket supporting the spine and a strap around the feet.
11 **Chair Sarvangasana** with the shoulders and neck supported.

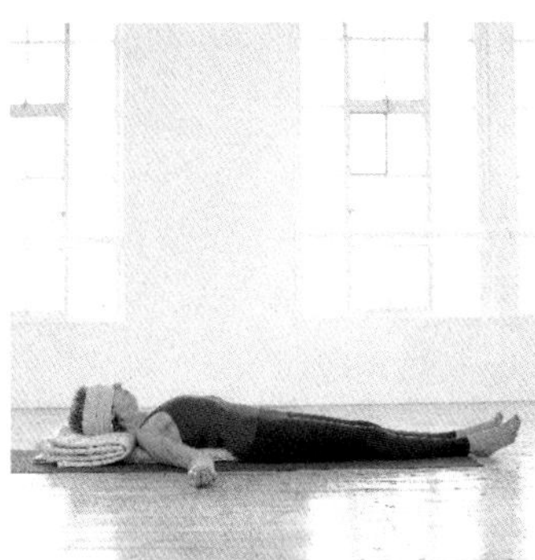

12 **Savasana** relaxing with a blanket supporting the head and neck.

Focus

- Flexibility is increased as a result of stretching the hamstring muscles.
- The seated postures create elasticity in the hip joints and can thus prevent the onset of arthritis.

Menstruation

Inversions and standing poses should be avoided when menstruating as one should not exert oneself physically during this time. Forward bends are extremely beneficial as they help to control the flow of blood and keep the brain quiet and passive.

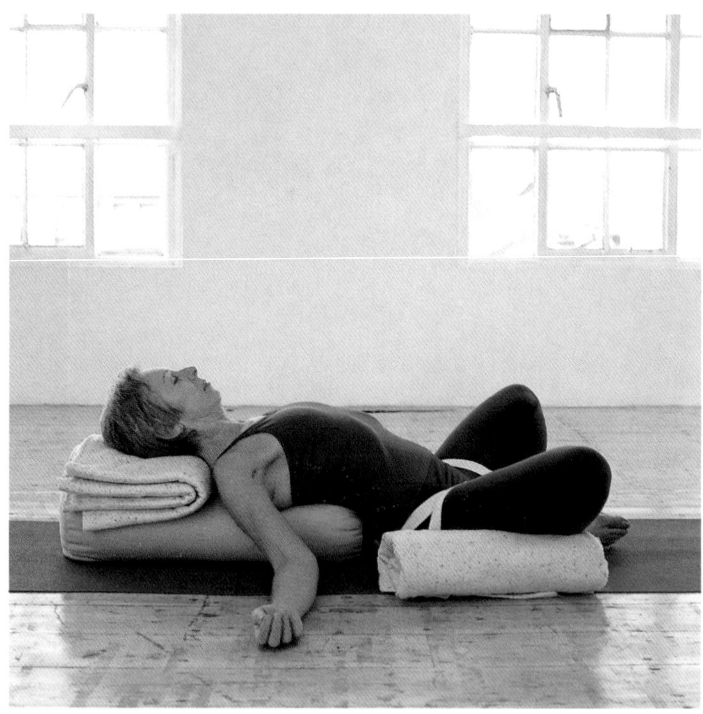

1 **Supta Baddhakonasana** using a bolster and folded blankets to support the head and trunk. Keep the strap around the hips to hold the feet in towards the groin and used rolled-up blankets to support the knees.

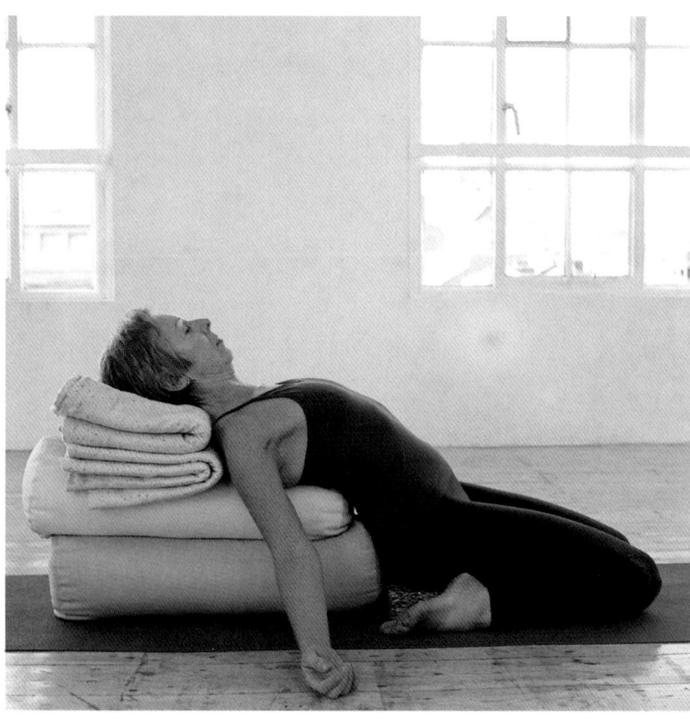

2 **Supta Virasana** using two bolsters and several blankets to support the head, neck and spine. The same effect can be acheived by using thick, rolled-up blankets, or cushions.

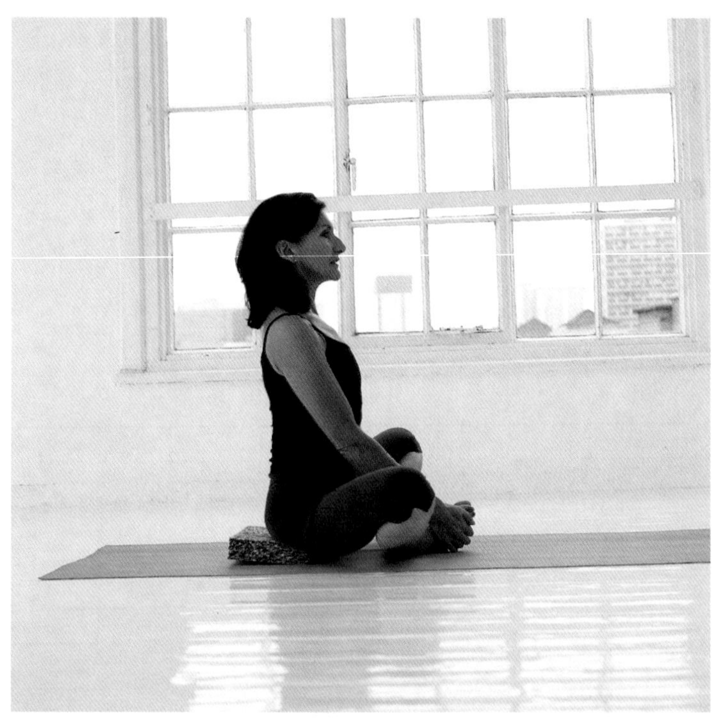

3 **Baddhakonasana** sitting on a support with the soles of the feet pressing together and the spine stretched up.

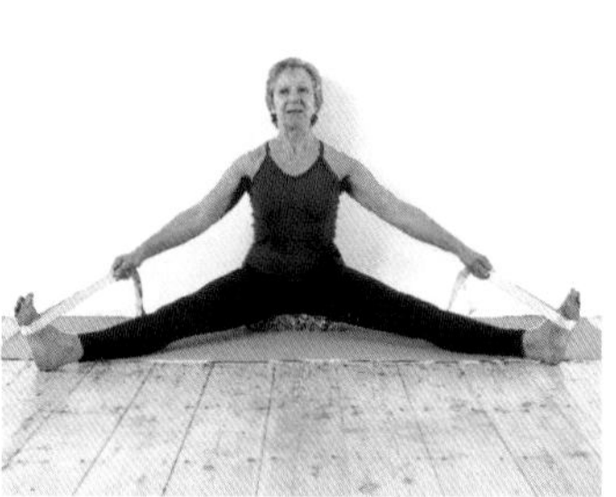

4 **Upavistakonasana** sitting on a support against the wall. Stretch the legs towards the heels.
5 **Adho Mukha Virasana** with a bolster and blanket supporting the head.

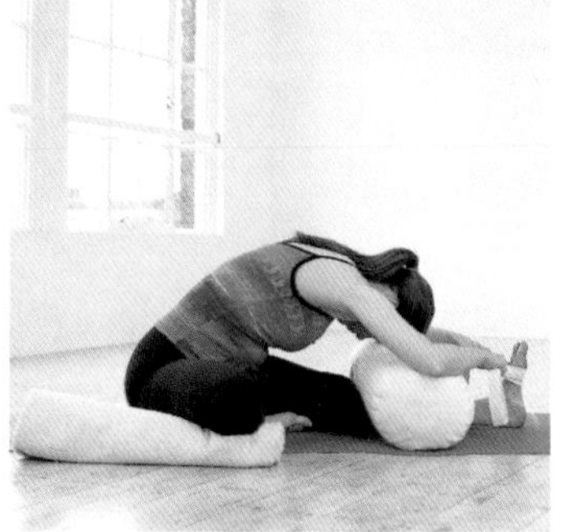

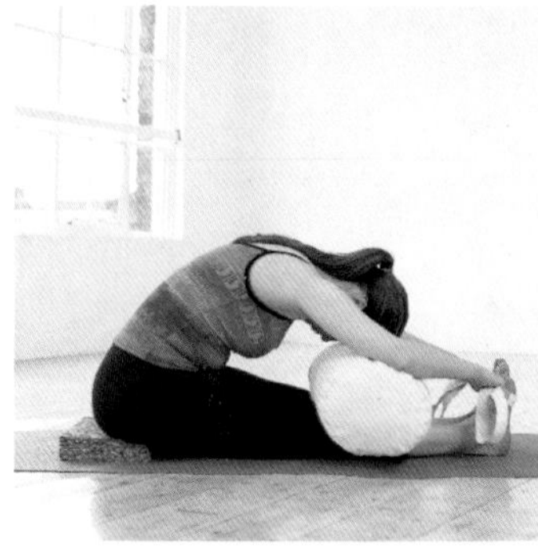

6 **Janusirsasana** with the head, arms and knee supported on a bolster.
7 **Pascimottanasana** sitting on a support, forehead on a bolster.

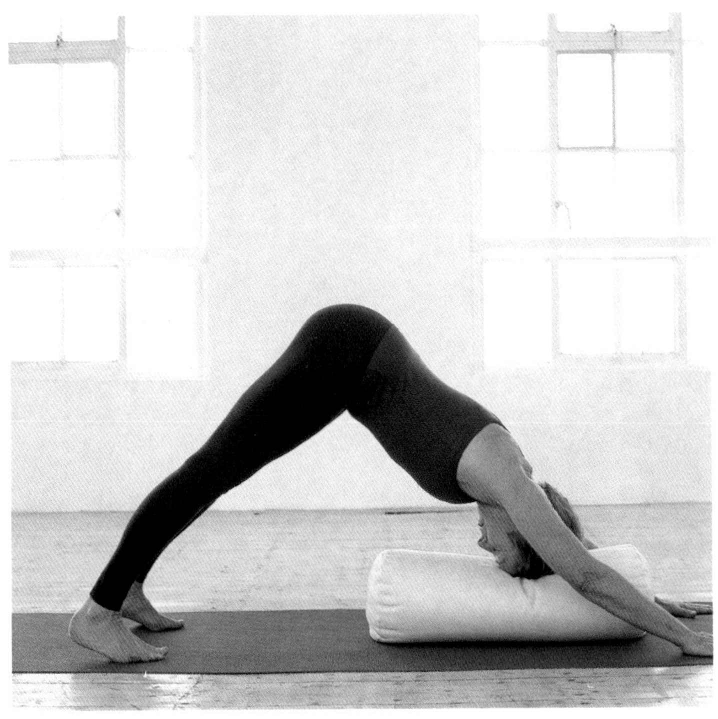

8 **Adho Mukha Svanasana** using a bolster or a pile of cushions to rest the head. Sitting bones should be stretched toward the ceiling, heels extending towards the floor.

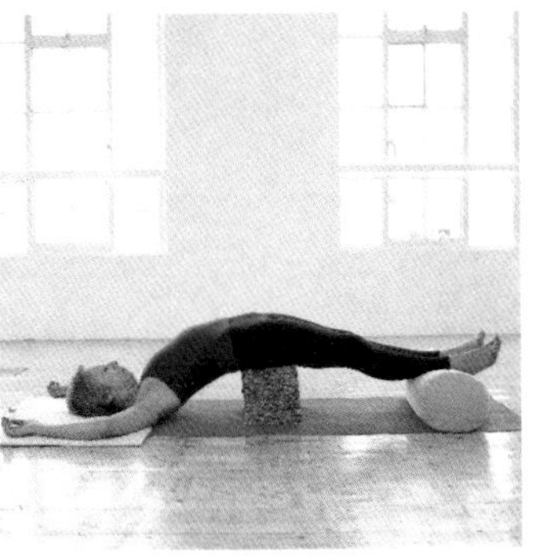

10 **Setu Bandha Sarvangasana** using four foam blocks to support the sacrum and raised feet.

Focus

- Menstruation is not an ailment but may cause discomfort in the form of backache, stomach cramps and bloating of the abdomen. Forward bends regulate menstrual flow, massage the reproductive organs, keep the brain passive and increase blood supply to the pelvic area.

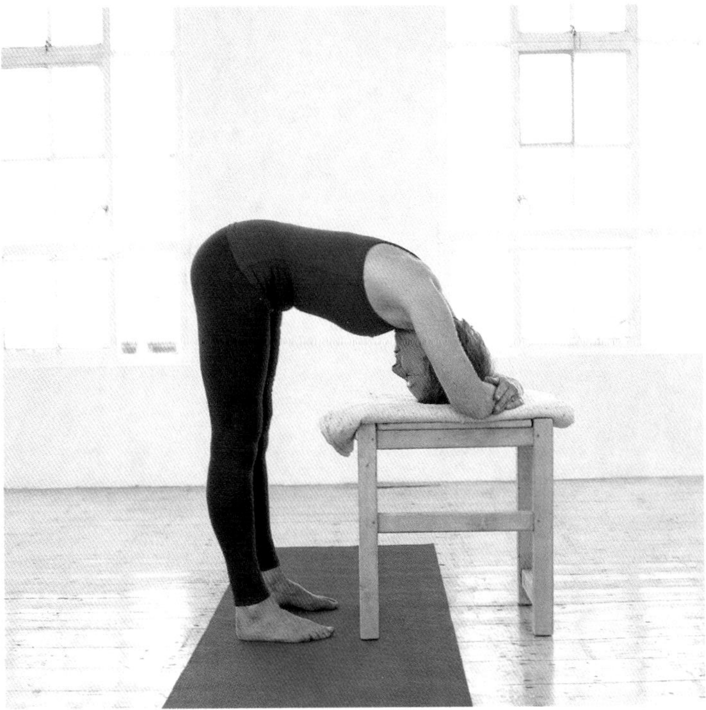

9 **Uttanasana I** with the head and arms supported on a blanket and stool. If the back is uncomfortable, or the hamstrings painful, increase the height of the support.

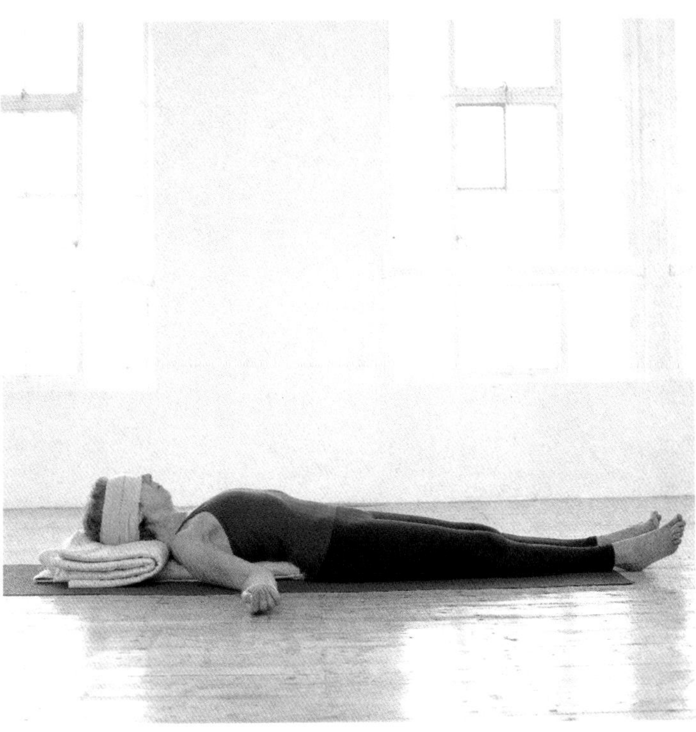

12 **Savasana** with the head and neck supported on a folded blanket and the eyes covered to keep the brain quiet. Use a specialist bandage, or a scarf or small bean-bag would be adequate.

Prolapsed Uterus

A prolapsed uterus occurs when muscles and ligaments of the pelvis weaken and the uterus changes position. The postures listed below strengthen the supporting ligaments and the forward bends create space in the pelvic area.

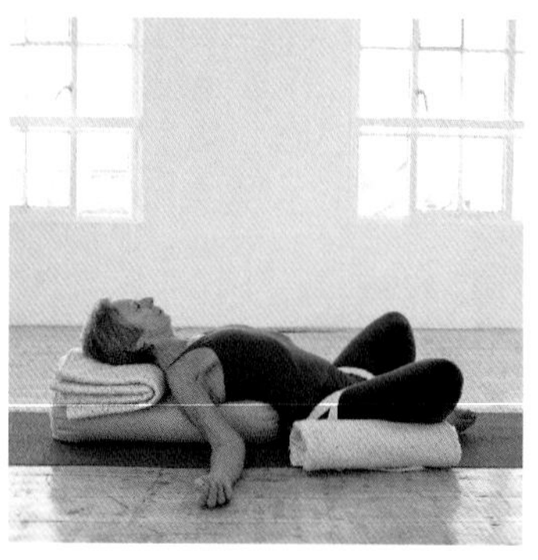

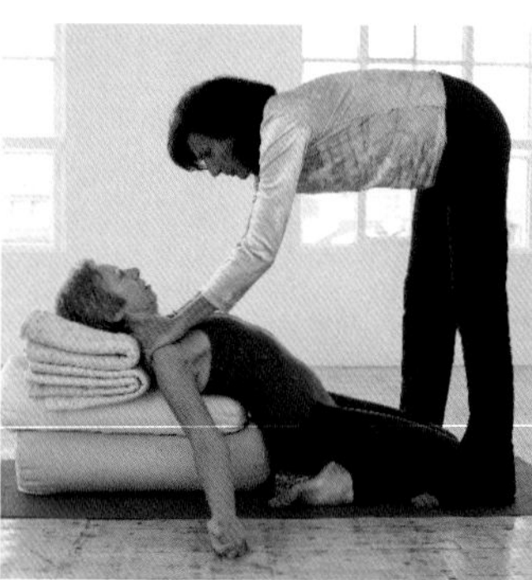

1 **Supta Baddhakonasana** with a bolster to support the body and rolled blankets under the knees.
2 **Supta Virasana** with bolsters and blankets to support the spine.

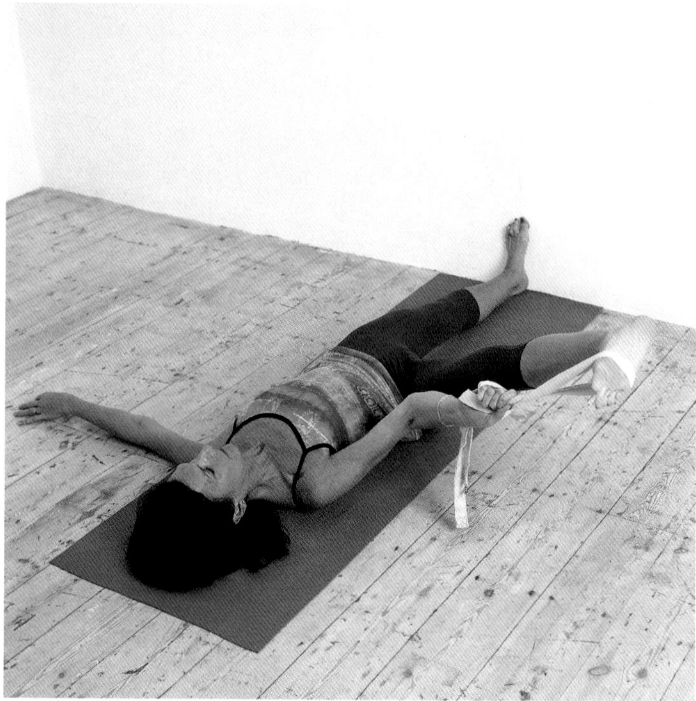

3 **Supta Padangustasana II** using a strap in one hand to reach the foot, keeping the opposite arm outstretched to keep the body flat on the floor.

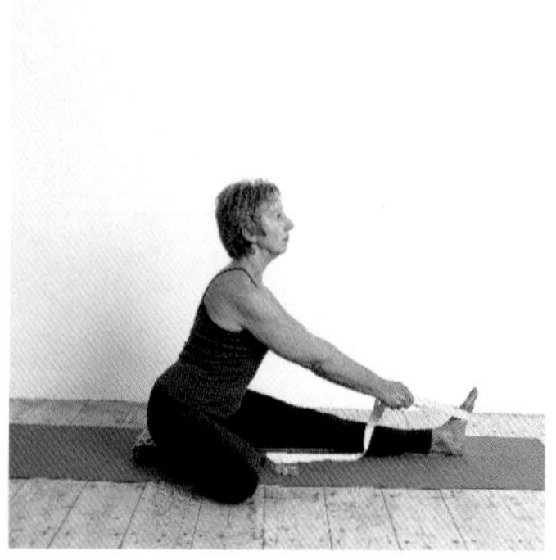

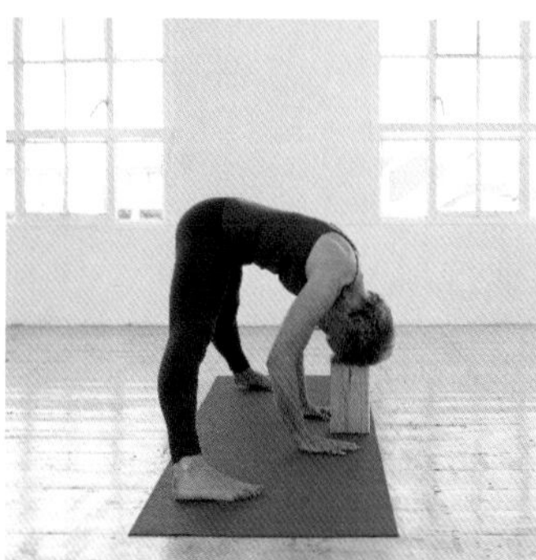

4 **Janusirsasana (concave)** keeping the back arched.
5 **Prasarita Padottanasana** with the head supported on a block (use more support if necessay).

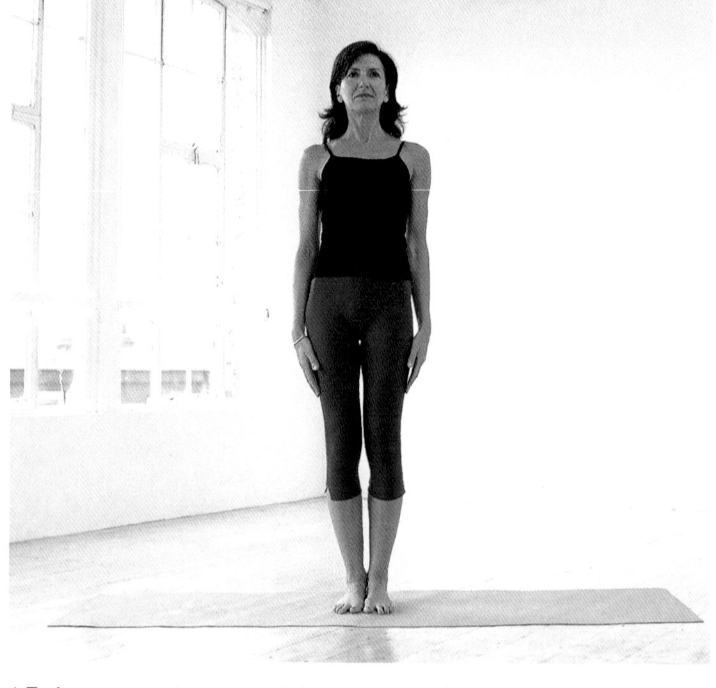

6 **Tadasana** stand up as straight as you can, drawing the crown of the head towards the ceiling. Keep the feet together, and the legs strong, knees lifted. Raise and open the chest, keeping shoulders down.

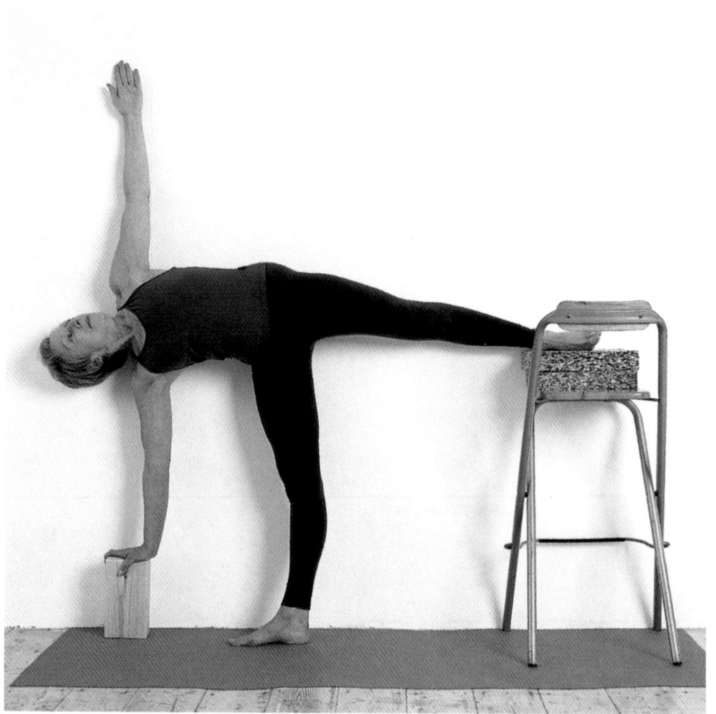

7 **Ardha Chandrasana** using the wall for support in this posture, keeping the foot supported on a stool with foam blocks raising it to the correct level for your height. The hand is supported on a wooden block.

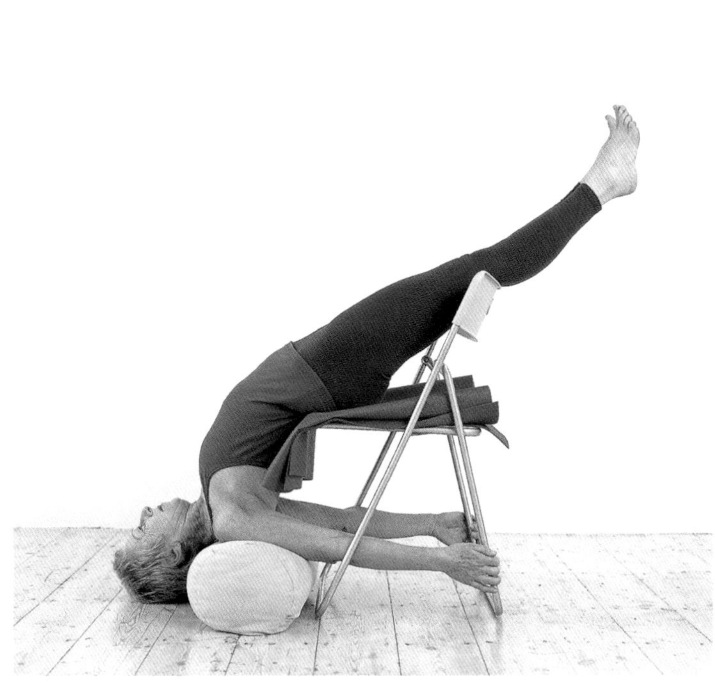

8 **Chair Sarvangasana** with the neck and shoulders on a bolster and the head on the floor. Reach the hands through to the back legs of the chair and use the pull to open the chest further.

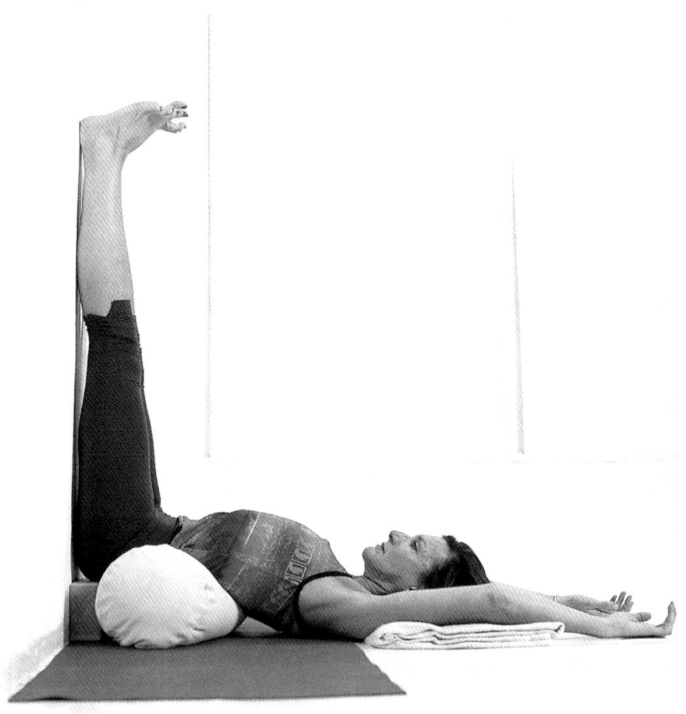

10 **Viparita Karani** pressing the legs against the wall and supporting the lumbar spine and sacrum with a block and a bolster. Arms stretched over the head, palms uppermost.

Focus

- Symptoms of a prolapsed uterus include a dragging sensation in the pelvic area and backache. In this sequence, the abdominal muscles are strengthened and the body is inverted, which improves this discomfort.
- The forward bends, done with a concave back, create space in the pelvic area and lift the uterus.

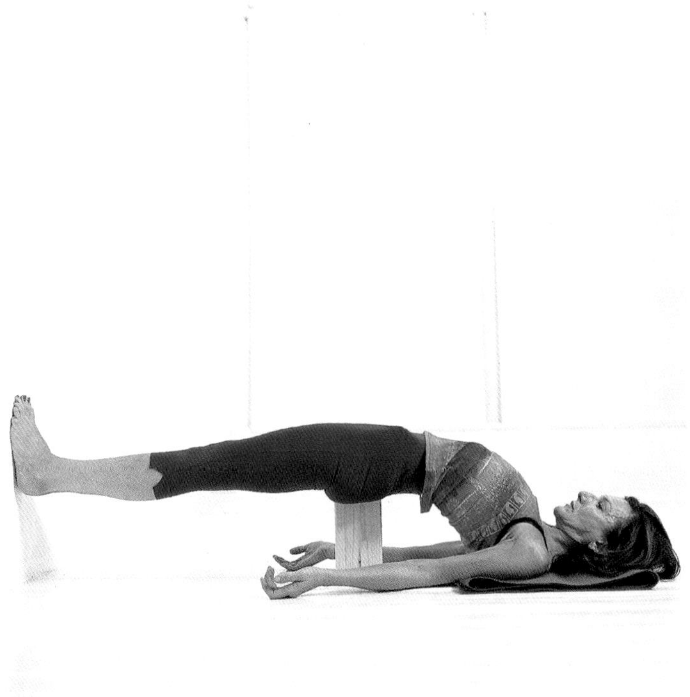

9 **Setu Bandha Sarvangasana** using a wooden block to support the sacrum, and both feet pressing into the wall. Make sure that the block is under the tailbone, not in your lower back.

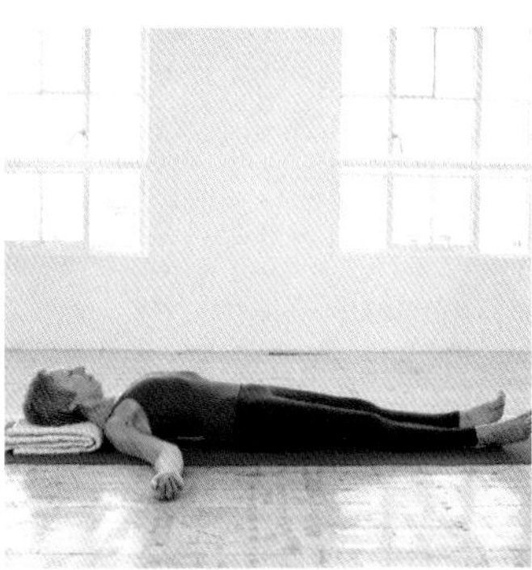

11 **Savasana** relaxing with a folded blanket to support the head and neck.

Menopause

The menopause occurs with changing hormonal balance. The following postures create a soothing sensation in the nerves, keep the brain passive, improve the flow of blood to the pelvic area and help to lessen many of the symptoms.

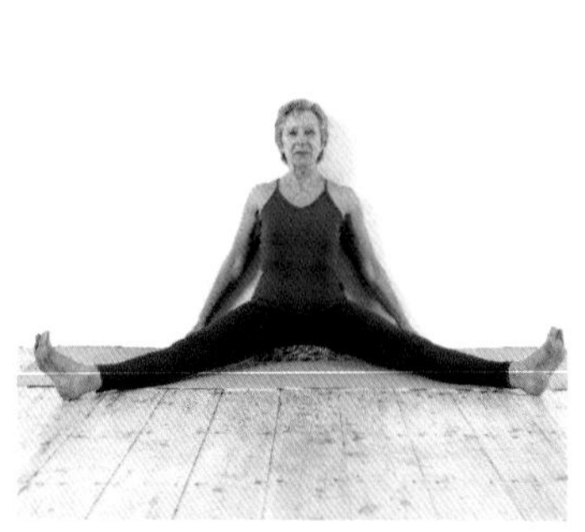

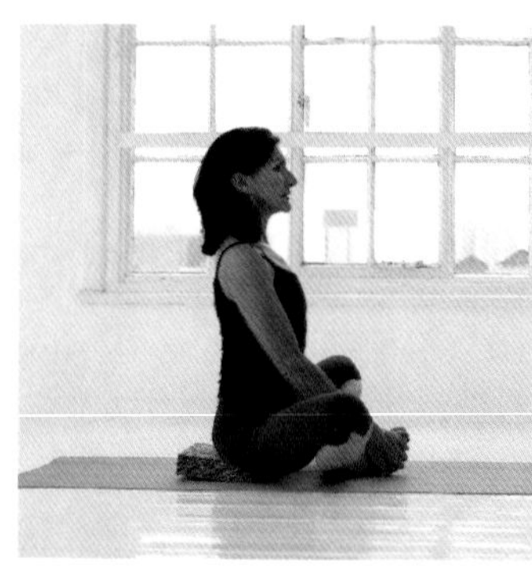

1 **Upavistakonasana** sitting on a support against the wall. Keep extending inner legs to heels.
2 **Baddhakonasana** sitting on a support with the soles of the feet together.

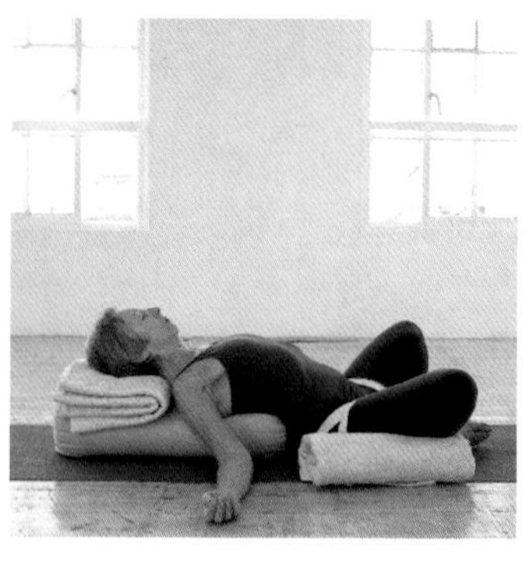

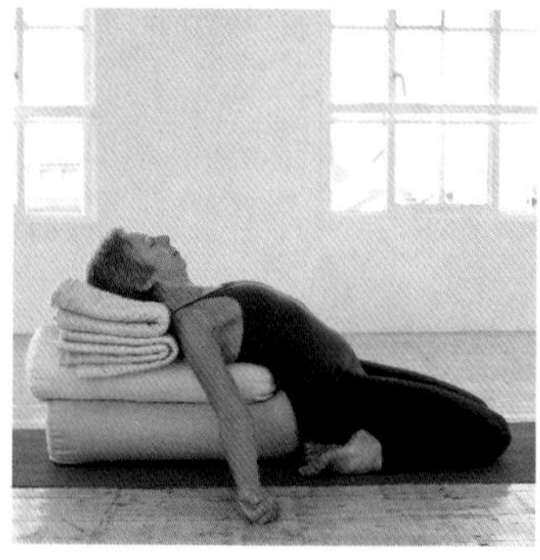

3 **Supta Baddhakonasana** with a bolster and blankets supporting the head, spine and knees.
4 **Supta Virasana** supporting the body on bolsters and blankets.

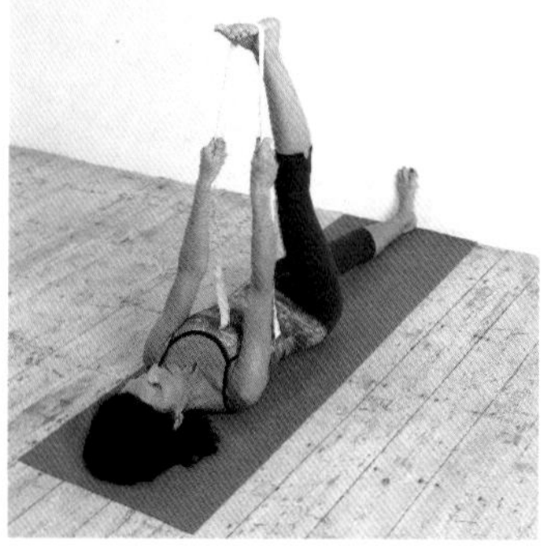

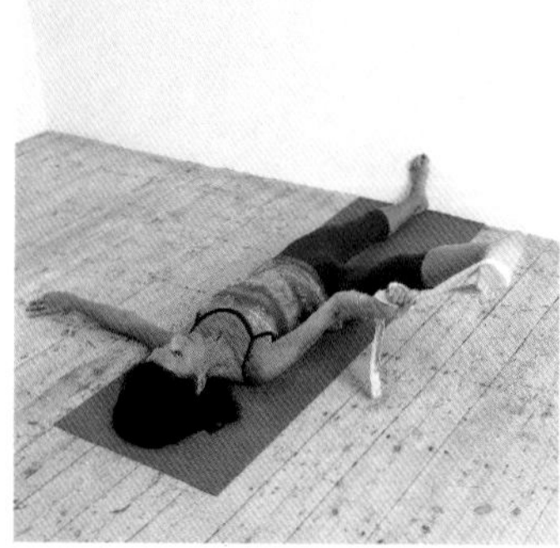

5 **Supta Padangusthasana I & II** holding a strap in one hand to reach the foot, stretching the leg up first, then out to the side for the second of the postures, while keeping the other foot against the wall.

Focus

• The menopause usually takes place between the ages of 45 and 55 and is accompanied by changes in the hormonal balance of the body. Symptoms include mood swings, depression, insomnia and hot flushes. Forward bends and inversions can be particularly beneficial.

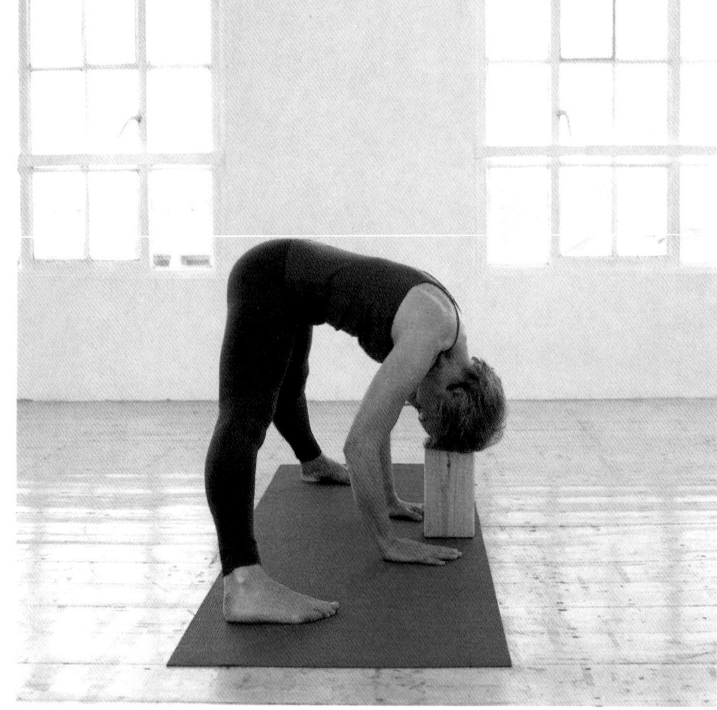

6 **Prasarita Padottanasana** with the head supported on a wooden block. If the hands do not reach the floor, put foam blocks under the hands so that the palms can press down.

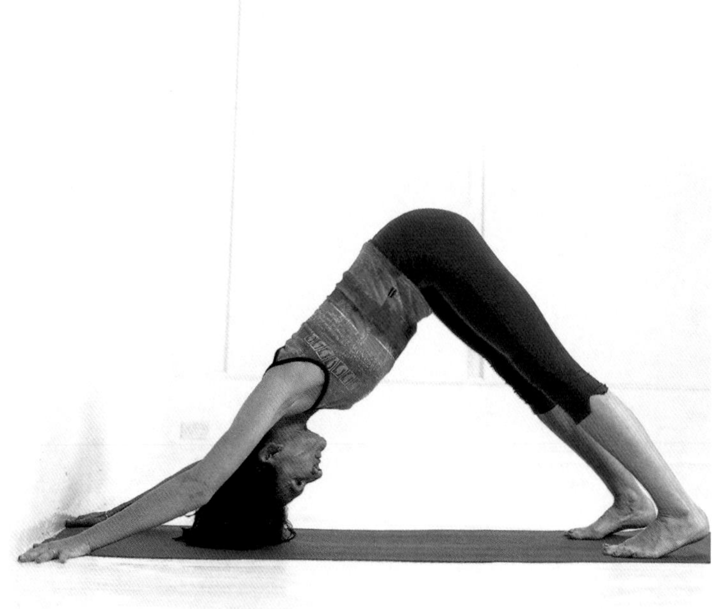

7 **Adho Mukha Svanasana** against the wall. Turn the hands out so that the thumbs and index fingers are pressing into the wall. Support the head with a bolster if necessary.

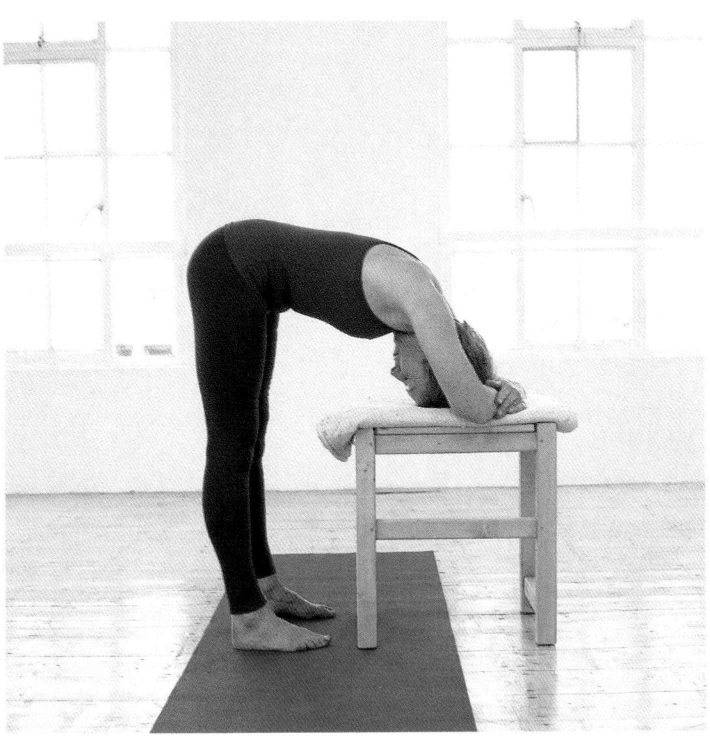

8 **Uttanasana I** with the head and forearms supported on a blanket and stool. Keep the feet parallel and hip-width apart, legs strong with the knees lifted.

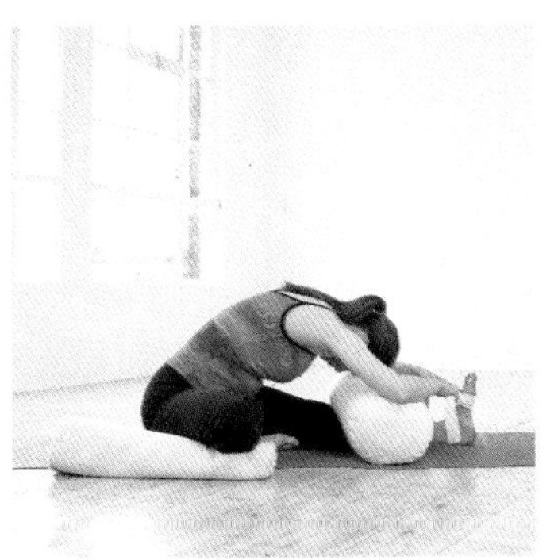

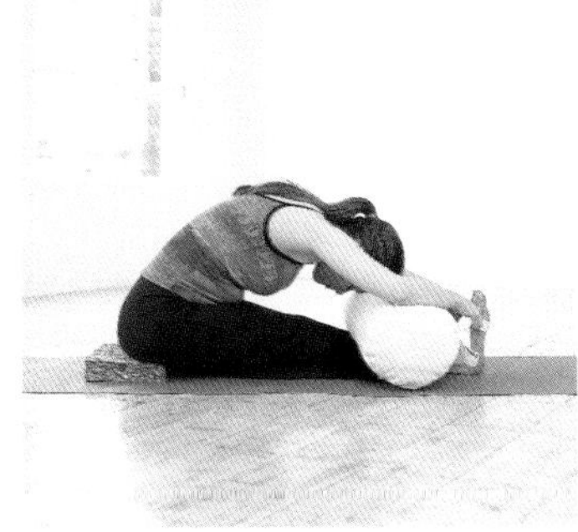

9 **Janusirsasana** sitting on a support and resting the head on a bolster.
10 **Pascimottanasana** with the head and arms supported on a bolster, and a strap around feet.

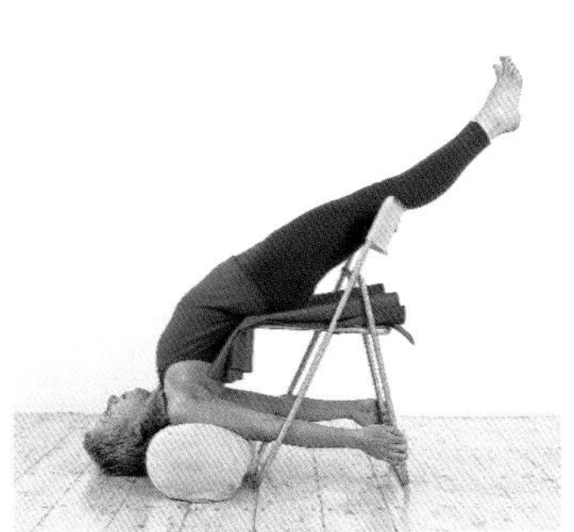

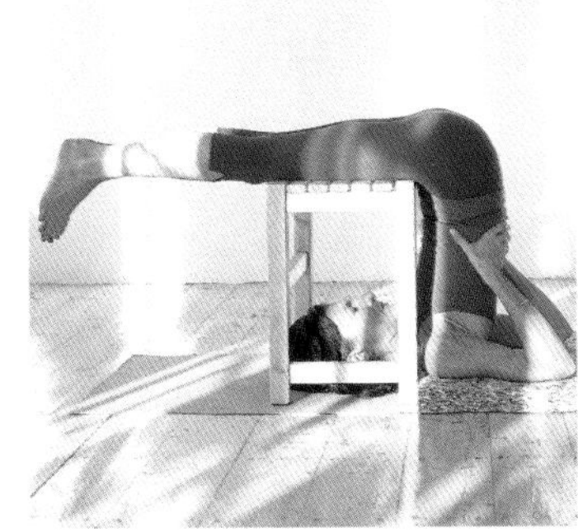

11 **Chair Sarvangasana** with the shoulders and neck on a bolster.
12 **Ardha Halasana** with the thighs supported on a stool.

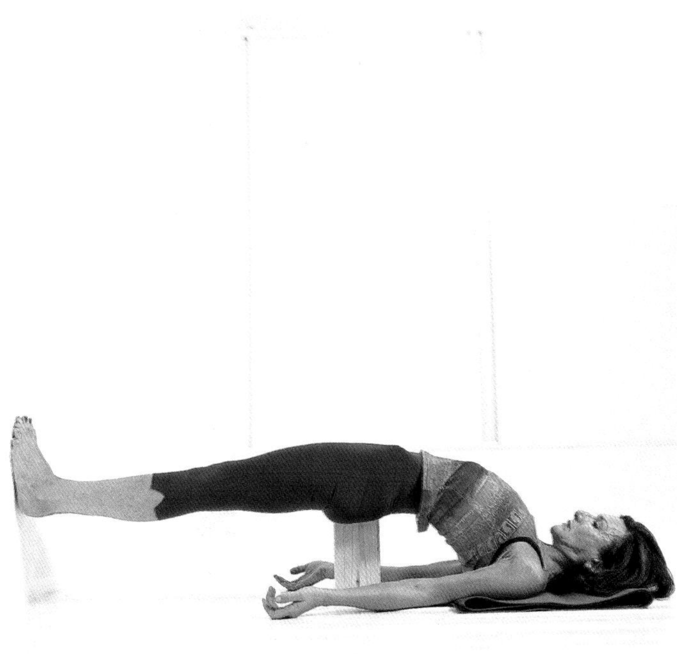

13 **Setu Bandha Sarvangasana** with a wooden block under the sacrum and the feet raised on the wall. Support the head and neck on a folded mat or blanket.

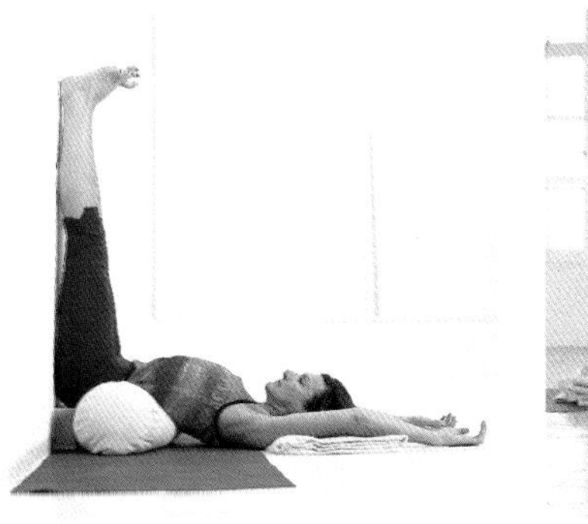

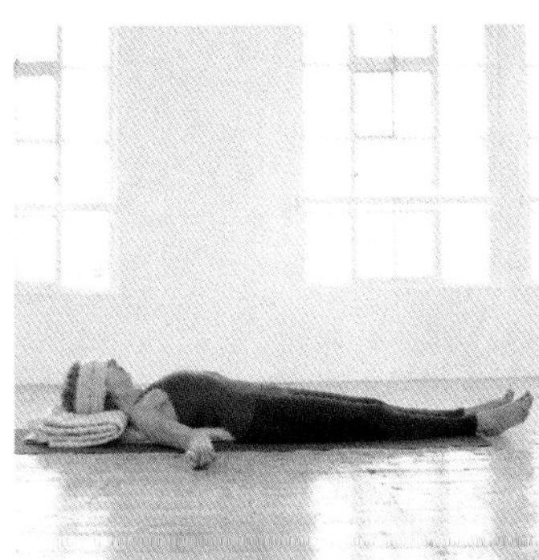

14 **Viparita Karani** with the legs raised and pressing into the wall. A wooden block and bolster support the lumbar spine. The arms are stretched along the floor, palms facing upwards.
15 **Savasana** relaxing with the head and neck supported on a folded blanket and the eyes covered.

Societies and Useful Addresses

Australia
BKS Iyengar Yoga Association of Australia
PO Box 130, Bayswater WA 6933
www.iyengaryoga.asn.au

Iyengar Yoga School of Kuringgai
113 Bent Street, Lindfield, Sydney, NSW 2070
tel 94165537
email willetts@dot.net.au

Canada
Canadian Iyengar Yoga Teacher's Association
www.iyengaryogacanada.com

India
Ramamani Iyengar Memorial Yoga Institute (RIMYI)
(the home institute)
Mr Pandurang Rao, Secretary
1107 B/1 Hare Krishna Mandir Road,
Shivaji Nagar, Pune 411 016,
tel. 91 20 565 6134
www.bksiyengar.com

Ireland
Christophe Mouze, The Healing Path
25a Nun's Island, Galway
tel. 353 87 2504845 fax 353 91 539420
www.yoga-ireland.com

New Zealand
The Iyengar Centre of Auckland, NZ
40 St Benedict Street, Newton, Auckland
tel. 021 2156 544
www.yogacentre.co.nz

The BKS Iyengar Association of New Zealand
PO Box 9278, Wellington
tel. 64 9 5713110 fax 64 9 5713101
www.iyengar-yoga.org.nz

Singapore
Anjani Shah
12 Amber Gardens, #12-05 King's Mansion Block-B, 439959.
tel. 4409156 email janaki@pacific.net.sg

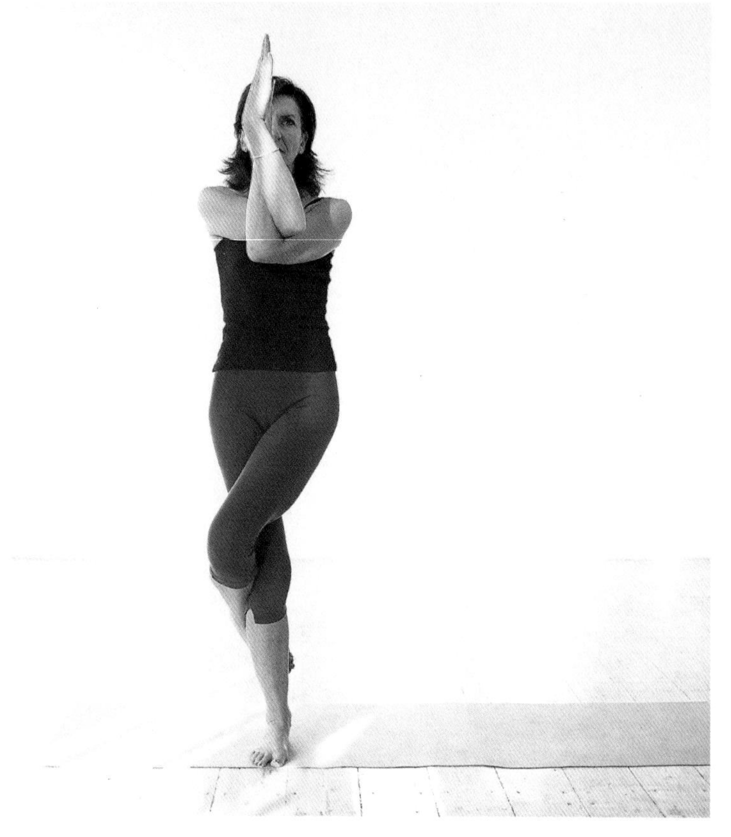

South Africa
BKS Iyengar Yoga Institute
58 Trelawney Road, Pietermaritzburg
KwaZulu Natal, 3102
tel. 27 331 62572

BKS Iyengar Yoga Institute of Southern Africa
104 Mowbray Road, Greenside, Gauteng, 2193
tel. 27 11 646 9687
email nmorris@iafrica.com
www.bksiyengar.co.za

United Kingdom
Iyengar Yoga Institute (Maida Vale)
223a Randolph Avenue, Maida Vale
London, W9 1NL
tel. 020 7624 3080
www.iyi.org.uk

BKS Iyengar Teacher's Association of the UK
email info@bksiyta.co.uk
www.bksiyta.co.uk

Manchester and District Institute of Iyengar Yoga (MDIIY)
134 King Street, Dukinfield SK16 4LG
tel. 0161 339 0748
email info@iyengar-yoga-mcr.org.uk
www.iyengar-yoga-mcr.org.uk

Triyoga
6 Erskine Road, Primrose Hill, London, NW3 3AJ
tel. 020 7483 3344 fax 020 7483 3346
www.triyoga.co.uk

Light on Yoga
105 Lower Thrift Street, Northampton, NN1 5HP
www,loya.ukf.net

West of Scotland Iyengar Yoga Group
23 Prospect Avenue, Glasgow G72 8 BW
tel. 0141 642 0476
email yogazone@net.ntl.com

United States

Abode of Iyengar Yoga
765 Monterey Boulvard
San Fransisco, CA 94127
tel. 415 469 9642

California Yoga Center
570 Showers Drive, Suite 5 (in San Antonio Center)
Mountain View, CA 94040
tel. 650 947 9642
e-mail Info@californiayoga.com
www.californiayoga.com

BKS Iyengar Yoga School of San Francisco
321 Divisadero Street, San Francisco, CA 94117
tel. 415 626 8441

Iyengar Yoga Institute of San Francisco
2404–27th Avenue, San Francisco, CA 94116
tel. 415 753 0909

BKS Iyengar Yoga National Assocation of the United States
1676 Hilton Head Ct., #2288, El Cajon, CA 92019
tel. 800 889 9642 www.iynaus.org

BKS Iyengar Yoga Institute of Los Angeles (IYILA)
8233 West Third Street, Los Angeles, CA 90048 4315
tel. 213 653 0357

BKS Iyengar Yoga Centers of San Diego
4704 East Mountain View Drive, San Diego, CA 92116
and 4869 Santa Monica Avenue, San Diego, CA 92107
tel. 619 226 2202

Iyengar Yoga Center of Boulder
1831 1/2 Pearl Street, Boulder, CO 80302
tel. 303 442 4048

YogaSpace
777 Federal Road, Brookfield, CT 06804
tel. 203 775 6220
email info@yogaspace-ct.com
www.yogaspace-ct.com

Iyengar Yoga School of Northern New Jersey
10 Franklin Turnpike, Waldwick, NJ 07463
tel. (201) 251 1001
email iysofnnj@juno.com
www.iyengaryogaschool.org

The Iyengar Yoga Association of Greater New York
27 West 24th Street, Suite 800
New York, NY 10010
tel. 212 691 9642 fax 212 255 1773
www.iyengarnyc.org

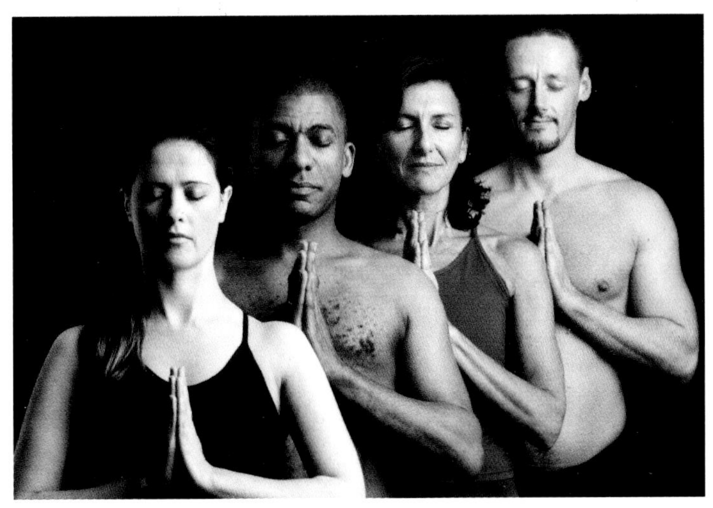

Acknowledgements

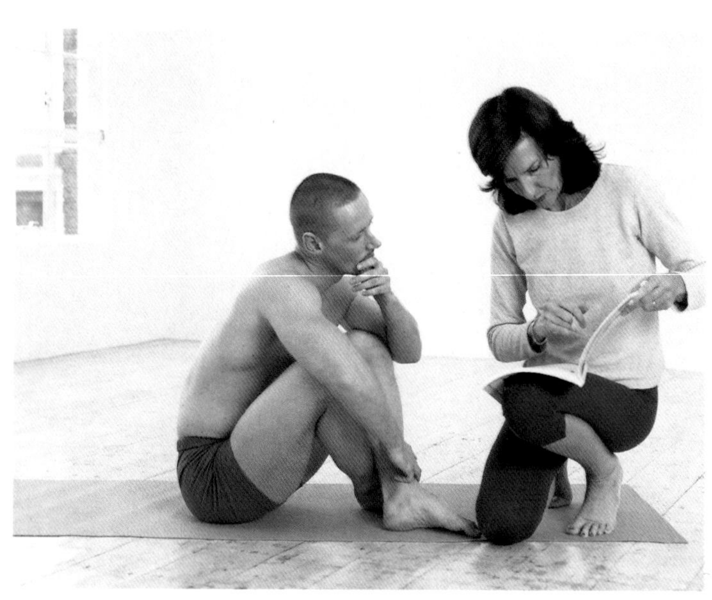

Author's Acknowledgements

I would like to give heartfelt thanks to my guru, Mr Iyengar, who has not only been a wonderfully patient teacher, but who also constantly inspires his students to delve deeper into the art, practice and science of yoga. His knowledge, intuition, intelligence and humour have motivated thousands of yoga practitioners all over the world, and for this we are eternally grateful.

Thank you to Jeanne Maslen for agreeing to write the foreword to this book.

I would also like to express my gratitude to Silvia Prescott and Penny Chaplin, my senior teachers. Their constant observations, excellent teaching and compassion have deepened my understanding, love and practice of yoga. Thanks to the models, Juliet, Jenny, David, Peter and Laura, for their enthusiasm and sense of humour while waiting for the sun to shine to achieve the best picture. Also, thank you to Paul Walker of Yoga Matters for the loan of the equipment and yoga wear. Many thanks also to Clare Park, who showed kindness, patience and understanding in trying to photograph the best possible version of each pose.

Lastly, I would like to express my love and gratitude to my husband, Rob, and my children, Matthew and Cassy, for their continual support and encouragement during this project.

Publisher's Acknowledgements

Thanks for the loan of props and mats to Paul Walker at Yoga Matters, suppliers of yoga mats, props and clothing.
32 Clarendon Road, London N8 0DJ
020 8888 8588 fax +44 (0)20 8888 0623
www.yogamatters.co.uk
for international sales www.yogapropshop.com

Thank you to Stuart Mackay at Beyond Hope for supplying the prAna clothing. Contact www.prana.com for stockists.

Further Reading

Light on Pranayama, BKS Iyengar, The Crossroad Publishing Company, 1995

Yoga: A Gem for Women, Geeta S. Iyengar, Timeless Books, 2002

Yoga: The Path to Holistic Health, BKS Iyengar, Dorling Kindersley, 2001

How to use Yoga, Mira Mehta, Lorenz Books 1994

Yoga: The Iyengar Way, Silva, Mira & Shyam Mehta Dorling Kindersley, 1990

Yoga Rahasya Volumes A & B – BKS Iyengar, RIMYI, Pune and Loy Research Trust, Mumbai, 1994. These two publications are a collection of Mr Iyengars speeches, question and answer sessions, and remedial talks.

A Matter of Health, Dr K Raman, Eastwest Books (Madras) Pvt Ltd, April 1998.

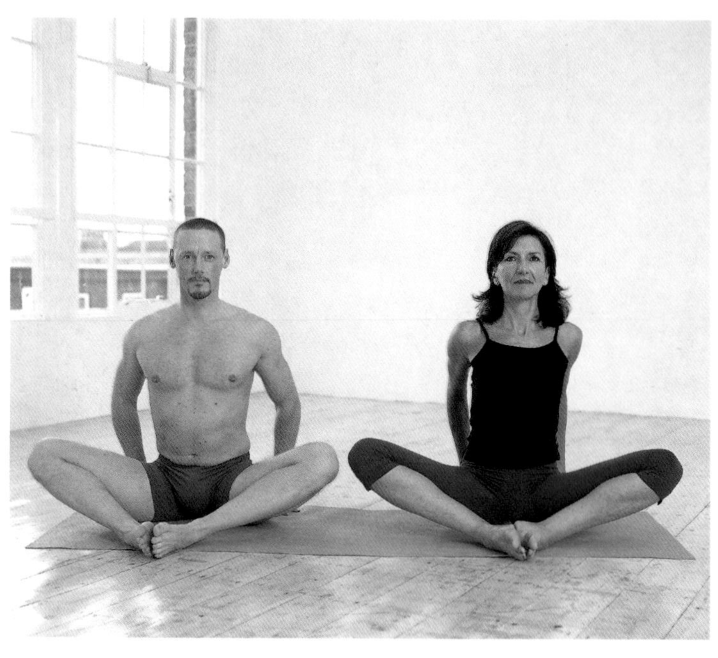

Index

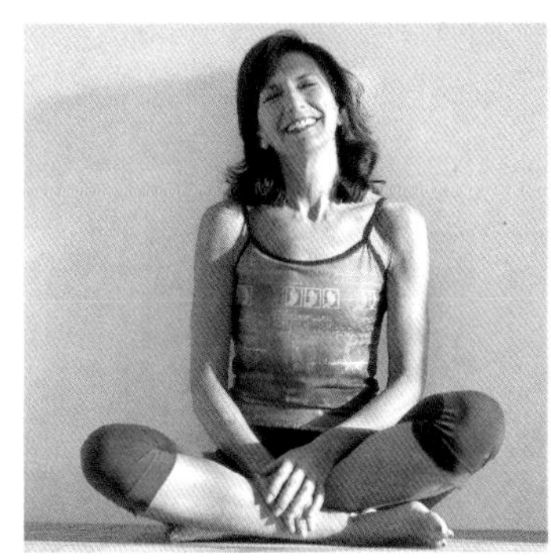

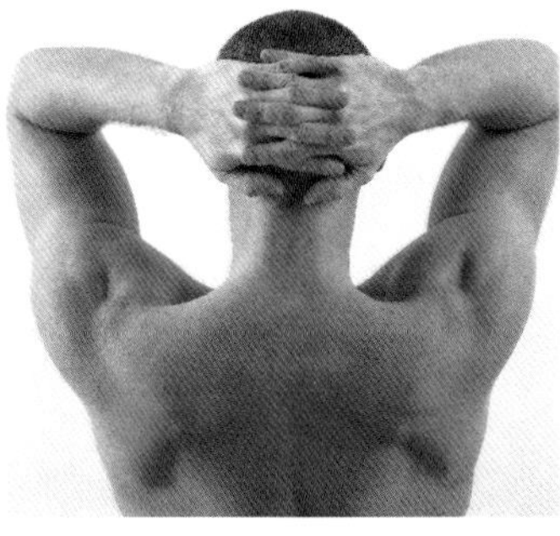

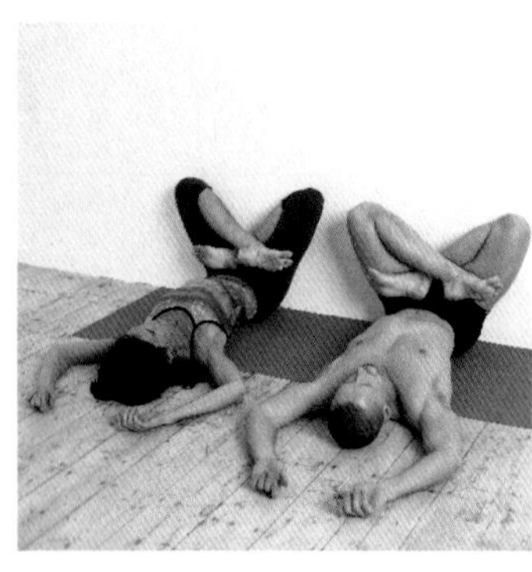

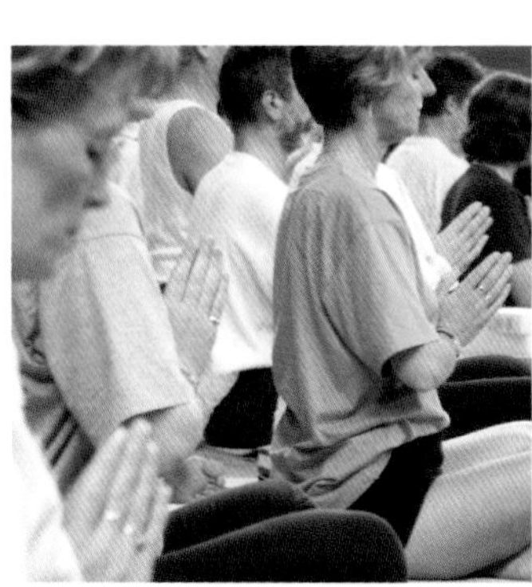

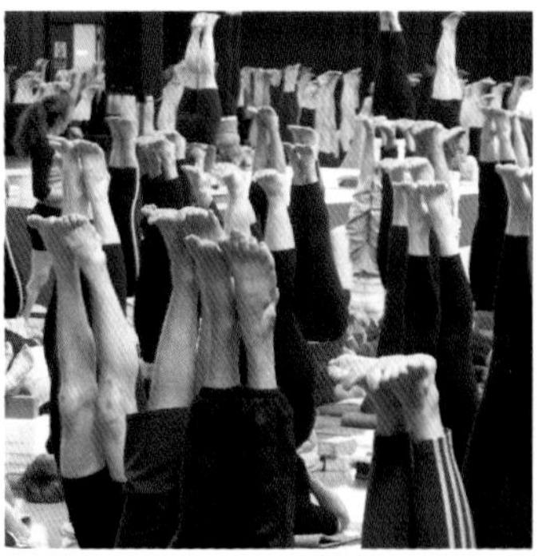